T0179424

STATISTICS IN
DRUG RESEARCH

Biostatistics: A Series of References and Textbooks

Series Editor

Shein-Chung Chow

President, U.S. Operations
StatPlus, Inc.
Yardley, Pennsylvania

Adjunct Professor
Temple University
Philadelphia, Pennsylvania

ADDITIONAL VOLUMES IN PREPARATION

STATISTICS IN DRUG RESEARCH

METHODOLOGIES AND RECENT DEVELOPMENTS

SHEIN-CHUNG CHOW

StatPlus, Inc.
Yardley, Pennsylvania
and Temple University
Philadelphia, Pennsylvania

JUN SHAO

University of Wisconsin–Madison
Madison, Wisconsin

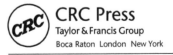

CRC Press
Taylor & Francis Group
Boca Raton London New York

CRC Press is an imprint of the
Taylor & Francis Group, an **informa** business

CRC Press
Taylor & Francis Group
6000 Broken Sound Parkway NW, Suite 300
Boca Raton, FL 33487-2742

First issued in paperback 2019

© 2002 by Taylor & Francis Group, LLC
CRC Press is an imprint of Taylor & Francis Group, an Informa business

No claim to original U.S. Government works

ISBN-13: 978-0-8247-0763-7 (hbk)
ISBN-13: 978-0-367-39633-6 (pbk)

Visit the Taylor & Francis Web site at
http://www.taylorandfrancis.com

and the CRC Press Web site at
http://www.crcpress.com

Series Introduction

The primary objectives of the Biostatistics series are to provide useful reference books for researchers and scientists in academia, industry, and government, and to offer textbooks for undergraduate and/or graduate courses in the area of biostatistics. This book series will provide comprehensive and unified presentations of statistical designs and analyses of important applications in biostatistics, such as those in biopharmaceuticals. A well-balanced summary will be given of current and recently developed statistical methods and interpretations for both statisticians and researchers/scientists with minimal statistical knowledge who are engaged in applied biostatistics. The series is committed to providing easy-to-understand state-of-the-art references and textbooks. In each volume, statistical concepts and methodologies will be illustrated through real examples.

Pharmaceutical research and development are lengthy and expensive processes, which involve discovery, formulation, laboratory work, animal studies, clinical studies, and regulatory submission. Research and development are necessary to provide substantial evidence regarding the efficacy and safety of a pharmaceutical entity under investigation prior to regulatory approval. In addition, they provide assurance that the pharmaceutical entity will possess good characteristics, such as identity, strength, quality, purity, and stability after regulatory approval. Statistics plays an important role in pharmaceutical research and development not only to provide a valid and fair assessment of the pharmaceuticals under investigation prior to regulatory approval, but also to ensure that the pharmaceutical entities possess good characteristics with desired accuracy and reliability. This volume covers several important topics in pharmaceutical research and development, such as pharmaceutical validation, including assay and process validation; dissolution testing and profile comparison; stability analysis; bioavailability and bioequivalence, including the assessment of *in vivo* population and individual bioequivalence and *in vitro* bioequivalence testing; and key statistical principles in clinical development, including randomization, blinding, substantial evidence, bridging studies, therapeutic equivalence/noninferiority trials, analysis of incomplete data, meta-analysis, quality of life, and medical imaging. This volume provides a challenge to biostatisticians, pharmaceutical scientists, and regulatory agents regarding statistical methodologies and recent developments in pharmaceutical research, especially for those issues that remain unsolved.

Shein-Chung Chow

Preface

Pharmaceutical research and development is a lengthy process involving drug discovery, laboratory development, animal studies, clinical development, regulatory registration, and postmarketing surveillance. To ensure the efficacy, safety, and good characteristics of pharmaceutical products, regulatory agencies have developed guidances and guidelines for good pharmaceutical practices to assist the sponsors and researchers in drug research and development. Even after a pharmaceutical product is approved, it must be tested for its identity, strength, quality, purity, and reproducibility before it can be released for use. This book provides not only a comprehensive and unified presentation of designs and analyses utilized at different stages of pharmaceutical research and development, but also a well-balanced summary of current regulatory requirements, methodology for design and analysis in pharmaceutical science, and recent developments in the area of drug research and development.

This book is a useful reference for pharmaceutical scientists and biostatisticians in the pharmaceutical industry, regulatory agencies, and academia, and other scientists who are in the related fields of pharmaceutical development and health. The primary focus of this book is on biopharmaceutical statistical applications that commonly occur during various stages of pharmaceutical research and development. This book provides clear, illustrated explanations of how statistical design and methodology can be used for the demonstration of quality, safety, and efficacy in pharmaceutical research and development.

The book contains 12 chapters, which cover various important topics in pharmaceutical research and development, such as pharmaceutical validations including assay and process validation, dissolution testing, stability analysis, bioavailability and bioequivalence, randomization and blinding, substantial evidence in clinical development, therapeutic equivalence/non-inferiority trials, analysis of incomplete data, meta-analysis, quality of life, and medical imaging. Each chapter is designed to be self-explanatory for readers who may not be familiar with the subject matter. Each chapter provides a brief history or background, regulatory requirements (if any), statistical design and methods for data analysis, recent development, and related references.

From Marcel Dekker, Inc., we thank Acquisitions Editor Maria Allegra, for providing us with the opportunity to work on this project, and Production Editor Theresa Stockton for her outstanding efforts in preparing this book for publication. We are deeply indebted to StatPlus, Inc. and the University of Wisconsin for their support. We would like to express our gratitude to Mrs. JoAnne Pinto of StatPlus, Inc. for her administrative assistance, and Mr. Yonghee Lee and Hansheng Wang of the University of Wisconsin for their considerable assistance in most of the numerical work during the preparation of this book.

Finally, we are fully responsible for any errors remaining in this book. The views expressed are those of the authors and are not necessarily those of their respective company and university. Any comments and suggestions that you may have are very much appreciated for the preparation of future editions of this book.

Shein-Chung Chow
Jun Shao

Contents

Chapter 1

Introduction

In recent years, a series of prescription drugs were pulled from the marketplace due to safety problems. Table 1.1.1 lists drugs recalled by the U.S. Food and Drug Administration (FDA) between 1993 and 2000, and their reasons for recall. As it can be seen from Table 1.1.1, the most commonly seen reasons for recalls were safety concerns regarding cardiac/ cardiovascular problems and liver toxicity/failure. This has renewed concerns that the drug development and regulatory approval process moves too quickly. In the United States, however, drug development is a lengthy and costly process. On average, it takes about 12 years to obtain regulatory approval for a new drug. The cost is estimated to be approximately 300 to 450 million U.S. dollars. In many cases (e.g., the development of drug products for severe or life-threatening diseases such as cancer and AIDS), it has been criticized that the drug development and regulatory process takes too long for a promising drug product to benefit patients with severe or life-threatening diseases. The lengthy and costly process of drug development is necessary, not only to ensure that the drug under investigation is efficacious and safe before it can be approved for use in humans, but also to assure that the drug product meets regulatory requirements for good drug characteristics of identity, strength (or potency), purity, quality, stability, and reproducibility after the drug is approved.

Drug development is not only used to efficiently identify promising compounds with fewer false negatives/positives, but it's also utilized to scientifically evaluate the safety and efficacy of these compounds with certain degrees of accuracy and reliability. To ensure the success of drug development, most regulatory agencies, such as the FDA, have issued numerous guidelines and/or guidances to assist the sponsors in fulfilling regulatory requirements of safety and efficacy, and good drug characteristics of identity, strength, purity, quality, stability, and reproducibility. The sponsors are strongly recommended to comply with the regulations and guidelines/guidances set forth by the regulatory agencies for best pharmaceutical practices. During the drug development process, practical issues in design, execution, analysis, report, and interpretation of studies that are necessarily conducted for regulatory submission, review, and approval are inevitably encountered. These practical issues may include violations or noncompliance of study protocol, invalid study design, misuse or abuse of statistics for data analysis, misinterpretations of the study results, and incorrectly addressed questions with wrong answers. These practical issues often result in a misleading conclusion for the evaluation of the drug under investigation.

A brief description of the process of drug development is given in §1.1. Regulatory requirements for obtaining drug approval is briefly introduced in §1.2. §1.3 reviews the concepts of good laboratory practice (GLP), good clinical practice (GCP), and current good manufacturing practices (cGMP) for good pharmaceutical practices. The role of good statistics practice (GSP) in good pharmaceutical practices is discussed in §1.4. The last section provides a description of the aim and scope of this book and an outline of a number of practical issues in various stages of the drug development process that are studied in the subsequent chapters.

Table 1.1.1. Recalled Drugs Between 1993-2000

Drug Name	Drug Type	Year	Reason for Recall
Propulsid	Heartburn	2000	Cardiac problems
Rezulin	Diabetes	2000	Liver toxicity
Raxar	Antibiotic	1999	Cardiovascular problems
Hismanal	Allergy	1999	Cardiac problems
Duract	Arthritis	1998	Liver failure
Posicor	Blood pressure	1998	Dangerous drug interaction
Seldane	Allergy	1998	Dangerous drug interaction
Redux	Diet	1997	Possible heart valve damage
Pondimin	Diet	1997	Possible heart valve damage
Manoplax	Congestive heart failure	1993	Increased risk of death

Source: U.S. Food and Drug Administration; compiled from AP wire reports

1.1 Process of Drug Development

The ultimate goal of the drug development process is to produce new drug products for marketing. The drug development process, involving drug discovery, formulation, laboratory development, animal studies for toxicity, clinical development, and regulatory registration, is a continual process. It consists of different phases of development, including nonclinical development (e.g., drug discovery, formulation, and laboratory development), preclinical development (e.g., animal studies), and clinical development (e.g., clinical studies). These phases may occur in sequential order or be overlapped during the development process. To provide a better understanding of the drug development process, critical stages or phases of drug development are briefly and separately outlined below.

1.1.1 Drug Discovery

Drug discovery consists of two phases, namely drug screening and drug lead optimization. The purpose of drug screening is to identify a stable and reproducible compound with fewer false-negative and false-positive results. At the drug screening phase, the mess compounds are necessarily screened to distinguish those that are active from those that are not. For this purpose, a multiple-stage procedure is usually employed. A compound must pass all stages to be active. The commonly encountered problem in drug screening for activity is the choice of dose. In practice, the dose is often chosen either too low to show activity or too high to exhibit a toxic effect. Drug screening for activities could be a general screening, based on pharmacological activities in animals or *in vitro* assays, or a targeted screening based on specific activities, such as that of an enzyme. Pharmacological activity is usually referred to as the selective biological activity of chemical substances on living matter. A chemical substance is called a drug if it has selective activity with medical value in the treatment of disease. Lead optimization is a process of finding a compound with some advantages over related leads based on some physical and/or chemical properties. To efficiently identify a stable and reproducible compound during the process of drug screening and lead optimization, statistical quality control based on some established standards for acceptance and rejection is critical. The success rate for identifying a promising active compound is relatively low. As a result, there may be only a few compounds that are identified as promising active compounds. These identified compounds have to pass the stages of laboratory development and animal studies before they can be used in humans. In practice, it is estimated that about one in 8 to 10 times 10^3 compounds screened may finally reach the stage of clinical development for human testing.

1.1.2   Formulation

When a new drug is discovered, it is important to develop an appropriate dosage form (or formulation) for the drug so that it can be delivered efficiently to the site of action of the body for the intended disease. It is necessary to develop appropriate formulation with an adequate dose to achieve optimal therapeutic effect in patients with the intended disease. The commonly seen pharmaceutical dosage forms include tablet, capsule, powder, liquid suspension, aerosol, cream, gel, solution, inhalation, lotion, paste, suspension, and suppository. Formulation is a synthesis of a new chemical entity, which modifies the structure to enhance biologic activity. At the initial development of formulation, a small amount of the drug product under development/investigation is usually produced for laboratory testing such as solubility and accelerated stability. The optimization of formulations usually occurs in a scale-up from the laboratory batch to commercial or production batch, process control, and validation. The purpose of the optimization of formulations is to optimize the responses of the drug delivery system by identifying critical formulations and/or process variables that can be manipulated or are controllable. The optimization of formulation helps in meeting regulatory requirements for identity, strength (or potency), quality, purity, stability, and reproducibility of the drug product.

1.1.3   Laboratory Development

During the drug development process, laboratory development usually applies to nonclinical safety studies, such as animal studies and *in vitro* assays studies. For each newly discovered compound, the FDA requires that analytical methods and test procedures be developed for determining the active ingredient(s) of the compound in compliance with USP/NF (United States Pharmacopedia and National Formulary) standards for the identity, strength, quality, purity, stability, and reproducibility of the compound. An analytical method is usually developed based on some instrument, such as high-performance liquid chromatography (HPLC). As a result, the establishment of the standard curve for calibration of an instrument is critical for the assurance of accuracy and reliability of the results obtained from the analytical method or test procedures. The FDA indicates that an instrument must be suitable for its intended purposes and be capable of producing valid results with a certain degree of accuracy and reliability. An analytical method is usually validated according to some performance characteristics such as accuracy, precision, linearity, range, specificity, limit of detection, limit of quantitation, and ruggedness as specified in the USP/NF standards. The instrument used for the development of an analytical method or test procedures must be calibrated, inspected, and checked routinely according to written procedures for suitability, sensitivity, and responsiveness.

1.1.4 Animal Studies

In drug development, because certain toxicities, such as the impairment of fertility, teratology, mutagenicity, and overdosage, cannot be investigated ethically in humans, the toxicity of the drug product is usually assessed in either *in vitro* assays or animal models. Animal models are often considered as a surrogate for human testing, under the assumption that they can be predictive of the results in humans. Animal studies involve dose selection, toxicological testing for toxicity and carcinogenicity, and animal pharmacokinetics. For the selection of an appropriate dose, dose-response (dose-ranging) studies in animals are usually conducted to determine an effective dose, such as the median effective dose (ED_{50}). In addition, drug interaction, such as potentiation, inhibition, similar joint action, synergism, and antagonism, are also studied. In general, animal toxicity studies are intended to alert the clinical investigators of the potential toxic effects associated with the investigational drugs so that those effects may be watched for during the clinical investigations. In most circumstances, acute and subacute toxicity studies are typically conducted in rodent and nonrodent mammalian species. It is necessary to conduct segments I, II, and III reproductive toxicity studies and chronic and carcinogenic studies to provide the complete spectrum of toxicological effects an investigational drug can elicit. In addition, it is necessary to perform absorption distribution, metabolism, and excretion (ADME) studies in animals in order to identify those pharmacokinetic parameters that are similar to those in humans and to verify the applicability of the animal species used in the toxicological tests.

1.1.5 Clinical Development

Clinical development involves phases 1-4 of clinical investigation. The primary objective of phase 1 is not only to determine the metabolism and pharmacologic activities of the drug in humans, the side effects associated with increasing doses, and the early evidence on effectiveness, but also to obtain sufficient information about the drug's pharmacokinetics and pharmacological effects to permit the design of well-controlled and scientifically valid phase 2 studies. Phase 2 studies are the first controlled clinical studies of the drug. The primary objectives of phase 2 studies are not only to first evaluate the effectiveness of a drug based on clinical endpoints for a particular indication or indications in patients with the disease or condition under study, but also to determine the dosing ranges and doses for phase 3 studies and the common short-term side effects and risks associated with the drug. Phase 3 studies are expanded controlled and uncontrolled trials. The primary objectives are to (a) gather additional information about the effectiveness and safety needed to evaluate the overall benefit-risk relationship of the drug, and (b) to provide an adequate basis for physician labeling. Phase 4 studies are usually conducted to further elucidate the incidence of adverse reactions and determine the effect of a drug on morbidity or mortality. Phase 4 studies are considered useful market-oriented comparison studies against competitor products.

According to the 1988 FDA guideline, the efficacy and safety of a study drug can only be established through the conduct of adequate and well-controlled clinical trials (FDA, 1988). Table 1.1.2 lists characteristics of an adequate and well-controlled study as specified in 21 CFR 314.126.

Table 1.1.2. Characteristics of an Adequate and Well-Controlled Study

Criterion	Characteristics
Objectives	Clear statement of investigation purpose
Methods of analysis	Summary of proposed or actual methods of analysis
Design	Valid comparison with a control to provide a quantitative assessment of drug effect
Selection of subjects	Adequate assurance of the disease or conditions under study
Assignment of subjects	Minimization of bias and assurance of comparability of groups
Participants of studies	Minimization of bias on the part of subjects, observations, and analysis
Assessment of responses	Well defined and reliable
Assessment of the effect	Requirements of appropriate statistical methods

1.1.6   Regulatory Registration

At the end of clinical development, the sponsor is required to submit all of the information collected from the studies conducted at different phases of drug development for regulatory review and approval. Regulatory review is a very intensive process, which involves reviewers from different disciplines such as chemistry, toxicology, clinical pharmacology, medicine, and biostatistics. The purpose of this intensive review is to make sure that there is substantial evidence to support the safety and efficacy of the drug product under investigation. In addition, the review assures that the proposed labeling for the investigational drug is appropriate for the target patient population with the intended indication. At the stage of regulatory registration, it is helpful to build up a communication with the FDA for advice on deficiencies or concerns regarding the safety and efficacy of the investigational drug. The FDA may approve the drug product if the sponsor has committed to conduct additional clinical studies to address the deficiencies and/or concerns/issues raised during the regulatory review/approval process. These additional clinical studies are usually referred to as phase 3B studies or pending approval clinical studies.

1.2 Regulatory Requirements

1.2.1 Regulatory Milestones

A century ago, the pharmaceutical industry in the United States was essentially unregulated. Drug companies could advertise their products as treatments for any and all diseases. The first effective legislation regarding drug products can be traced back to the Biologics Act of 1902. This was precipitated by a tragedy involving diptheria antitoxin contaminated with tetanus, which resulted in the death of 12 children and subsequently led to the passage of the Pure Food and Drugs Act of 1906. The purpose of this act was to prevent misbranding and adulteration of food and drugs and yet the scope is rather limited. In 1912, the Sherley Amendment to the act was passed to prohibit the labeling of medicines with false and fraudulent claims. The concept of testing marketed drugs in human subjects did not become a public issue until the Elixir Sulfanilamide disaster occurred in the late 1930s. The disaster was regarding a liquid formulation of a sulfa drug, which had never been tested in humans before its marketing. This drug caused more than 100 deaths and raised the safety concern that led to the passing of the Federal Food, Drug, and Cosmetic Act in 1938. This act extended regulatory regulation to cosmetics and therapeutic devices. More importantly, it requires the pharmaceutical companies to submit full reports of investigations regarding the safety of new drugs. In 1962, a significant Kefauver-Harris Drug Amendment was passed, which not only strengthened the safety requirements for new drugs, but also established an efficacy requirement for new drugs for the first time. In 1984, Congress passed the Price Competition and Patent Term Restoration Act to provide an increased patent protection to compensate for patent life lost during the approval process. Based on this act, the FDA was authorized to approve generic drugs only based on bioavailability and bioequivalence trials on healthy subjects.

1.2.2   International Conference on Harmonization

For the marketing approval of pharmaceutical entities, the regulatory process and requirements may vary from country (region) to country (region). The necessity to standardize these similar and yet different regulatory requirements has been recognized by both regulatory authorities and the pharmaceutical industry. Hence, the International Conference on Harmonization (ICH), which consists of the European Community (EC), Japan, and the United States, was organized to provide an opportunity for important initiatives to be developed by regulatory authorities as well as industry associations for the promotion of international harmonization of regulatory requirements. The ICH, however, is only concerned with tripartite harmonization of technical requirements for the registration of pharmaceutical products among the three regions of the EC, Japan, and the United States. That is, the information generated in any of the three areas of the EC, Japan and the United States would be acceptable to the other two areas. Basically, the ICH consists of six parties that operate in these three regions, which include the European Commission of the European Union, the European Federation of Pharmaceutical Industries' Association (EFPIA), the Japanese Ministry of Health and Welfare (MHW), the Japanese Pharmaceutical Manufacturers Association (JPMA), the Center for Drug Evaluation and Research (CDER) of FDA, and the Pharmaceutical Research and Manufacturers of America (PhRMA). To assist sponsors in the drug development process, the ICH has issued a number of guidelines and draft guidances. These guidelines and guidances are summarized in Table 1.2.1.

1.2.3   U.S. Regulations

In this section, for illustration purposes, we focus on the regulatory process and requirements currently adopted in the United States. The current regulations for conducting studies, regulatory submission, review, and approval of results for pharmaceutical entities (including drugs, biological products, and medical devices under investigation) in the United States can be found in the Code of Federal Regulations (CFR). Table 1.2.2 lists the most relevant regulations with respect to drug development and approval. The Center for Drug Evaluation and Research (CDER) of the FDA has jurisdiction over the administration of regulations and the approval of pharmaceutical products classified as drugs. These regulations include investigational new drug application (IND) and new drug application (NDA) for new drugs, orphan drugs, and over-the-counter (OTC) human drugs and abbreviated new drug application (ANDA) for generic drugs.

Table 1.2.1. ICH Clinical Guidelines and Draft Guidelines

Guidelines
Safety
1 S1A: The need for long-term rodent carcinogenicity studies of pharmaceuticals
2 S1B: Testing for carcinogenicity of pharmaceuticals
3 S1C: Dose selection for carcinogenicity studies of pharmaceuticals
4 S1C(R): Guidance on dose selection for carcinogenicity studies of pharmaceuticals: Addendum on a limit dose and related notes
5 S2A: Specific aspects of regulatory genotoxicity tests for pharmaceuticals
6 S2B: Genotoxicity: A standard battery for genotoxicity testing of pharmaceuticals
7 S3A: Toxicokinetics: The assessment of systemic exposure in toxicity studies
8 S3B: Pharmacokinetics: Guideline for repeated dose tissue distribution studies
9 S4A: Duration of chronic toxicity testing in animals (rodent and nonrodent toxicity testing)
10 S5A: Detection of toxicity to reproduction for medicinal products
11 S5B: Detection of toxicity to reproduction for medicinal products: Addendum on toxicity to male fertility
12 S6: Preclinical safety evaluation of biotechnology — derived pharmaceuticals
Joint Safety/Efficacy
1 M4: Common technical document
Efficacy
1 E1A: The extent of population exposure to assess clinical safety for drugs intended for long-term treatment of non-life-threatening conditions
2 E2A: Clinical safety data management: Definitions and standards for expedited reporting
3 E2B:Data elements for transmission of individual case report forms
4 E2C: Clinical safety data management: Periodic safety update reports for marketed drugs
5 E3: Structure and content of clinical studies

Table 1.2.1. (Continued)

Efficacy	
6	E4: Dose-response information to support drug registration
7	E5: Ethnic factors in the acceptability of foreign clinical data
8	E6: Good clinical practice: Consolidated guideline
9	E7: Studies in support of special populations: Geriatrics
10	E8: General considerations for clinical trials
11	E9: Statistical principles for clinical trials
12	E11: Clinical investigation of medicinal products in the pediatric population

Quality	
1	Q1A: Stability testing of new drug substances and products
2	Q1B: Photostability testing of new drug substances and products
3	Q1C: Stability testing for new dosage forms
4	Q2A: Test on validation of analytical procedures
5	Q2B: Validation of analytical procedures: Methodology
6	Q3A: Impurities in new drug substances
7	Q3B: Impurities in new drug products
8	Q3C: Impurities: Residual solvents
9	Q5A: Viral safety evaluation of biotechnology products derived from cell lines of human or animal origin
10	Q5B: Quality of biotechnology products: analysis of the expression construct in cells used for production of r-DNA derived protein products
11	Q5C: Quality of biotechnology products: Stability testing of biotechnological/biological products
12	Q5D: Quality of biotechnology/biological products: Derivation and characterization of cell substrates used for production of biotechnological/biological products
13	Q6A: Specifications: Test procedures and acceptance criteria for new drug substances and new drug products: Chemical substances
14	Q6B: Test procedures and acceptance criteria for biotechnological/biological products

Table 1.2.1. (Continued)

Draft Guidelines
Safety
1   S7: Safety pharmacology studies for human pharmaceuticals
Efficacy
1   E10: Choice of control group in clinical trials
2   E12A: Principles for clinical evaluation of new antihypertensive drugs
Quality
1   Q1A(R): Stability testing of new drug substances and products
2   Q3A(R): Impurities in new drug substances
3   Q3B(R): Impurities in new drug products
4   Q7A: Good manufacturing practice for active pharmaceutical ingredients

Table 1.2.2. U.S. Codes of Federal Regulation (CFR) for Clinical Trials Used to Approve Pharmaceutical Entities

CFR Number	Regulations
21 CFR 50	Protection of human subjects
21 CFR 56	Institutional review boards (IRB)
21 CFR 312	Investigational new drug application (IND)
Subpart E	Treatment IND
21 CFR 314	New drug application (NDA)
Subpart C	Abbreviated applications
Subpart H	Accelerated approval
21 CFR 601	Establishment license and product license applications (ELA and PLA)
Subpart E	Accelerated approval
21 CFR 316	Orphan drugs
21 CFR 320	Bioavailability and bioequivalence requirements
21 CFR 330	Over-the-counter (OTC) human drugs
21 CFR 812	Investigational device exemptions (IDE)
21 CFR 814	Premarket approval of medical devices (PMA)
21 CFR 60	Patent term restoration
21 CFR 201	Labeling
21 CFR 202	Prescription drug advertsing

1.2.4   Institutional Review Board (IRB)

Since 1971, the FDA has required that all proposed clinical studies be reviewed both by the FDA and an institutional review board (IRB). The responsibilities of an IRB are to evaluate the ethical acceptability of the proposed clinical research and to examine the scientific validity of the study to the extent needed to be confident that the study does not expose its subjects to an unreasonable risk. The composition and function of an IRB are subject to the FDA requirements. Section 56.107 in Part 56 of 21 CFR states that each IRB should have at least five members with varying backgrounds to promote a complete review of research activities commonly conducted by the institution. Note that in order to avoid conflict of interest and to provide an unbiased and objective evaluation of scientific merits, ethical conduct of clinical trials, and protection of human subjects, the CFR enforces a very strict requirement for the composition of members of an IRB. These strict requirements include (i) no IRB is entirely composed of one gender, (ii) no IRB may consist entirely of members of one profession, (iii) each IRB should include at least one member whose primary concerns are in the scientific area and at least one member whose primary concerns are in nonscientific area, and (iv) no IRB should have a member participate in the IRB's initial or continuous review of any project in which the member has a conflicting interest, except to provide information requested by the IRB.

1.2.5   Investigational New Drug Application (IND)

Before a drug can be studied in humans, its sponsor must submit an IND to the FDA. Unless notified otherwise, the sponsor may begin to investigate the drug 30 days after the FDA has received the application. The IND requirements extend throughout the period during which a drug is under study. By the time an IND is filed, the sponsor should have sufficient information about the chemistry, manufacturing, and controls of the drug substance and drug product to ensure the identity, strength, quality, purity, stability, and reproducibility of the investigational drug covered by the IND. In addition, the sponsor should provide adequate information about pharmacological studies for absorption, distribution, metabolism, and excretion (ADME), and acute, subacute, and chronic toxicological studies and reproductive tests in various animal species to support that the investigational drug is reasonably safe to be evaluated in humans.

1.2.6 New Drug Application (NDA)

For the approval of a new drug, the FDA requires that at least two adequate well-controlled clinical studies be conducted in humans to demonstrate substantial evidence of the effectiveness and safety of the drug. Substantial evidence can be obtained through adequate and well-controlled clinical investigations. Section 314.50 of 21 CFR specifies the format and content of an NDA, which contains the application form (365H), index, summary, technical sections, samples and labeling, and case report forms and tabulations. The technical sections include chemistry, manufacturing, and controls (CMC), nonclinical pharmacology and toxicology, human pharmacology and bioavailability, microbiology (for anti-infective drugs), clinical data, and statistics. As a result, the reviewing disciplines include chemistry reviewers for the CMC section; pharmacology reviewers for nonclinical pharmacology and toxicology; medical reviewers for clinical data section; and statistical reviewers for statistical technical section.

1.2.7 Advisory Committee

The FDA has also established advisory committees in designated drug classes and subspecialities each consisting of clinical, pharmacological, and statistical experts and one consumer advocate (not employed by the FDA). The responsibilities of the committees are to review the data presented in the NDAs and to advise the FDA as to whether there exists substantial evidence of safety and effectiveness based on adequate and well-controlled clinical studies. As a result, the advisory committees address the following questions posted by the FDA followed by an intensive discussion at the end of the advisory committee meeting:

1. *Are there two or more adequate and well-controlled trials?*

2. *Have the patient populations been well enough characteristized?*

3. *Has the dose-response relationship been sufficiently characterized?*

4. *Do you recommend the use of the drug for the indication sought by the sponsor for the intended patient population?*

Note that the FDA usually follows the recommendations made by the advisory committee for marketing approval, though they do not have to legally.

1.3 Good Pharmaceutical Practices

To ensure the success of drug development in compliance with regulatory requirements for approval, good pharmaceutical practices have to be implemented. Good pharmaceutical practices are established standards to assure the drug under investigation meets the requirements of the Federal Food, Drug, and Cosmetic Act related to safety and efficacy before marketing approval and drug characteristics of identity, strength, quality, purity, stability, and reproducibility after approval. Good pharmaceutical practices include good laboratory practice (GLP), good clinical practice (GCP), and current good manufacturing practice (cGMP). GLP, GCP, and cGMP are regulations governing the conduct of preclinical safety studies and *in vitro* studies, clinical studies, and the conduct of manufacturing operations, respectively. GLP, GCP, and cGMP are briefly described in the subsequent sections.

1.3.1   Good Laboratory Practice (GLP)

Good laboratory practice (GLP) for nonclinical laboratory studies is codified in 21 CFR 58. GLP applies to animal and *in vitro* studies for safety assessment. Similar to cGMP, GLP covers regulations with respect to requirements for organization and personnel, facilities, equipment, testing facilities operations, test and control articles, protocol for and conduct of a nonclinical laboratory study, records and reports, and disqualification of testing facilities. GLP requires the existence of a quality assurance unit (QAU). The QAU's responsibilities include that (i) sampling plan, test procedure, acceptance/rejection criteria are properly documented, (ii) any identified deviations from standard operating procedure (SOP) or protocol are properly corrected and documented, (iii) internal audits are properly conducted and documented, and (iv) form 483 notice of observations as the result of an FDA's inspection are properly addressed and documented.

1.3.2   Good Clinical Practice (GCP)

Good clinical practice (GCP) is usually referred to as a set of standards for clinical studies to achieve and maintain high-quality clinical research in a sensible and responsible manner. The FDA, the Committee for Proprietary Medicinal Products (CPMP) for the European Community, the Ministry of Health and Welfare of Japan, and agencies in other countries have each issued guidelines on good clinical practices. For example, the FDA promulgated a number of regulations and guidelines governing the conduct of clinical studies from which data was to be used to support applications for marketing approval of drug products. The FDA regulations referring to GCP are specified in CFR parts 50 (protection of human subjects), 56 (institutional review boards, IRB), 312 (investigational new drug application, IND), and 314 (new drug application, NDA). Note that in 1992, Dr. A. B. Lisook at the FDA assembled a GCP packet to assist sponsors in the planning, execution, data analysis, and submission of results to the FDA (Lisook, 1992). On the other hand, the European Community established principles for their own GCP standards in all four phases of clinical investigation of medicinal products in July 1990. The ICH also issued the Guideline on Good Clinical Practice: Consolidated Guideline. This guideline defines the responsibilities of sponsors, monitors, and investigators in the initiation, conduct, documentation, and verification of clinical studies to establish the credibility of data and to protect the rights and integrity of study participants.

In essence, GCP deals with patients' protection and the equality of data used to prove the efficacy and safety of a drug product. GCP ensures that all data, information, and documents related to a clinical study can be confirmed as being properly generated, recorded, and reported through the institution by independent audits.

1.3.3 Current Good Manufacturing Practice (cGMP)

cGMP was promulgated in 1962 as part of the Federal Food, Drug and Cosmetic Act to afford greater consumer protection during the manufacture of pharmaceutical products. cGMP is now codified in 21 CFR 211, which provides minimum requirements for the manufacture, processing, packing, and holding of a drug product. Its purpose is to assure that the drug product meets the requirements of safety, identity, strength, quality, and purity characteristics that it purports to possess. cGMP covers regulations with respect to requirements for organization and personnel, buildings and facilities, equipment, control of components and drug product containers and closures, production and process control, packing and process control, holding and distribution, laboratory controls, records and reports, and returned and salvaged drug products. Failure to comply with cGMP renders the drug adulterated and the person responsible subject to regulatory action.

Record retention is an important part of cGMP. The FDA suggests that record retention should follow the principles of (i) two years after FDA approval of research or marketing permit, (ii) five years after application for IND, and (iii) two years if no application filed.

1.3.4 FDA Inspection

One of the FDA's major responsibilities is to enforce the Federal Food, Drug, and Cosmetic Act for the protection of public health. This is often done through the FDA Facility Inspection Program, which is to assure that the manufacturer is in compliance with all applicable FDA regulations. The purpose of an FDA inspection is multifold. First, it is to determine and to evaluate a firm's adherence to the concepts of cGMP. Second, it is to ensure that production and control procedures include all reasonable precautions to ensure the identity, strength, quality, purity, stability, and reproducibility of the finished products. In addition, it is to identify deficiencies that could lead to the manufacturing and distribution of products in violation of the Federal Food, Drug, and Cosmetic Act. Furthermore, it is to obtain correction of those deficiencies and to ensure that new drugs are manufactured by essentially the same procedures and the same formulations as the products used as the basis for approval.

Basically, the FDA may initiate different types of inspections depending upon the circumstances at different stages of drug research and development. These types of inspections include routine scheduled/unscheduled, survey, compliant, recall, bioresearch monitoring, government contract, and preapproval inspections. The process of a FDA inspection usually begins with a notice of inspection (form 482). The sponsor should be prepared for an FDA inspection upon the receipt of 482. After the inspection, the FDA inspector(s) will prepare an establishment inspection report (EIR) including 483 notice of observations. The sponsor should address 483 issues fully in response to the FDA Local Field Office. If no action is required as the result of the sponsor's response to 483 and EIR, the sponsor is considered to have met the requirement of the FDA's inspection. However, if an action is required, samples will be sent to the FDA District Office Compliance Office and a warning letter will be issued. Failure to comply with cGMP, GLP, and/or GCP could subject the sponsor to a regulatory action, such as seizure, injunction, prosecution, citation (483 notice of observations), detention (hold of shipment), fine, affection of license or permits, or import detention. For a better understanding, Figure 1.3.1 provides a flowchart for the FDA inspection process.

In the FDA's inspection for GLP, cGMP, and GCP, some commonly observed errors should be avoided. These errors inlcude (i) document not signed, (ii) incomplete records, e.g., missing date, time, specification number, batch number, and anything else left blank, etc., (iii) correction not signed, (iv) out of specific condition, e.g., not performed at proper time as specified in the study protocol, (v) incorrect sampling plan, e.g., samples were not uniformly and randomly selected from the target population to constitute a representative sample, (vi) incorrect information, e.g., wrong calculation and typos in date and transposed number, etc., and (vii) incorrect techniques, e.g., inappropriate use of pencil, blue ink, white out/liquid paper, and crossed out mistakes. The FDA inspection for GLP, cGMP, and GCP assures not only that the sponsor is in compliance with all applicable FDA regulations during the drug development process, but also that the drug product meets regulatory requirements for the good drug characteristics of identity, strength, quality, purity, stability, and reproducibility.

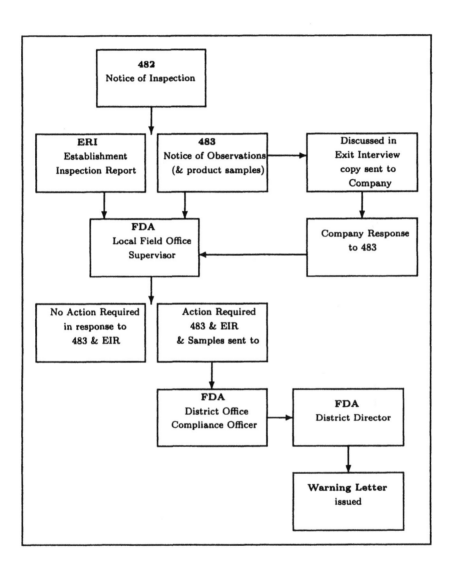

Figure 1.3.1. FDA Inspection Process

1.4   Good Statistics Practice

Good statistics practice (GSP) is defined as a set of statistical principles
for the best pharmaceutical practices in design and analysis of studies conducted at various stages of drug research and development (Chow, 1997a).
The purpose of GSP is not only to minimize bias but also to minimize
variability that may occur before, during, and after the conduct of the
studies. More importantly, GSP provides a valid and fair assessment of
the drug product under study. The concept of GSP can be seen in many
guidelines and guidances that were issued by the FDA at various stages
of drug research and development. These guidelines and guidances include
good laboratory practice (GLP), good clinical practice (GCP), current good
manufacturing practice (cGMP), and good regulatory practice (GRP). Another example of GSP is the guideline on *Statistical Principles in Clinical
Trials* recently issued by the International Conference on Harmonization
(ICH, 1998b). As a result, GSP can not only provide accuracy and reliability of the results derived from the studies, but also assure the validity and
integrity of the studies.

The implementation of GSP in pharmaceutical research and development is a team project that requires mutual communication, confidence,
respect, and cooperation among statisticians, pharmaceutical scientists in
the related areas, and regulatory agents. The implementation of GSP involves some key factors that have an impact on the success of GSP. These
factors include (i) regulatory requirements for statistics, (ii) the dissemination of the concept of statistics, (iii) appropriate use of statistics, (iv)
effective communication and flexibility, and (v) statistical training. These
factors are briefly described below.

In the pharmaceutical development and approval process, regulatory requirements for statistics are the key to the implementation of GSP. They
not only enforce the use of statistics but also establish standards for statistical evaluation of the drug products under investigation. An unbiased
statistical evaluation helps pharmaceutical scientists and regulatory agents
in determining (i) whether the drug product has the claimed effectiveness
and safety for the intended disease, and (ii) whether the drug product
possesses good drug characteristics such as the proper identity, strength,
quality, purity, and stability.

In addition to regulatory requirements, it is always helpful to dissemi-
nate the concept of statistical principles described above whenever possible.
It is important for pharmaceutical scientists and regulatory agents to rec-
ognize that (i) a valid statistical inference is necessary to provide a fair
assessment with certain assurance regarding the uncertainty of the drug
product under investigation, (ii) an invalid design and analysis may result
in a misleading or wrong conclusion about the drug product, and (iii) a

larger sample size is often required to increase statistical power and precision of the studies. The dissemination of the concept of statistics is critical to establish the pharmaceutical scientists and regulatory agents' brief in statistics for scientific excellence.

One of the commonly encountered problems in drug research and development is the misuse or sometimes the abuse of statistics in some studies. The misuse or abuse of statistics is critical, which may result in either having the right question with the wrong answer or having the right answer for the wrong question. For example, for a given study, suppose that a right set of hypotheses (the right question) is established to reflect the study objective. A misused statistical test may provide a misleading or wrong answer to the right question. On the other hand, in many clinical trials, point hypotheses for equality (the wrong question) are often wrongly used for establishment of equivalence. In this case, we have right answer (for equality) for the wrong question. As a result, it is recommended that appropriate statistical methods be chosen to reflect the design which should be able to address the scientific or medical questions regarding the intended study objectives for implementation of GSP.

Communication and flexibility are important factors to the success of GSP. Inefficient communication between statisticians and pharmaceutical scientists or regulatory agents may result in a misunderstanding of the intended study objectives and consequently an invalid design and/or inappropriate statistical methods. Thus, effective communications among statisticians, pharmaceutical scientists and regulatory agents is essential for the implementation of GSP. In addition, in many studies, the assumption of a statistical design or model may not be met due to the nature of the drug product under investigation, experimental environment, and/or other causes related/unrelated to the studies. In this case, the traditional approach of doing everything by the book does not help. In practice, since concerns from a pharmaceutical scientist or the regulatory agent may translate into a constraint for a valid statistical design and appropriate statistical analysis, it is suggested that a flexible and yet innovative solution be developed under the constraints for the implementation of GSP.

Since regulatory requirements for the drug development and approval process vary from drug to drug and country to country, various designs and/or statistical methods are often required for a valid assessment of a drug product. Therefore, it is suggested that statistical continued/advanced education and training programs be routinely held for both statisticians and nonstatisticians including pharmaceutical scientists and regulatory agents. The purpose of such a continued/advanced education and/or training program is threefold. First, it enhances communications within the statistical community. Statisticians can certainly benefit from such a training and/or educational program by acquiring more practical experience and knowledge. In addition, it provides the opportunity to share/exchange information, ideas and/or concepts regarding drug development between professional societies. Finally, it identifies critical practical and/or regulatory issues that are commonly encountered in the drug development and regulatory approval process. A panel discussion from different disciplines may result in some consensus to resolve the issues, which helps in establishing standards of statistical principles for implementation of GSP.

1.5 Aim of the Book and Outline of Practical Issues

1.5.1 The Aim and Scope of the Book

As indicated earlier, drug development is a lengthy and costly process. The purpose of this lengthy and costly process is not only to ensure the safety and efficacy of the drug under investigation before approval, but also to assure the drug possesses some good drug characteristics such as identity, strength, quality, purity, and stability after approval. Statistics plays an important role in the process of drug research and development. In the process of drug development, misusing, abusing, or not using statistics often results in misleading results/conclusions and inflating the false positive/negative rates. Appropriate use of statistics provides a fair and unbiased assessment of the drug under investigation with a certain degree of accuracy and reliability. The concept of good statistics practice in design, analysis, and interpretation of studies conducted during the drug development process is the key to the success of drug development.

This book is intended to provide a well-balanced summarization of current and emerging practical issues and the corresponding statistical methodologies in various stages of drug research and development. Our emphasis is on recent development in regulatory requirement and statistical methodology for these practical issues. It is our goal to fill the gap between pharmaceutical and statistical disciplines and to provide a comprehensive reference book for pharmaceutical scientists and biostatisticians in the area of drug research and development.

The scope of this book covers practical issues from nonclinical, preclinical, and clinical areas. Previous sections of this chapter provide an introduction to the drug development process and regulatory requirement for approving a drug product and an overview of good pharmaceutical practices and good statistics practice. Nonclinical and preclinical applications are presented in Chapter 2 through Chapter 5. Practical issues that are commonly seen in clinical development are discussed in Chapter 6 through

Chapter 12.

The following is an outline of the practical issues covered in this book and what each of Chapters 2–12 covers.

1.5.2 Pharmaceutical Validation

As indicated by Bergum and Utter (2000), pharmaceutical validation started in the early 1970s with assay verification. However, most of the FDA's attention was directed toward the validation of sterile processes of injectable products. In the early 1980s, the FDA began to focus on the validation of nonsterile processes such as solid dosage, semisolid dosage, liquids, suspensions, and aerosols. Basically, pharmaceutical validation includes the validation of laboratory instruments, such as gas chromatography (GC), and high-performance liquid chromatography (HPLC), or analytical methods developed based on these instruments and manufacturing processes for specific compounds. The cGMP requires that the sponsors establish the reliability of test results through the appropriate validation of the test results at appropriate intervals (21 CFR 210 and 211). More specifically, the cGMP requires that the accuracy and reliability of the test results be established and validated. The purpose of analytical method validation is to ensure that the assay result meets the proper standards of accuracy and reliability, while the purpose of the manufacturing process is to ensure that the manufacturing process does what it purports to do (Chow, 1997b).

The USP/NF defines the validation of analytical methods as the process by which it is established, in laboratory studies, that performance characteristics of the methods meet the requirements for the intended analytical application (USP/NF, 2000). The analytical application could be a drug potency assay for potency and stability studies, immunoassay for the *in vitro* activity of an antibody or antigen, or a biological assay for the *in vivo* activity. The performance characteristics include accuracy, precision, selectivity (or specificity), linearity, range, limit of detection, limit of quantitation, and ruggedness which are useful measures for the assessment of the accuracy and reliability of the assay results. In practice, the selection of a model and/or weights for the standard curve in calibration is critical for assurance of the accuracy and reliability of the assay results. Statistical methods for evaluation of the analytical method based on each performance characteristic under the selected model with appropriate weight are necessarily developed and justified in compliance with regulatory requirements for good validation practice.

The FDA defines process validation as establishing documented evidence which provides a high degree of assurance that a specific process will consistently produce a product meeting its predetermined specifications and quality characteristics (FDA, 1987a). A manufacturing process is necessarily validated to ensure that it does what it purports to do. A valid process assures that the final product has a high probability of meeting the standards for identity, strength, quality, purity, stability, and reproducibility of the drug product. A manufacturing process is a continuous process involving a number of critical stages. A manufacturing process is considered validated if at least three batches (or lots) pass the required USP/NF tests. A batch is considered to pass the USP/NF tests if each critical stage and the final product meet the USP/NF specifications for identity, strength, quality, purity, stability, and reproducibility. USP/NF tests are referred to as tests for potency, content uniformity (weight variation), disintegration, dissolution, and stability, which are usually conducted according to the testing plan, sampling plan, and acceptance criteria as specified in the USP/NF. In practice, it is of interest to establish in-house specification limits for each USP/NF tests at each critical stage of the manufacturing process, so that if the test results meet the in-house specification limits, there is a high probability that future batches (lots) will also meet the USP/NF specifications prior to the expiration dating period.

More details regarding regulatory requirements and statistical issues for selection of an appropriate standard curve in calibration for assay development and validation are given in Chapter 2. Also included in Chapter 2 are the concept of in-process controls and process validation and statistical methods for establishment of in-house specification limits.

1.5.3   Dissolution Testing

For oral solid dosage forms of drug products, dissolution testing is usually conducted to assess the rate and extent of drug release. The purpose of dissolution testing is multifold. First, it is to ensure that a certain amount of the drug product will be released at a specific time point after administration in order for the drug to be efficiently delivered to the site of action for optimal therapeutic effect. Second, it is to ensure that the dissolution of the drug product meets the acceptance limits for quality assurance before the drug product is released to the marketplace. Finally, it is to monitor whether the dissolution of the drug product meets the product specification limits prior to the expiration dating period (or shelf-life) of the drug product. For a valid and fair assessment of the dissolution of the drug product, specific sampling plan, acceptance criteria, and testing procedure are necessarily conducted in order to meet regulatory requirements for accuracy and reliability (USP/NF, 2000). The USP/NF suggests that a three-stage sampling plan be adopted. At each stage, a set of criteria must be met in order to pass the test. A set of in-house specification limits is usually considered to ensure that there is a high probability of passing the USP/NF dissolution test if the test results meet the in-house specification limits.

Recently, the *in vitro* dissolution testing has often been considered a surrogate for *in vivo* bioequivalence testing, which in turn serves as a surrogate for clinical outcomes. When two drug products are bioequivalent to each other, it is assumed that they reach the same therapeutic effect or that they are therapeutically equivalent. Under the assumption that there is a correlation between the *in vitro* dissolution testing and the *in vivo* bioequivalence testing, the FDA requires that dissolution profiles between the two drug products be compared, in addition to the usual USP test for dissolution. The FDA recommends a similarity factor, which is known as the f_2 similarity factor, be evaluated to determine whether two drug products have similar dissolution profiles. The use of the f_2 similarity factor has received much criticism since it was introduced by the FDA.

In practice, it is of interest to evaluate the probability of passing dissolution testing according to the sampling plan and acceptance criteria as specified by the USP/NF. The information is useful for the construct of in-house specification limits for the quality control and assurance of future batches of the drug product. In addition, it is of particular interest to study the statistical properties of the f_2 similarity factor as suggested by the FDA for dissolution profile comparison.

Chapter 3 provides an extensive discussion regarding the evaluation of the probability of passing the USP/NF dissolution test and statistical assessment of similarity between dissolution profiles, including a review of the f_2 similarity factor and a discussion of some recently developed methods.

1.5.4 Stability Analysis

For each drug product on the market, the FDA requires that an expiration dating period (or shelf-life) be indicated on the immediate container of the drug product. The expiration dating period (or shelf-life) is defined as the interval at which the drug characteristics remain unchanged. As indicated in the FDA Stability Guideline (FDA, 1987b) and in the stability guideline published by the International Conference on Harmonization (ICH, 1993), the shelf-life can be determined as the time interval at which the lower product specification intersects the 95% confidence lower bound of the average degradation curve of the drug product. In practice, stability studies are usually conducted to characterize the degradation curve of the drug product under appropriate storage conditions. The FDA and ICH stability guidelines require that at least three batches (lots) and preferably more batches be tested for the establishment of a single shelf-life for the drug product. It is suggested that stability testing be performed at a three-month interval for the first year, a six-month interval for the second year, and yearly after that. Stability test results can be combined for the establishment of a single shelf-life if there is no batch-to-batch variation. A preliminary test for batch similarity should be performed at the 25% level of significance before the data can be combined for analysis.

In recent years, the study of the effectiveness and safety of combination drug products, which may or may not have been approved by regulatory agencies, has attracted much attention. The relative proportions of individual drug products in the combination drug product and the potential drug-to-drug interaction (over time) may have an impact on the stability of the combined drug product. A typical approach is to consider the minimum of the shelf-lives observed from the individual drug products based on the percent of label claim. This method, however, is not only too conservative to be of practical interest, but it also lacks statistical justification. Therefore, how to establish the shelf-life of a combination drug product has become an interesting scientific question. This question also applies to Chinese herbal medicines, which often contain a number of active ingredients with different ratios. In practice, it is, therefore, of interest to explore statistical methods for the shelf-life estimation of drug products with multiple components. Other statistical issues related to stability include the development of statistical methods for shelf-life estimation of frozen drug products, practical issues and considerations in stability design and analysis (such as the use of matrixing) and bracketing designs and shelf-life estimation with discrete responses.

Chapter 4 provides a comprehensive review of statistical designs and methods for stability analysis. In addition, statistical methods and recent development for two phase shelf-life estimation of frozen drug products, stability analysis with discrete responses, and shelf-life estimation of drug products with multiple components are discussed.

1.5.5 Bioavailability and Bioequivalence

When a brand-name drug is going off patent, the sponsors can file an abbreviated new drug application (ANDA) for generic approval. For approval of generic copies of a brand-name drug, the FDA requires that a bioequivalence trial be conducted to provide evidence of bioequivalence in drug absorption (FDA, 1992; 2000a). The FDA indicates that an approved generic copy of a brand-name drug can serve as the substitute of the brand-name drug. However, the FDA does not indicate that two approved generic copies of the same brand-name drugs can be used interchangeably. As more generic drugs become available, the safety of drug interchangeability among generic drugs of the same brand-name drug is of great concern to consumers and the regulatory agencies as well.

The concept of drug interchangeability can be divided into prescribability and switchability. Prescribability is referred to as a physician's choice for prescribing an appropriate drug between the brand-name drug and its generic copies, while switchability is the switch from a brand-name drug or its generic copies to its generic copies within the same patient. The FDA suggests that the population bioequivalence be assessed to address prescribability. For switchability, the concept of individual bioequivalence is recommended. In practice, it is of interest to explore the statistical properties of the bioequivalence criteria for both population bioequivalence and individual bioequivalence, as proposed by the FDA.

In a recent FDA guidance on population bioequivalence and individual bioequivalence, the FDA recommends the method proposed by Hyslop, Hsuan, and Holder (2000) for assessment of population bioequivalence and individual bioequivalence (FDA, 2001). In addition, the FDA recommends that a two-sequence, four-period (2×4) crossover design be used and that a two-sequence, three-period (2×3) crossover design may be used as an alternative to the 2×4 crossover design if necessary. Although a detailed statistical procedure for assessment of individual bioequivalence under a 2×4 crossover design is provided in the FDA draft guidance, little or no information regarding statistical procedures for (i) assessment of individual bioequivalence under a 2×3 crossover design and (ii) assessment of population bioequivalence under either a 2×2, 2×3, or 2×4 crossover design is given.

Chapter 5 provides details of recent development on criteria and statistical methods for assessment of population bioequivalence and individual bioequivalence under various crossover designs. In addition, statistical methods for assessment of *in vitro* bioequivalence are also discussed.

1.5.6 Randomization and Blinding

The ultimate goal of most clinical trials is to demonstrate the safety and efficacy of the study drug products. A typical approach is to first show that there is a significant difference between the study drug product with the control (e.g., a placebo or an active control agent) with some statistical assurance. Power for detection of a clinically meaningful difference is then obtained to determine the chance of correctly detecting the difference when such a difference truly exists. Statistical inference or assurance on the uncertainties regarding the drug products under investigation can only be obtained under a probability structure of the uncertainties. The probability structure cannot be established without randomization. As a result, randomization plays an important role in clinical trials. If there is no randomization, then there is no probability structure, and hence, there is no statistical inference on which the uncertainties can be drawn. Randomization not only generates comparable groups of patients who constitute representative samples from the intended patient population, but also enable valid statistical tests for clinical evaluation of the study drug product.

In clinical trials, bias often occurs due to the knowledge of the identity of treatment. To avoid such a bias, blinding is commonly employed to block the indentity of treatments. In practice, it is of interest to determine the integrity of blinding based on the probability of correctly guessing the treatment codes. When the integrity of blinding is questionable, adjustment should be made in statistical inference on the efficacy of the study drug.

In Chapter 6, the concept of randomization, randomization models and methods, and blinding are introduced, followed by discussions of practical issues related to randomization and blinding, such as the selection of the number of study centers in a multicenter trial, the effect of mixed-up randomization schedule, assessment of integrity of blinding, and inference under breached blindness.

1.5.7   Substantial Evidence in Clinical Development

For the approval of a new drug product, the FDA requires that substantial evidence regarding the safety and efficacy of the drug product be provided through the conduct of at least two adequate and well-controlled clinical trials. The purpose for having at least two adequate and well-controlled clinical trials is not only to ensure that the clinical results observed from the two clinical trials are reproducible, but also to provide valuable information regarding generalizability of the results to a similar but different patient population.

In recent years, regulatory agencies are constantly challenged for scientific justification of the requirement that at least two adequate and well-controlled clinical trials are necessary for generalizability and reproducibility. In some cases, the variability associated with a powered clinical trial may be relatively small, and/or the observed p-value is relatively small. These facts are often used to argue against the requirement of at least two adequate and well-controlled trials. Note that, under certain circumstance, the FDA Modernization Act of 1997 includes a provision to allow data from one adequate and well-controlled clinical trial investigation and confirmatory evidence to establish effectiveness for risk/benefit assessment of drug and biological candidates for approval. Thus, if one can show a high probability of observing a significant result in future studies given that a significant result has been observed in a clinical trial that is similar to future studies, then the observed result from one clinical trial may be sufficient to fulfill the regulatory requirement.

The concept of reproducibility probability and generalizability probability of a positive clinical result is introduced in Chapter 7. Several statistical methods for evaluation of these probabilities based on observed clinical results are proposed. Applications such as bridging studies are also included.

1.5.8 Therapeutic Equivalence and Noninferiority

In drug research and development, therapeutic equivalence and noninferiority trials have become increasingly popular. Therapeutic equivalence/ noninferiority trials usually involve the comparison of a test drug with a control. The assessment of therapeutic equivalence/noninferiority depends upon the choice of a clinically meaningful difference which may vary from indication to indication and from therapy to therapy.

For the establishment of the safety and efficacy of a new drug product, the FDA prefers that placebo-control clinical trials be considered if possible. However, in many cases, placebo-control clinical trials may not be feasible, such as with anti-infective agents. In addition, it may not be ethical to conduct placebo-control clinical trials for patients with severe or life-threatening diseases, such a cancer or AIDS. As a result, active control trials are preferred in these situations as alternative clinical trials over placebo-control clinical trials.

Basically, the primary objective of an active control trial is either to show noninferiority or therapeutic equivalence. Without the inclusion of a placebo, the active control trial could lead to the conclusion that the test drug and the active control agent are either both effective or both ineffective. In practice, it is then of particular interest to develop an appropriate statistical methodology for providing direct evidence of the safety and efficacy of the study drug provided that the safety and efficacy information of the active control agent as compared to a placebo is available.

Chapter 8 introduces the concepts of therapeutic equivalence and noninferiority tests in clinical research, including the selection of controls, interval hypotheses for equivalence/noninferiority, and equivalence limit or noninferiority margin. Two commonly used statistical methods for assessment of therapeutic equivalence/noninferiority, the two one-sided tests procedure and the confidence interval approach, are introduced and some related statistical issues are discussed. Also included in this chapter are discussions on active control trials and active control equivalence trials in clinical development. Statistical methods for determination of direct evidence of efficacy of a test drug product relative to a placebo in an active control trial are studied.

1.5.9   Analysis of Incomplete Data

In clinical trials, dropouts and missing values may occur due to medical evaluations, administrative considerations, or other reasons unrelated to the conduct of the trials. As a result of dropouts or missing values, the observed clinical data are incomplete. When dropouts or missing values are not related to the main response variable used to evaluate treatment effects, i.e., a dropout or missing value is at random, statistical inference can be made by conditioning on the observed incomplete data. Chapter 9 studies the effect of the rate of missing values on the statistical power of the tests for treatment effects. The result is useful for the determination of sample size in planning a clinical trial to account for possible missing values in order to achieve the desired power. In some cases, information provided by auxiliary variables can be used to improve the statistical power, which is also discussed in Chapter 9.

When dropouts or missing values are related to the main response variable used to evaluate treatment effects, the evaluation of treatment effects between patients who stay and patients who drop out is necessary to provide a fair and unbiased assessment of the treatment effect. As indicated in the ICH guideline, the primary analysis of clinical trials should be the one based on the intention-to-treat population. The analysis of this kind is referred to as the intention-to-treat analysis. For efficacy evaluation, the intention-to-treat population is usually defined as all randomized patients who have at least one post-treatment assessment regardless of noncompliance and dropouts. For safety assessment, the intention-to-treat population includes all randomized patients who take any amount of study medications. When dropouts occur during the conduct of clinical trials with repeated measurements, the approach using the concept of last observation carried forward (LOCF) is recommended. The validity of this approach has been challenged by many researchers. Chapter 9 provides a comprehensive evaluation of the LOCF analysis. Some other methods providing valid statistical inference in analysis of last observation and analysis of longitudinal data, which are useful when the LOCF analysis fails, are also introduced in Chapter 9.

1.5.10   Meta-Analysis

Meta-analysis is a systematic reviewing strategy that combines results from a number of independent studies to address some scientific questions of interest individually. These independent studies could be either too small or inconclusive in addressing the questions of interest. The purpose of a meta-analysis is not only to reduce bias, but also to increase the power of an overall assessment of the treatment effect. The concept of meta-analysis is well accepted by regulatory agencies provided that the selection bias has been appropriately addressed and the studies are combinable (i.e., there is no significant treatment-by-study interaction). A meta-analysis is often confused with a multicenter trial, when each study is treated as a center. It should be noted that, unlike in a multicenter trial, the study protocols, inclusion/exclusion criteria, patient populations, dosages and routes of administration, trial procedure, and duration may be different from study to study in a meta-analysis. However, statistical methods applicable to meta-analysis are also applicable to multicenter trials.

Chapter 10 introduces some traditional methods for meta-analysis as well as some new developments in testing treatment-by-study interaction in a meta-analysis (or treatment-by-center in a multicenter trial), in assessment of bioequivalence, and in comparison of multiple drug products.

1.5.11 Quality of Life

In recent years, the assessment of quality of life (QOL) has become very popular in clinical trials. It is a debate whether it is more important to prolong life than to enhance life for patients with chronic, severe, or life-threatening disease. Smith (1992) considered QOL as how a person feels in daily activity. QOL is usually assessed through an instrument, which is a questionnaire containing a number of questions regarding several domains of QOL, such as general well-being and emotional status.

Since QOL is assessed by a rather subjective questionnaire, the validation of the instrument is necessary to ensure the validity and reliability of the instrument. An instrument is considered validated if it meets some pre-specified criteria of performance characteristics such as validity, reliability (e.g., internal consistency and reproducibility), sensitivity, and responsiveness. It practice, it is of interest to explore statistical methods for the validation of a QOL instrument, the assessment of parallel questionnaires, and the calibration of the QOL score against life events.

Chapter 11 provides a comprehensive review of quality of life assessment in clinical trials. In addition, statistical methods for validation of a QOL instrument, the assessment of parallel questionnaires and the calibration of QOL score against life events are explored.

1.5.12 Statistics in Medical Imaging

In recent years, the development of medical imaging agents has become increasingly important. The intention of a medical imaging agent is twofold. First, it is to delineate nonanatomic structures such as tumors or abscesses. Second, it is to detect disease or pathology within an anatomic structure. Hence, the indications of medical imaging drugs include structure delineation (normal or abnormal), functional, physiological, or biochemical assessment, disease or pathology detection or assessment, and diagnostic or therapeutic patient management. Although medical imaging agents are generally governed by the same regulations as other drugs or biological products, the FDA requires special considerations in clinical trials designed to establish or support the efficacy of a medical imaging agent. These special considerations include subject selection, imaging condition and evaluation, including appropriate blinded-reader imaging evaluation procedures, the use of truth standards (or gold standards), the analysis of receiver operating characteristic (ROC), and comparison between groups.

Chapter 12 attempts to provide a comprehensive overview of these issues that are commonly encountered in medical imaging studies.

Chapter 2

Pharmaceutical Validation

In drug research and development, pharmaceutical validations are implemented to ensure that the drug product under investigation meet specifications for identity, strength, quality, purity, stability and reproducibility of the drug product. Basically, pharmaceutical validations include *assay validation* of analytical methods and *process validation* of manufacturing processes. Note that pharmaceutical validation started in the early 1970s with assay validation (Bergum and Utter, 2000). However, most of the FDA's attention was directed toward the validation of sterile processes of injectable products. In early 1980s, the FDA began to focus on the validation of nonsterile processes. The purpose of the validation of an analytical method or a testing procedure is to assure the accuracy and reliability of the test results obtained from the analytical method or the testing procedure. The objective of the validation of a manufacturing process is to ensure that the manufacturing process does what it purports to do. A validated process assures that the final product has a high probability of meeting the standards for the identity, strength, quality, purity, stability, and reproducibility of the drug product.

Regulatory requirements for assay and process validations are described in §2.1. Statistical methods for establishment of the standard curve in calibration for assay validation are introduced in §2.2. §2.3 discusses calibration for obtaining assay results and its statistical validity (bias and mean squared error). §2.4 provides a summary of statistical methods for assessment of performance characteristics for assay validation as described in the USP/NF. The concept of in-process controls and process validation is introduced in §2.5. Multiple stage tests for establishment of in-house specification limits in in-process controls and validation are discussed in §2.6.

2.1   Regulatory Requirements

When a new pharmaceutical compound is discovered, the FDA requires that an analytical method or test procedure for quantitation of the active ingredients of the compound be developed and validated before it can be applied to animal and/or human subjects (FDA, 1987a). The current good manufacturing practice (cGMP) requires that test methods, which are used for assessing compliance of pharmaceutical products with established specifications, must meet proper standards of accuracy and reliability. The General Chapter of the USP/NF defines the validation of analytical methods as the process by which it is established, in laboratory studies, that performance characteristics of the methods meet the requirements for the intended analytical application (USP/NF, 2000). The performance characteristics include accuracy, precision, limit of detection, limit of quantitation, selectivity (or specificity), linearity, range, and ruggedness. These performance characteristics are often used for assessment of accuracy and reliability of the test results obtained from the analytical methods or the test procedures. The analytical application may be referred to as a drug potency, which is usually based on gas chromatography (GC) or high-performance liquid chromatography (HPLC) for potency and stability studies, immunoassays such as radioimmunoassay (RIA) for the *in vitro* activity of an antibody or antigen, or a biological assay for the *in vivo* activity such as median effective dose (ED_{50}).

For the evaluation of a manufacturing process of a drug product, subpart F of part 210 for cGMP in 21 CFR describes the requirements of sampling plans and test procedures for in-process control and process validation. cGMP requires that drug manufacturers establish and follow written procedures for in-process controls and process validations. For the establishment of written procedures of in-process controls and process validations, the cGMP indicates that some minimum requirements should be established. These requirements include adequacy of mixing to assure uniformity and homogeneity, dissolution time and rate, disintegration time, tablets or capsule weight variation, and clarity, completeness, or pH of solution. As a result, content uniformity testing of dosage form, dissolution testing, and disintegration testing as described in the USP/NF are often conducted to determine whether the in-process materials and the final product conform to these minimum requirements. These tests are usually referred to as USP/NF tests. A manufacturing process is a continuous process involving a number of critical stages such as initial blending, mill, primary blending, final blending, compression, and coating stages for tablets manufacturing. A manufacturing process is considered to pass the USP/NF tests if each critical stage of the manufacturing process and the final product meet the required USP/NF specifications for the identity, strength, quality, purity, stability, and reproducibility of the drug product. A manufacturing process is considered validated if at least three validation batches (or lots) pass all required USP/NF tests.

2.2   Standard Curve

As mentioned earlier, when a new pharmaceutical compound is discovered, analytical methods or test procedures are necessarily developed for determining the active ingredients of the compound in compliance with USP/NF standards for the identity, strength, quality, purity stability, and reproducibility of the compound. An analytical method or test procedure is usually developed based on instruments such as HPLC. cGMP indicates that an instrument must be suitable for its intended purposes and be capable of producing valid results with certain degrees of accuracy and reliability. Therefore, the instrument must be calibrated, inspected, and checked routinely according to written procedures. As a result, instrument calibration is essential in order to meet the established written procedures or specifications.

A typical approach to instrument calibration is to have a number of known standard concentration preparations $\{x_i, i = 1, ..., n\}$ put through the instrument to obtain the corresponding responses $\{y_i, i = 1, ..., n\}$. Based on $\{x_i, y_i, i = 1, ..., n\}$, an estimated calibration curve can be obtained by fitting an appropriate statistical model between y_i and x_i. The estimated calibration curve is usually referred to as the *standard curve*. For a given unknown sample x_0 with a response of y_0, the concentration of x_0 can be estimated based on the established standard curve by the x-value that corresponds to y_0 (see §2.3). Alternatively, an estimate of x_0 can also be obtained by applying the inverse regression with x_i and y_i switched. Chow and Shao (1990) studied the difference between the estimates of x_0 obtained by using the standard curve and the inverse regression.

2.2.1   Model Selection

For an analytical method or a test procedure, the precision and reliability of the assay result or the test result of an unknown sample rely on the validity and efficiency of the established standard curve that is constructed based on the selected statistical model. Therefore, it is critical to select an appropriate statistical model for instrument calibration. Let x_i be the ith standard concentration preparation and y_i be the corresponding response from the instrument, $i = 1, ..., n$. In practice, the following models are commonly used for establishment of standard curve:

Model	Description
1	$y_i = \alpha + \beta x_i + e_i$
2	$y_i = \beta x_i + e_i$
3	$y_i = \alpha + \beta_1 x_i + \beta_2 x_i^2 + e_i$
4	$y_i = \alpha x_i^\beta e_i$
5	$y_i = \alpha e^{\beta x_i} e_i$

where α, β, β_1, and β_2 are unknown parameters and e_i's are independent random errors with $E(e_i) = 0$ and finite $\text{Var}(e_i)$ in models 1-3, and $E(\log e_i) = 0$ and finite $\text{Var}(\log e_i)$ in models 4-5.

Model 1 is a simple linear regression model which is probably the most commonly used statistical model for establishment of standard curves. When the standard curve passes through the origin, model 1 reduces to model 2. Model 3 indicates that the relationship between y_i and x_i is quadratic. When there is a nonlinear relationship between y_i and x_i, models 4 and 5 are useful. As a matter of fact, both model 4 and model 5 are equivalent to a simple linear regression model after a logarithmic transformation. It can be seen that under each of the above models, although the standard curve can be obtained by fitting an ordinary linear regression, the resultant estimates of the concentration of the unknown sample are different. Thus, how to select an appropriate model among the five models has been a challenge for scientists in this area. For example, Box and Hill (1967) used a Bayesian approach to determine the *true* model out of several candidate models. Some statistical tests of hypotheses for discriminating among models were developed by Cox (1961, 1962) and Atkinson (1969). Akaike (1973) suggested an information measure to discriminate among several models. Borowiak (1989) gave a comprehensive discussion on the general issues of model discrimination for nonlinear regression models.

Since models 1-4 are polynomials and model 5 can be approximated by a polynomial, Ju and Chow (1996) recommended the following ad hoc procedure for model selection using a sequential hypotheses testing approach:

Step 1: If the number of levels of standard concentration is less than 4, go to the next step; otherwise, start with the following polynomial regression model

$$y_i = \alpha + \beta_1 x_i + \beta_2 x_i^2 + \beta_3 x_i^3 + \beta_4 x_i^4 + e_i. \tag{2.2.1}$$

Let p_{34} be the p-value for testing

$$H_{034} : \beta_3 = \beta_4 = 0,$$

based on the ordinary least squares fitting of model (2.2.1). If p_{34} is greater than a predetermined level of significance, go to the next step; otherwise, go to Step 4.

Step 2: Since β_3 and β_4 are not significantly different from zero, model (2.2.1) reduces to

$$y_i = \alpha + \beta_1 x_i + \beta_2 x_i^2 + e_i. \tag{2.2.2}$$

We then select a model among models 1 to 3. Let p_2 be the p-value for testing

$$H_{02} : \beta_2 = 0.$$

If p_2 is greater than a predetermined level of significance, model 3 is chosen; otherwise, go to the next step.

Step 3: If β_2 is not significantly different from zero, model (2.2.2) reduces to

$$y_i = \alpha + \beta_1 x_i + e_i.$$

In this case, we select a model between models 1 and 2 by testing

$$H_{01} : \beta_1 = 0.$$

If the p-value for testing H_{01} is smaller than the predetermined level of significance, model 1 is chosen; otherwise, model 2 is selected.

Step 4: We select model 4 or model 5. Since models 4 and 5 have the same number of parameters, we would select the model with a smaller residual sum of squares.

Alternatively, Tse and Chow (1995) proposed a selection procedure based on the R^2 statistic and the mean squared error of the resultant calibration estimator of the unknown sample. Their idea can be described as follows. First, fit the five candidate models using data $\{x_i, y_i, i = 1, ..., n\}$. Then, eliminate those candidate models that fail the lack-of-fit test or significance test. For the remaining models, calculate the corresponding R^2 value, where

$$R^2 = \frac{\text{SSR}}{\text{SSR} + \text{SSE}},$$

and SSR and SSE are the sum of squares due to the regression and the sum of squares of residuals, respectively. The R^2 represents the proportion of the total variability of the responses explained by the model. It is often used as an indicator for the goodness of fit of the selected statistical model in analytical research in drug research and development (Anderson-Sprecher, 1994). Let R_{max}^2 be the maximum of the R^2 values among the remaining models. For each model, define $r = R^2/R_{\text{max}}^2$. Eliminate those models with r-value less than r_0 where r_0 is a predetermined critical value. For the remaining models, identify the best model by comparing the mean squared errors of the calibration estimator of the unknown concentration at x_0 based on the candidate models that would produce a given target response y_0. Some formulae for the mean squared errors of calibration estimators are given in §2.3.

2.2.2   Weight Selection

For establishment of standard curve in calibration of an instrument, larger
variability is often observed in the response of a higher standard concentration preparation. If this is the case, the ordinary least squares estimators may not be efficient. Alternatively, a weighted least squares
method is often considered to incorporate the heterogeneity of the variability. Let $Y = (y_1, ..., y_n)'$ and $\varepsilon = (e_1, ..., e_n)'$ under models 1-3 and
$Y = (\log y_1, ..., \log y_n)'$ and $\varepsilon = (\log e_1, ..., \log e_n)'$ under models 4-5. Then,
the five models described in §2.2.1 can be written as

$$Y = X\theta + \varepsilon,$$

where θ is a p-vector of parameters, X is the $n \times p$ matrix whose ith row is
X_i, and θ and X_i for each model are given below.

Model	θ	X_i
1	$(\alpha, \beta)'$	$(1, x_i)'$
2	β	x_i
3	$(\alpha, \beta_1, \beta_2)'$	$(1, x_i, x_i^2)'$
4	$(\log \alpha, \beta)'$	$(1, \log x_i)'$
5	$(\log \alpha, \beta)'$	$(1, x_i)'$

Let W be the $n \times n$ diagonal matrix whose ith diagonal element is the
weight w_i. Then a weighted least squares estimator of θ is

$$\hat{\theta}_W = (X'WX)^{-1}X'WY. \tag{2.2.3}$$

Appropriate weights are usually selected so that the variance of the response at each standard concentration preparation is stabilized. Selection
of an appropriate weight depends on the pattern of the standard deviation
of the response at each standard concentration preparation. Let SD_x be
the standard deviation of the response corresponding to the standard concentration preparation x. In practice, the following three types of weights
are commonly employed for establishment of standard curve:

SD_x	Weight
σ_e	1
$\sigma_e\sqrt{x}$	$1/x$
$\sigma_e x$	$1/x^2$

where $\sigma_e > 0$ is an unknown parameter. When SD_x is a constant across
all standard concentration preparations under study, no weight is necessary
and $W =$ the identity matrix, in which case $\hat{\theta}_W$ in (2.2.3) is the same as the

ordinary least squares estimator. If SD_x is proportional to $\sqrt{x}$ (or x), an appropriate choice for w_i is $1/x_i$ (or $1/x_i^2$). For each of these three weights, the weighted least squares estimator $\hat{\theta}_W$ is an unbiased estimator of θ with

$$\text{Var}(\hat{\theta}_W) = (X'WX)^{-1}X'W\text{Var}(\varepsilon)WX(X'WX)^{-1}, \qquad (2.2.4)$$

which reduces to $\sigma_e^2(X'WX)^{-1}$ if the correct weight is used (e.g., $SD_x = \sigma_e\sqrt{x}$ and $w_i = 1/x_i$ is chosen).

Ju and Chow (1996) suggested to use the following model for weight selection:

$$|r_i| = \gamma_0 + \gamma_1\sqrt{x_i} + \gamma_2 x_i + u_i, \quad i = 1, ..., n,$$

where r_i is the ith residual from the ordinary least squares estimation of θ and γ_j's are unknown parameters. If we fail to reject the null hypothesis of

$$H_0 : \gamma_1 = \gamma_2 = 0,$$

then no weight is necessary. When the above null hypothesis is rejected, we select the weight of $1/x^2$ if

$$SS(b_2|b_0, b_1) > SS(b_1|b_0, b_2),$$

where $SS(b_2|b_0, b_1)$ is the extra sum of squares due to the inclusion of the term $\gamma_2 x$ provided that γ_0 and $\gamma_1\sqrt{x}$ are already in the model. $SS(b_1|b_0, b_2)$ is similarly defined. Otherwise, we select the weight of $1/x$.

Alternatively, we may select a weight function by minimizing an estimated $\text{Var}(\hat{\theta}_W)$ given by (2.2.4), since the true variance of $\hat{\theta}_W$ is minimized when the correct weight is selected. Let W_j, $j = 0, 1, 2$, be the weight matrix W corresponding to the selection of weight functions 1, $1/x$, $1/x^2$, respectively. An approximately unbiased estimator of $\text{Var}(\hat{\theta}_{W_j})$ is

$$D_j = (X'W_jX)^{-1}X'W_j\hat{V}W_jX(X'W_jX)^{-1},$$

where $\hat{V}$ is the $n \times n$ diagonal matrix whose ith diagonal element is r_i^2 and r_i is the ith residual from the ordinary least squares estimation. Then the weight function corresponding to W_j is selected if $D_j = \min\{D_0, D_1, D_2\}$. It will be shown in §2.3 that choosing W by minimizing $\text{Var}(\hat{\theta}_W)$ leads to the most efficient calibration.

Note that weight selection affects the efficiency, not the bias of the estimation of θ, since any weighted least squares estimator is unbiased as long as a correct model is chosen. On the other hand, if a wrong model is used, then all weighted least squares estimators are biased, and they are not good estimators even if the best weights are used. Thus, weight selection can be performed after a suitable model is chosen and at the model selection stage, the ordinary least squares method can be used for simplicity.

2.3   Calibration and Assay Results

For a given unknown sample concentration x_0 with a response of y_0, the *assay result* of the unknown sample, denoted by $\hat{x}_0$, is the estimated value of x_0 obtained by finding the x-value corresponding to y_0 on the established standard curve. For example, if model 1 in §2.2.1 is used, then

$$\hat{x}_0 = (y_0 - \hat{\alpha})/\hat{\beta},$$

where $\hat{\alpha}$ and $\hat{\beta}$ are the ordinary or weighted least squares estimators of α and β. In general,

$$\hat{x}_0 = h(y_0, \hat{\theta}_W),$$

where $\hat{\theta}_W$ is the weighted least squares estimator of θ given by (2.2.3) under one of the five models in §2.2.1 and h is a function depending on the model. The functions h for the five models in §2.2.1 are given as follows:

Model	θ	$h(y_0, \theta)$
1	$(\alpha, \beta)'$	$(y_0 - \alpha)/\beta$
2	β	y_0/β
3	$(\alpha, \beta_1, \beta_2)'$	$[-\beta_1 \pm \sqrt{\beta_1^2 - 4\beta_2(\alpha - y_0)}]/(2\beta_2)$
4	$(\log \alpha, \beta)'$	$(y_0/\alpha)^{1/\beta}$
5	$(\log \alpha, \beta)'$	$(\log y_0 - \log \alpha)/\beta$

Note that under model 3, there may be two x-values corresponding to a single y_0. One of these x-values, however, is usually outside of the study range of x and, thus, the other x-value is $\hat{x}_0$.

In general, $\hat{x}_0$ is not exactly equal to x_0 because of two sources of variability: the variation due to the response y_0 and the statistical variation in the construction of the standard curve. The variability of an estimator is usually assessed by its bias and mean squared error. For $\hat{x}_0$, however, its exact first and second moments may not exist, since h is a nonlinear function of θ. Thus, we use asymptotic (large n) bias and mean squared error of $\hat{x}_0$ (see, e.g., Shao, 1999, §2.5) to assess its variability. The asymptotic bias of $\hat{x}_0$ is

$$\text{bias}_{x_0} = E_{y_0}[h(y_0, \theta)] - x_0,$$

where E_{y_0} is the expectation with respect to y_0. Under models 1-2, h is linear in y_0 and, hence,

$$\text{bias}_{x_0} = h(E(y_0), \theta) - x_0 = 0,$$

i.e., $\hat{x}_0$ is asymptotically unbiased. Similarly, $\hat{x}_0$ is asymptotically unbiased under model 5. Under model 3 or 4, $\hat{x}_0$ is slightly biased, since h is nonlinear in y_0. Similarly, the asymptotic mean squared error of $\hat{x}_0$ is

$$\text{mse}_{x_0} = E_{y_0}[h(y_0, \theta) - x_0]^2 + E_{y_0}[H(y_0, \theta)'\text{Var}(\hat{\theta}_W)H(y_0, \theta)], \quad (2.3.1)$$

where $H(y_0, \theta) = \partial h(y_0, \theta)/\partial \theta$. Under model 1, for example,

$$\text{mse}_{x_0} = \frac{1}{\beta^2} \left\{ \text{Var}(y_0) + E_{y_0} \left[\left(1, \tfrac{y_0 - \alpha}{\beta}\right) \text{Var}(\hat{\theta}_W) \left(1, \tfrac{y_0 - \alpha}{\beta}\right)' \right] \right\}$$

and in the case of constant weight function, it reduces to

$$\text{mse}_{x_0} = \frac{\sigma_e^2}{\beta^2} \left[1 + \frac{1}{n} + \frac{(x_0 - \bar{x})^2 + \sigma_e^2/\beta^2}{S_{xx}} \right], \qquad (2.3.2)$$

where $\bar{x}$ is the average of x_i's and $S_{xx} = \sum_{i=1}^{n}(x_i - \bar{x})^2$. A result similar to (2.3.2) is given by Buonaccorsi (1986).

Formula (2.3.1) also indicates that we should select the weight matrix W by minimizing $\text{Var}(\hat{\theta}_W)$, which yields the most efficient estimator $\hat{x}_0$. Note that Formula (2.3.1) is still valid even if an incorrect weight function is used. However, this formula is not valid if a wrong model is selected.

Formula (2.3.1) or (2.3.2) can be used to determine the sample size n in establishing the standard curve. For example, Buonaccorsi and Iyer (1986) suggested three criteria for choosing n: V-optimality, which concerns mse_{x_0}; AV-optimality, which concerns an average of mse_{x_0} over x_0 with respect to a distribution of x_0; and M-optimality, which concerns the maximum of mse_{x_0} over a range of x_0.

When there are some independent replicates at x_0, which yield several estimates of x_0, the asymptotic mean squared error of $\hat{x}_0$ can be estimated (see, e.g., §2.4). Without replicates, we can still estimate mse_{x_0}, but some derivations are necessary. We illustrate this in the following example.

Example 2.3.1. Table 2.3.1 contains 12 standard concentration preparations and their corresponding absorbances (the y-responses) in a potency test of a drug product. The response y_0 corresponding to the unknown sample concentration x_0 is also included in Table 2.3.1. The results in Table 2.3.1 are in the actual order of the runs.

Ju and Chow's model and weight selection procedure described in §2.2 was applied to select a model and weight function, which results in model 1 with constant variance. The standard curve is

$$y = -2.358 + 5.429x$$

with $R^2 = 0.966$ and $\hat{\sigma}_e = 3.987$. With $y_0 = 90.044$, we obtain that

$$\hat{x}_0 = 17.020.$$

Note that under model 1 with constant variance, $\hat{x}_0$ is asymptotically unbiased with mse_{x_0} given by (2.3.2). mse_{x_0} can be estimated by replacing

σ_e^2/β^2 in (2.3.2) by $\hat{\sigma}_e^2/\hat{\beta}^2 = 3.987^2/5.429^2 = 0.539$. The formula in (2.3.2) also involves x_0. If x_0 in (2.3.2) is replaced by $\hat{x}_0$, then we obtain the following estimate of mse_{x_0}:

$$\widehat{\text{mse}}_{x_0} = \frac{\hat{\sigma}_e^2}{\hat{\beta}^2}\left[1 + \frac{1}{n} + \frac{(\hat{x}_0 - \bar{x})^2 + \hat{\sigma}_e^2/\hat{\beta}^2}{S_{xx}}\right] = 0.674.$$

A slightly different estimator according to Buonaccorsi (1986) is

$$\widetilde{\text{mse}}_{x_0} = \frac{\hat{\sigma}_e^2}{\hat{\beta}^2}\left[1 + \frac{1}{n} + \frac{(\hat{x}_0 - \bar{x})^2}{S_{xx}}\right] = 0.672,$$

which is motivated by the fact that

$$\begin{aligned}
E_{y_0}(\hat{x}_0 - \bar{x})^2 &= E_{y_0}\left(\frac{y_0 - \hat{\alpha}}{\hat{\beta}} - \bar{x}\right)^2 \\
&= \frac{E_{y_0}(y_0 - \hat{\alpha} - \hat{\beta}\bar{x})^2}{\hat{\beta}^2} \\
&\approx \frac{E_{y_0}(y_0 - \alpha - \beta\bar{x})^2}{\beta^2} \\
&= (x_0 - \bar{x})^2 + \sigma_e^2/\beta^2.
\end{aligned}$$

Note that $\widehat{\text{mse}}_{x_0}$ is slightly more conservative than $\widetilde{\text{mse}}_{x_0}$.

Table 2.3.1. Calibration Data (Example 2.3.1)

Concentration ($\mu g \ ml^{-1}$)	Absorbance (area)
17.65 (L)	97.485
17.65 (L)	95.406
22.06 (M)	121.200
22.06 (M)	121.968
26.47 (H)	142.346
26.47 (H)	145.464
x_0	90.044
26.47 (H)	141.835
26.47 (H)	135.625
22.06 (M)	113.814
22.06 (M)	112.890
17.65 (L)	89.872
17.65 (L)	90.964

2.4 Assay Validation

As indicated by the USP/NF, the validation of an analytical method or a test procedure can be carried out by assessing a set of performance characteristics or analytical validation parameters. These validation parameters include accuracy, precision, limit of detection, limit of quantitation, selectivity, range, linearity, and ruggedness. Shah et al. (1992) recommended that an analytical method be considered validated in terms of accuracy if the mean value is within ±15% of the actual value. Similarly, it is also suggested that the analytical method be considered validated in terms of precision if the precision around the mean value does not exceed a 15% coefficient of variation (CV). One may use the same 15% criterion for other validation parameters, except for the limit of quantitation (LOQ), where it should not deviate from the actual value by more than 20%.

In practice, the validation of an analytical method is usually carried out by the following steps. First, it is important to develop a prospective protocol, which clearly states the validation design, sampling procedure, acceptance criteria for the performance characteristics to be evaluated, and how the validation is to be carried out. Second, collect the data and document the experiment, including any violations from the protocol that may occur. The data should be audited for quality assurance. The collected data are then analyzed based on appropriate statistical methods. Appropriate statistical methods are referred to as those methods which can reflect the validation design and meet the study objective. Finally, draw a conclusion regarding whether the analytical method is validated based on the statistical inference drawn about the accuracy, precision, and ruggedness of the assay results. In this section, we define each validation parameter and provide a description of standard statistical method for assessment of the validation parameter.

2.4.1 Accuracy

The accuracy of an analytical method or a test procedure is defined as the closeness of the result obtained by the analytical method or the test procedure to the true value. In practice, the bias is often considered as the primary measure for closeness in the assessment of assay accuracy.

In the validation of an analytical method, the accuracy of an analytical method is usually assessed through the conduct of a recovery study. In a recovery study, the analytical method is applied to samples or mixtures of excipients, which usually consist of known amounts of analyte that are added both above and below the normal levels expected in the samples. The analytical method employed recovers the active ingredients from the excipients. The recovered added amount of active ingredients are usually expressed as a percent of a label claim. A recovery study is typically conducted on three separate days and three assay results are obtained on each day. Let y_{ij} be the assay result obtained by the analytical method when the known amount of analyte is x_{ij}, where i is the index for day. The percent recovery of x_{ij} is defined to be $z_{ij} = y_{ij}/x_{ij}$, which is assumed to follow a one way random effects model

$$z_{ij} = \mu_z + D_i + e_{ij}, \quad i = 1, 2, 3, j = 1, 2, 3, \qquad (2.4.1)$$

where μ_z is an unknown parameter, D_i's are independently distributed as $N(0, \sigma_D^2)$, e_{ij}'s are independently distributed as $N(0, \sigma_e^2)$, and D_i's and e_{ij}'s are mutually independent. Note that σ_D^2 and σ_e^2 are known as the between day (or day-to-day) variability and the within day (or intra-day) variability, respectively.

Using the criteria recommended by Shah et al. (1992), the analytical method is validated in terms of accuracy if $85\% < \mu_z < 115\%$. Thus, if a 95% confidence interval based on the recovery data is within the interval $(85\%, 115\%)$, then the analytical method is considered validated. In practice, the largest possible bias (i.e., either the lower or upper limit of the 95% confidence interval for the mean) is often reported in assay validation for accuracy.

Since model (2.4.1) is a balanced one way random effects model, the best unbiased estimator of μ_z is $\bar{z} = \sum_{i,j} z_{ij}/9$. A 95% confidence interval for μ_z is

$$\left(\bar{z} - t_{0.975;2} s_D/\sqrt{3}, \ \bar{z} + t_{0.975;2} s_D/\sqrt{3} \right),$$

where $s_D^2 = \sum_{i=1}^{3} (\bar{z}_i - \bar{z})^2$, $\bar{z}_i = \sum_{i=1}^{3} z_i/3$, and $t_{0.975;r}$ is the 97.5th percentile of the t-distribution with r degrees of freedom.

The accuracy of an analytical method can also be assessed by a statistical analysis of the standard curve corresponding to the analytical method (see §2.2). For example, when the standard curve is given by a simple linear regression model, i.e.,

$$y_i = \alpha + \beta x_i + e_i,$$

Bohidar (1983) and Bohidar and Peace (1988) suggested that the accuracy of an analytical method be assessed by testing the following hypotheses:

$$
\begin{array}{llll}
H_{01} : \beta = 0 & \text{versus} & H_{11} : \beta \neq 0, \\
H_{02} : \beta = 1 & \text{versus} & H_{12} : \beta \neq 1, \\
H_{03} : \alpha = 0 & \text{versus} & H_{13} : \alpha \neq 0.
\end{array}
$$

The first set of hypotheses is used to quantify a significant linear relationship between recovered (or found) and added amounts (input). This is because an analytical method cannot be validated if no relationship between found and input exists. The second set of hypotheses is used to verify whether the change in one unit of the added amount will result in the change in one unit of the recovered amount. The third set of hypotheses is to make sure that the analytical method does not recover any active ingredient if it is not added.

2.4.2 Precision

The precision of an analytical method or a test procedure is referred to as the degree of closeness of the result obtained by the analytical method or the test procedure to the true value. In practice, the total variability associated with the assay result is often considered as the primary measure for the assessment of assay precision.

The assessment of assay precision can be carried out by using the data from the recovery study described in §2.4.1. Under model (2.4.1), the total variability, the between day (or day-to-day) variability, and the within day variability of the analytical method can be estimated. Using the method of analysis of variance (ANOVA), we obtain the following estimator of within day variance σ_e^2:

$$\hat{\sigma}_e^2 = \frac{1}{6} \sum_{i=1}^{3} \sum_{j=1}^{3} (z_{ij} - \bar{Z}_i)^2,$$

and the following estimator of between day variance σ_D^2:

$$\hat{\sigma}_D^2 = s_D^2 - \hat{\sigma}_e^2/3.$$

Since an ANOVA estimate may lead to a negative estimate for the between day variance σ_D^2, the method of restricted maximum likelihood (REML), which truncates the ANOVA estimate at zero, is usually considered as an alternative to the ANOVA estimate. To avoid a negative estimate, it is recommended that the method proposed by Chow and Shao (1988) be used.

The total variability of an analytical method, $\sigma_T^2 = \sigma_D^2 + \sigma_e^2$, can be estimated by

$$\hat{\sigma}_T^2 = \frac{1}{8} \sum_{i,j} (z_{ij} - \bar{z})^2.$$

If an analytical method is considered validated in terms of precise when the total variability is less than a predetermined σ_0^2, then we may claim that the analytical method is validated if $8\hat{\sigma}_T^2/\chi_{0.95;8}^2 < \sigma_0^2$, where $\chi_{0.95;r}^2$ is the 95th percentile of the chi-square distribution with r degrees of freedom and $8\hat{\sigma}_T^2/\chi_{0.95;8}^2$ is a 95% confidence bound for σ_T^2.

2.4.3   Other Performance Characteristics

Other performance characteristics of an analytical method or a test procedure that are commonly considered in assay validation include ruggedness, specificity, linearity, range, limit of detection, and limit of quantification. These performance characteristics are briefly described below. More details can be found in USP/NF (2000), Bohidar (1983), Bohidar and Peace (1988), Chow and Liu (1995), and Schofield (2000).

The ruggedness of an analytical method usually refers to the degree of reproducibility of the analytical results obtained by analysis of the same sample under a variety of normal test conditions such as different laboratories, different instruments, different analysts, different lots of reagents, different elapse times, different assay temperatures, and different days. Ruggedness is often used to assess the influence of uncontrollable factors or the degree of reproducibility on assay performance. Typical approaches for assessing assay ruggedness include the one-way nested random effects model and the two-way crossed-classification mixed model. For the assessment of assay ruggedness, it should be noted, however, that the classical analysis of variance method may produce negative estimates for the variance components and that the sum of best estimates of variance components may not be the best estimate of the total variability. In these situations, methods proposed by Chow and Shao (1988) and Chow and Tse (1991) are useful.

The specificity, which is also known as selectivity, is defined as the ability of an analytical method to measure the analyte accurately and specifically in the presence of components that may be expected to be present in the sample matrix. Specificity is often expressed as the difference in assay results obtained by analysis of samples containing added impurities, degradation products, related chemical compounds, or placebo ingredients to those from samples without added substances. Hence, specificity is a measure of the degree of interference in analysis of complex sample matrix. An acceptable method should be free of any significant interference by substances known to be present in the drug product.

The linearity of an analytical method is defined as the ability to elicit assay results that are directly proportional to the concentration of analyte in samples within a given range. The range of an analytical method is the interval between the upper and lower levels (inclusive) of analyte that have been determined with accuracy, precision, and linearity using the method as written.

The limit of detection (LOD) is defined as the lowest concentration of analyte in a sample that can be detected, but not necessarily quantitated, under the experimental conditions specified. In other words, LOD denotes the amount of analyte that can be reliably distinguished from background with certain assurance. Let x be the amount of analyte and y be the response. Suppose that $x = 0$ corresponds to the background and the standard curve passes through the origin. Then, the following $100(1 - a)\%$ upper confidence limit of the mean response at background,

$$LC = z_{1-a}\sigma_0,$$

can be viewed as a critical limit (LC) for detecting an analyte from background, where z_{1-a} is the $(1-a)$th quantile of the standard normal distribution and σ_0^2 is the variance of a response at background. An amount of analyte x is considered to be detectable from the background if and only if the probability that a response at x falls below the critical limit is less than a. Thus, the limit of detection, LOD, for a given analyte is the x value corresponding to $LC + z_{1-a}\sigma_D$, i.e.,

$$LOD = \frac{LC + z_{1-a}\sigma_D}{\beta}, \qquad (2.4.2)$$

where β is the slope of the calibration curve and σ_D is the standard deviation of the response at the detectable analyte in the sample. To provide a better understanding, a graphical interpretation for determination of LOD is given in Figure 2.4.1. Alternatively, the ICH guideline for validation of analytical procedures suggests that the concept of the signal-to-noise ratio be applied for estimating the detection limit (ICH, 1996). The concept of the signal-to-noise ratio is to compare signals obtained from samples with known low concentrations of analyte with those of blank (background) samples and establishing the minimum concentration at which the analyte can be reliably detected. The ICH guideline indicates that a signal-to-noise ratio of 3.3:1 is generally considered acceptable for establishing the detection limit. This leads to

$$LOD = \frac{3.3\sigma_D}{\beta}, \qquad (2.4.3)$$

where β is the slope of the calibration curve. It should be noted that (2.4.2) is equivalent to (2.4.3) if $a = 5\%$ and $\sigma_0 = \sigma_D$.

The limit of quantitation (LOQ) is the lowest concentration of an analyte in a sample that can be determined with acceptable precision and accuracy under the experimental condition specified. In practice, the lowest concentration of an analyte in a sample is usually defined as that for which the relative standard deviation is 10%. This leads to a signal-to-noise ratio of 0.1. As a result, the limit of quantitation can be obtained by

$$LOQ = \frac{10\sigma_D}{\beta}.$$

It, however, should be noted that although a relative standard deviation of 10% is considered an acceptable standard in chemical assays in practice,

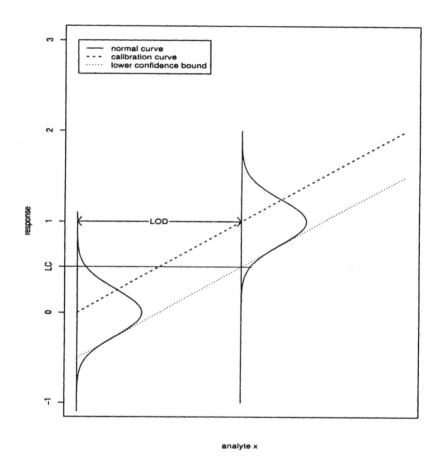

Figure 2.4.1. Limit of Detection

10% RSD is often unachievable in biological assays. About 20-25% variability is generally sought in binding assays, while much higher levels are more realistic in bioassay.

2.5 In-process Controls and Validation

As indicated earlier, the objective of in-process controls and validation of a manufacturing process is to ensure that the manufacturing process does what it purports to do. A validated process assures that the final product has a high probability of meeting the standards for the identity, strength, quality, purity, stability, and reproducibility of the drug product. A manufacturing process is a continuous process involving a number of critical stages. For example, for the manufacturing of tablets, the process may include initial blending, mill, primary blending, final blending, compression, and coating stages. At each critical stage, some problems may occur. For example, the ingredients may not be uniformly mixed at the primary blending stage, the segregation may occur at the final blending stage, and the weight of tablets may not be suitably controlled during the compression stage. Therefore, in practice, it is important to evaluate the performance of the manufacturing at each critical stage by testing in-process and/or processed materials for potency, dosage uniformity, dissolution, and disintegration according to sampling plans and acceptance criteria as stated in the USP/NF.

A manufacturing process is considered to pass the USP/NF tests if each critical stage of the manufacturing process and the final product meet regulatory requirements for the identity, strength, quality, purity, stability, and reproducibility of the drug product. A manufacturing process is considered validated if at least three validation batches (or lots) pass all required USP/NF tests. In-process controls and validation usually refer to as the establishment of documented evidence that a process does what it purports to do. A typical approach is to develop a protocol which describes how the in-process controls and validation will be carried out. A complete protocol should address the issues such as (i) critical stages, (ii) equipment to be used at each critical stage, (iii) possible problems, (iv) USP/NF tests to be performed, (v) sampling plans, (vi) testing plans, (vii) acceptance criteria, (viii) pertinent information, (ix) test or specification to be used as reference, and (x) validation summary with project scientists to acquire a good understanding of the manufacturing process.

Basically, there are four different types of manufacturing process validations in the pharmaceutical industry: prospective, concurrent, retrospective, and re-validation. Prospective validation establishes documented evidence that a process does what it purports to do based on a preplanned protocol. Prospective validation is usually performed in the situations where (i) historical data are not available or sufficient and in-process and end-product testing data are not adequate, (ii) new equipment or components are used, (iii) a new product is reformulated from an existing product, or there are significant modifications or changes in the manufacturing process, and (iv) the manufacturing process is transferred from development laboratory to full-scale production. Retrospective validation provides documented evidence based on review and analysis of historical information, which is useful when there is a stable process with a larger historical database. One of the objectives of the retrospective validation is to support the confidence of the process. Concurrent validation evaluates the process based on information generated during actual implementation of the process. In some situations where (i) a step of the process is modified, (ii) the product is made infrequently, and (iii) a new raw material must be introduced, a concurrent validation is recommended. In practice, a well-established manufacturing process may need to be revalidated when there are changes in critical components (e.g., raw materials), changes/replacement of equipment, changes in facility/plant (e.g., location or size), and a significant increase and/or decrease in batch size.

2.6 Multiple-Stage Tests

For a validated process, there is no guarantee that if the test is performed again it will have a desired probability of meeting regulatory requirement for good characteristics of a drug product. Thus, it is of interest to conduct some in-house acceptance limits (specifications) which guarantee that future batches produced by the process will pass the USP/NF test with a high probability. A common approach to process validation is to obtain a single sample and test the attributes of interest to see whether the USP/NF specifications are met. Bergum (1990) proposed constructing acceptance limits that guarantee that future samples from a batch will meet a given product specification a given percentage of times. The idea is to construct acceptance limits based on a multiple-stage test. If the criteria for the first stage are met, the test is passed. If the criteria for the first stage are not met, then additional stages of testing are done. If the criteria at any stages are met, the test is passed. Acceptance limits for a validation sample are then constructed based on sampled test results to assure that a future sample will have at least a certain chance of passing a multiple-stage test. More details about in-house specification limits can be found in Bergum (1990) and Chow and Liu (1995).

In establishing in-house specification limits, it is necessary to evaluate and estimate the probability of passing the USP/NF test. Let S_i denote the event that the ith stage of a k-stage USP/NF test is passed and let C_{ij} be the event that the jth criterion for the ith stage is met, where $j = 1, ..., m_i$, and $i = 1, ..., k$. Then

$$S_i = C_{i1} \cap C_{i2} \cap \cdots \cap C_{im_i}, \quad i = 1, ..., k$$

and the probability of passing the USP/NF test is

$$P = P(S_1 \cup S_2 \cup \cdots \cup S_k). \tag{2.6.1}$$

In some cases, the probability in (2.6.1) can be evaluated by simulation. For establishment of in-house specification limits, it may be more effective to consider a lower bound of P in terms of some probabilities (such as $P(C_{ij})$)

that can be easily evaluated or estimated. A simple but rough lower bound for P in (2.6.1) is given in the following:

$$P \geq \max\{P(S_i), i = 1, ..., k\}$$

$$\geq \max\left\{0, \sum_{j=1}^{m_i} P(C_{ij}) - (m_i - 1), i = 1, ..., k\right\}.$$

For a particular test, however, an improved lower bound may be obtained. In the following discussion we consider as an example the test of the uniformity of dosage units. Another example, dissolution testing, will be discussed in §3.1-3.2.

The uniformity of dosage units is usually demonstrated either by weight variation testing or content uniformity testing (USP/NF, 2000). We consider weight variation testing. Content uniformity testing is similar. Weight variation testing is a two stage test. In the first stage, 10 dosage units are randomly sampled and weighted individually. From the result of the assay, as directed in the individual monograph, the content of the active ingredient in each of the 10 units are calculated. Homogeneous distribution of the active ingredient is assumed. The requirements for dosage uniformity are met if the amount of active ingredient in each of the 10 dosage units lies within the range 85% to 115% of label claim and the coefficient of variation is less than 6%. If one unit is outside the range 85% to 115% of label claim and no units is outside the range 75% to 125% of label claim, or if the coefficient of variation is greater than 6%, or if both conditions prevail, then 20 additional units are sampled and tested in the second stage. The requirements are met if not more than one unit of the 30 units is outside the range 85% to 115% of label claim and no unit is outside the range 75% to 125% of label claim and the coefficient of variation of the 30 units does not exceed 7.8%.

Let y_i be the active ingredient of the ith sampled unit and CV_n be the sample coefficient of variation based on $y_1, ..., y_n$, $n = 10$ or 30. Define

$$C_{11} = \{85 \leq y_i \leq 115, i = 1, ..., 10\},$$
$$C_{12} = \{CV_{10} < 6\},$$
$$C_{21} = \{75 \leq y_i \leq 125, i = 1, ..., 30\},$$
$$C_{22} = \{\text{no more than one of } y_i\text{'s} < 85 \text{ or} > 115, 1 \leq i \leq 30\},$$
$$C_{23} = \{CV_{30} < 7.8\},$$
$$S_1 = C_{11} \cap C_{12},$$
$$S_2 = C_{21} \cap C_{22} \cap C_{23}.$$

Then, the probability of passing the USP/NF test for dosage uniformity by weight variation is equal to

$$P_{\text{DU}} = P(S_1 \cup S_2) = P\left((C_{11} \cap C_{12}) \cup (C_{21} \cap C_{22} \cap C_{23})\right). \qquad (2.6.2)$$

If the distribution of y_i is known or estimated based on previously sampled test results, then the probability P_{DU} in (2.6.2) can be evaluated by simulation. That is, we generate N sets of data from the distribution of y_i and perform the USP/NF test based on each generated data set. Then

$$P_{\text{DU}} \approx \frac{\text{the number of times the USP/NF test is passed}}{N}. \qquad (2.6.3)$$

For example, if y_i is normally distributed with mean μ and variance σ^2, then data sets can be generated from $N(\hat{\mu}, \hat{\sigma}^2)$, where $\hat{\mu}$ and $\hat{\sigma}^2$ are the sample mean and sample variance, respectively, based on some previously sampled test results.

We now introduce a lower bound of P_{DU} derived in Chow, Shao, and Wang (2001a). Define

$$
\begin{aligned}
P_1 &= P(85 \leq y_i \leq 115), \\
P_2 &= P(75 \leq y_i \leq 85) + P(115 \leq y_i \leq 125), \\
P_3 &= P(\text{CV}_{10} \geq 6), \\
P_4 &= P(\text{CV}_{30} \geq 7.8).
\end{aligned}
$$

Let A^c denote the complement of the event A. Note that

$$
\begin{aligned}
P_{\text{DU}} &= P(S_1 \cup S_2) \\
&= P(S_1) + P(S_1^c \cap S_2) \\
&= P(C_{11} \cap C_{12}) + P(S_1^c \cap C_{21} \cap C_{22} \cap C_{23}) \\
&\geq P(C_{11}) - P(C_{12}^c) + P(C_{11}^c \cap C_{21} \cap C_{22}) - P(C_{23}^c) \\
&= P_1^{10} + 10 P_1^{29} P_2 - P_3 - P_4,
\end{aligned}
$$

where the last equality follows from the fact that y_i's are independent and identically distributed and

$$P(C_{11}^c \cap C_{21} \cap C_{22}) = 10 P \left(\begin{array}{l} 75 \leq y_1 < 85 \text{ or } 115 < y_1 \leq 125 \\ 85 \leq y_i \leq 115, i = 2, ..., 30 \end{array} \right).$$

On the other hand,

$$
\begin{aligned}
P_{\text{DU}} &= P(S_1 \cup S_2) \\
&\geq P(S_1) \\
&\geq P(C_{11}) - P(C_{12}^c) \\
&= P_1^{10} - P_3
\end{aligned}
$$

and

$$P_{DU} = P(S_1 \cup S_2)$$
$$\geq P(S_2)$$
$$\geq P(C_{21} \cap C_{22}) - P(C_{23})$$
$$= P_1^{30} + 30P_1^{29}P_2 - P_4.$$

Hence, a lower bound for P_{DU} is

$$\underline{P_{DU}} = \max(0, P_1^{10} + 10P_1^{29}P_2 - P_3 - P_4, P_1^{10} - P_3, P_1^{30} + 30P_1^{29}P_2 - P_4).$$

This lower bound is a function of P_j, $j = 1, ..., 4$, which can be easily evaluated if P_j's are known or estimated. If y_i is normally distributed with known mean μ and variance σ^2, then

$$P_1 = \Phi\left(\frac{115 - \mu}{\sigma}\right) - \Phi\left(\frac{85 - \mu}{\sigma}\right),$$

$$P_2 = \Phi\left(\frac{125 - \mu}{\sigma}\right) - \Phi\left(\frac{75 - \mu}{\sigma}\right) - P_1,$$

$$P_3 = T_9\left(\frac{\sqrt{10}}{6}\middle|\frac{\sqrt{10}\mu}{\sigma}\right) - T_9\left(-\frac{\sqrt{10}}{6}\middle|\frac{\sqrt{10}\mu}{\sigma}\right)$$

and

$$P_4 = T_{29}\left(\frac{\sqrt{30}}{7.8}\middle|\frac{\sqrt{30}\mu}{\sigma}\right) - T_{29}\left(-\frac{\sqrt{30}}{7.8}\middle|\frac{\sqrt{30}\mu}{\sigma}\right),$$

where Φ is the standard normal distribution function and $T_n(\cdot|\theta)$ is the noncentral t-distribution function with n degrees of freedom and the noncentrality parameter θ. If μ and σ^2 are estimated by $\hat{\mu}$ and $\hat{\sigma}^2$, respectively, then P_j's can be estimated with μ and σ^2 replaced by $\hat{\mu}$ and $\hat{\sigma}^2$, respectively.

A numerical comparison of P_{DU} and its lower bound $\underline{P_{DU}}$ is shown in Figure 2.6.1 for the case where y_i's are from $N(\mu, \sigma^2)$ with some values of μ and σ. The true probability P_{DU} is obtained by using approximation (2.6.3) with $N = 10,000$. It can be seen from Figure 2.6.1 that $\underline{P_{DU}}$ is close to P_{DU} when $\sigma \leq 5$ or $\mu \leq 105$. Note that the computation of $\underline{P_{DU}}$ is much quicker than that of P_{DU}. Even with $N = 10,000$, the curve of P_{DU} against σ computed using approximation (2.6.3) is still not smooth.

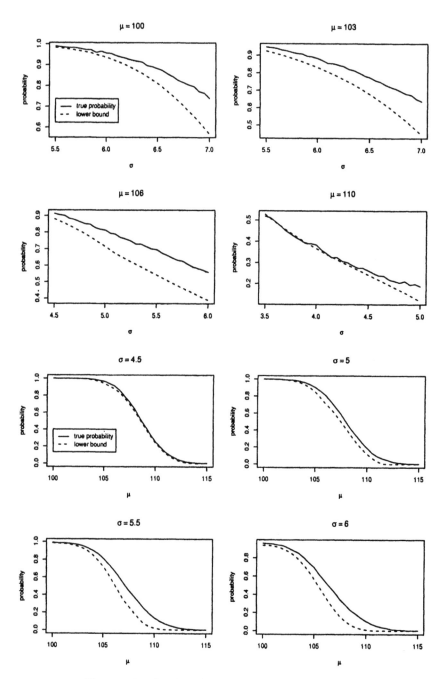

Figure 2.6.1. Probability of Passing the USP/NF Test
and Its Lower Bound

Chapter 3

Dissolution Testing

In the pharmaceutical industry, *in vitro* dissolution testing is one of the primary USP/NF tests that is often performed to ensure that a drug product meets the USP/NF standards for identity, strength, quality, purity, stability, and reproducibility. *In vitro* dissolution testing is usually conducted with materials drawn at some critical stages of a manufacturing process for in-process controls. At the end of the manufacturing process, the finished product is also tested for the purpose of quality assurance. The FDA requires that a drug product should not be released for human use if it fails to pass the USP/NF acceptance criteria for dissolution testing.

In 1984, the FDA was authorized to approve generic drugs of a brand-name drug based on evidence of bioequivalence in the rate and extent of drug absorption between the generic drugs and the brand-name drug. In practice, *in vitro* dissolution testing is a rapid technique for determining the rate and extent of drug release of a drug product. For some drug products, the FDA indicates that an *in vitro* dissolution test could serve as a surrogate for an *in vivo* bioequivalence test by comparing the dissolution profiles between drug products. Two drug products are said to have a similar drug absorption profile if their dissolution profiles are similar. These drug products include (i) pre-1962 classified "AA" drug products; (ii) lower strength products (in the same application or as strength extension in separate application); (iii) scale-up and postapproval change (e.g., components and composition changes, site change, scale-up or down, manufacturing equipment or process changes, new product versus marketed product; see SUPAC-IR, 1995); and (iv) products demonstrating *in vitro* and *in vivo* correlation (IVIVC). Dissolution testing is an integral part of drug products approval process.

In §3.1, the sampling plan and acceptance criteria for dissolution testing as specified in the USP/NF are introduced. The probability of passing the USP/NF dissolution test is studied in §3.2. Section 3.3 describes various proposed models for characterizing dissolution profiles and the concepts of local similarity and global similarity between dissolution profiles of two drug products. Statistical methods for assessment of similarity between dissolution profiles of two drug products including the method based on the f_2 similarity factor suggested by the FDA are given in §3.4. Sections 3.5 and 3.6 contain some recent development in methods for the assessment of similarity between dissolution profiles based on the time series approach proposed by Chow and Ki (1997).

3.1   USP/NF Dissolution Test

Dissolution testing is typically performed by placing a dosage unit in a transparent vessel containing a dissolution medium. A variable-speed motor rotates a cylindrical basket containing the dosage unit. The dissolution medium is then analyzed to determine the percentage of the drug dissolved. Dissolution testing is usually performed on six units simultaneously. The dissolution medium is routinely sampled at various predetermined time intervals to form a dissolution profile.

For dissolution testing, USP/NF (2000) contains an explanation of the test for acceptability of dissolution rates. The requirements are met if the quantities of active ingredient dissolved from the units conform to the USP/NF acceptance criteria. Let Q be the amount of dissolved active ingredient specified in the individual monograph of USP/NF. The USP/NF dissolution test is a three-stage testing procedure. For the first stage, six units are sampled and tested. The product passes the USP/NF dissolution test if each unit is not less than $Q + 5\%$. If the product fails to pass at stage one, an additional six units are sampled and tested at the second stage. The product passes the USP/NF dissolution test if the average of the 12 units from two stages is no smaller than Q and if no unit is less than $Q - 15\%$. If the product fails to pass at stage two, an additional 12 units are sampled and tested at the third stage. If the average of all 24 units from three stages is no smaller than Q, no more than two units are less than $Q - 15\%$, and no unit is less than $Q - 25\%$, the product has passed the USP/NF dissolution test; otherwise the product fails to pass the test.

Tsong et al. (1995) investigated the operating characteristic (OC) curves of the three-stage dissolution test as stated in the USP/NF. They found that the three-stage test procedure is rather liberal and is incapable of rejecting a lot with a high fraction of units dissolved less than Q and with an average amount dissolved just slightly larger than Q. Alternatively, they suggested two modified multiple-stage tests for dissolution. The first modified multiple-stage test is to change $Q - 15\%$ at stages 2 and 3 of the USP/NF dissolution test to a more stringent limit of $Q - 5\%$. The second is a three-stage test based primarily on the results of sample mean and sample standard deviation and some prespecified limits.

Regulatory requirements and/or specifications for dissolution testing may vary from drug product to drug product. To assist the sponsors in preparing NDA/ANDA submission for approval of drug products, the FDA has issued a number of guidances since 1995. These guidances include SUPAC-IR for immediate-release oral solid dosage forms (SUPAC-IR, 1995), SUPAC-MR for extended-release oral solid dosage forms (SUPAC-MR, 1997), SUPAC-SS for solutions and semisolid dosage forms (SUPAC-SS, 1997), and SUPAC-TDS for transdermal drug delivery system. According to these guidances, dissolution testing may be performed at a single time point or multiple time points. For example, three cases (cases A, B, and C) of dissolution testing are considered in SUPAC-IR. Case A requires that dissolution testing be performed at one time point using one medium (i.e., $Q = 85\%$ in 15 minutes in 900 ml of 0.1N HCl), while multiple time points dissolution tests at 15, 30, 45, and 120 minutes or until asymptotes is reached are recommended for case B. Case C suggests multiple time points dissolution tests be performed in water, 0.1N HCl, and USP/NF buffer media at pH values of 4.5, 6.5, and 7.5 for proposed and currently accepted formulations. Adequate sampling should be done at 15, 30, 45, 60, and 120 minutes or until as asymptote is reached.

3.2 Probability of Passing the Dissolution Test

In practice, it is of interest to evaluate P_{DT}, the probability of passing the USP/NF dissolution test, according to the sampling plan and acceptance criteria described in §3.1. Knowledge about P_{DT} is useful in establishing a set of in-house specification limits for dissolution testing (Chow and Liu, 1995). Since P_{DT} does not have an explicit form, we may consider a simulation approximation similar to that in the test for the uniformity of dosage units (see §2.6). An alternative is to consider a lower bound of P_{DT} which is a simple function of some probabilities whose evaluation can be done much easier than the direct evaluation of P_{DT}.

Bergum (1990) provided the following lower bound for P_{DT}:

$$P_B = P_{Q-15}^{24} + 24P_{Q-15}^{23}(P_{Q-25} - P_{Q-15})$$
$$+ 276P_{Q-15}^{22}(P_{Q-25} - P_{Q-15})^2 - P(\bar{y}_{24} \leq Q) \qquad (3.2.1)$$

(P_B is replaced by 0 if it is negative), where

$$P_x = P(y \geq x),$$

y is the dissolution testing result expressed as a percentage of label claim, and $\bar{y}_{24}$ is the average of the dissolution testing results from all three stages. Note that probabilities P_x and $P(\bar{y}_{24} \leq Q)$ are easy to compute. The lower bound P_B, however, is somewhat conservative. In what follows, we introduce a better lower bound proposed in Chow, Shao, and Wang (2001a).

Let y_i, $i = 1, ..., 6$, be the dissolution testing results from the first stage, y_i, $i = 7, ..., 12$, be the dissolution testing results from the second stage, y_i, $i = 13, ..., 24$, be the dissolution testing results from the third stage, and $\bar{y}_k$ be the average of $y_1, ..., y_k$. Define the following events:

$$S_1 = \{y_i \geq Q + 5, i = 1, ..., 6\},$$
$$S_{21} = \{y_i \geq Q - 15, i = 1, ..., 12\},$$
$$S_{22} = \{\bar{y}_{12} \geq Q\},$$
$$S_{31} = \{y_i \geq Q - 25, i = 1, ..., 24\},$$
$$S_{32} = \{\text{no more than two } y_i\text{'s} < Q - 15\},$$
$$S_{33} = \{\bar{y}_{24} \geq Q\},$$
$$S_2 = S_{21} \cap S_{22},$$
$$S_3 = S_{31} \cap S_{32} \cap S_{33}.$$

Then

$$P_{\text{DT}} = P(S_1 \cup S_2 \cup S_3).$$

Note that Bergum's lower bound P_B in (3.2.1) is obtained by using the inequalities

$$P(S_1 \cup S_2 \cup S_3) \geq P(S_3)$$

and

$$P(S_{31} \cap S_{32} \cap S_{33}) \geq P(S_{31} \cap S_{32}) - P(S_{33}^c),$$

where A^c denotes the complement of the event A, and the fact that $S_3 = S_{31} \cap S_{32} \cap S_{33}$ and y_i's are independent and identically distributed. When the probability $P(S_{33}^c)$ is not small, these inequalities are not sharp enough.

From the equation

$$P_{\text{DT}} = P(S_3) + P(S_2 \cap S_3^c) + P(S_1 \cap S_2^c \cap S_3^c),$$

a lower bound for P_{DT} can be obtained by deriving a lower bound for each of $P(S_3)$, $P(S_2 \cap S_3^c)$, and $P(S_1 \cap S_2^c \cap S_3^c)$. We take Bergum's bound P_B in (3.2.1) as the lower bound for $P(S_3)$. For $P(S_2 \cap S_3^c)$, consider the fact that

$$
\begin{aligned}
P(S_2 \cap S_3^c) &= P(S_{21} \cap S_{22} \cap S_3^c) \\
&\geq P(S_{21} \cap S_3^c) - P(S_{22}^c) \\
&= P(S_{21} \cap S_{31}^c) + P(S_{21} \cap S_{31} \cap S_{32}^c)
\end{aligned}
$$

$$+ P(S_{21} \cap S_{31} \cap S_{32} \cap S_{33}^c) - P(\bar{y}_{12} < Q)$$
$$\geq P(S_{21} \cap S_{31}^c) + P(S_{21} \cap S_{31} \cap S_{32}^c) - P(\bar{y}_{12} < Q).$$

Since y_i's are independent and identically distributed,

$$P(S_{21} \cap S_{31}^c) = P(S_{21}) - P(S_{21} \cap S_{31})$$
$$= P_{Q-15}^{12} - P_{Q-15}^{12} P_{Q-25}^{12}.$$

Note that

$$P(S_{21} \cap S_{31} \cap S_{32}) = P\,(y_i \geq Q - 15, i = 1, ..., 24)$$
$$+ 12P \left(\begin{array}{c} y_i \geq Q - 15, i = 1, ..., 23 \\ Q - 25 \leq y_{24} < Q - 15 \end{array} \right)$$
$$+ \binom{12}{2} P \left(\begin{array}{c} y_i \geq Q - 15, i = 1, ..., 22 \\ Q - 25 \leq y_i < Q - 15, i = 23, 24 \end{array} \right)$$
$$= P_{Q-15}^{24} + 12P_{Q-15}^{23}(P_{Q-25} - P_{Q-15})$$
$$+ 66P_{Q-15}^{22}(P_{Q-25} - P_{Q-15})^2.$$

Hence,

$$P(S_{21} \cap S_{31} \cap S_{32}^c) = P(S_{21} \cap S_{31}) - P(S_{21} \cap S_{31} \cap S_{32})$$
$$= P_{Q-15}^{12} P_{Q-25}^{12} - P_{Q-15}^{24} - 12P_{Q-15}^{23}(P_{Q-25} - P_{Q-15})$$
$$- 66P_{Q-15}^{22}(P_{Q-25} - P_{Q-15})^2.$$

Thus, a lower bound for $P(S_2 \cap S_3^c)$ is

$$P_C = P_{Q-15}^{12} - P_{Q-15}^{24} - 12P_{Q-15}^{23}(P_{Q-25} - P_{Q-15})$$
$$- 66P_{Q-15}^{22}(P_{Q-25} - P_{Q-15})^2 - P(\bar{y}_{12} < Q). \qquad (3.2.2)$$

This lower bound is good when $P(\bar{y}_{12} < Q)$ is small. On the other hand,

$$P(S_2 \cap S_3^c) = P(S_{21} \cap S_{22} \cap (S_{31} \cap S_{32} \cap S_{33})^c)$$
$$\geq P(S_{21} \cap S_{22} \cap S_{33}^c)$$
$$\geq P(S_{22} \cap S_{33}^c) - P(S_{21}^c)$$
$$= P(\bar{y}_{12} \geq Q, \bar{y}_{24} < Q) - (1 - P_{Q-15}^{12}).$$

The previous two inequalities provide an accurate lower bound if $P(S_{21}^c)$ and $P(S_{21} \cap S_{31}^c \cup S_{32}^c)$ are small. Thus, a better lower bound for $P(S_2 \cap S_3^c)$ is the larger of P_C in (3.2.2) and

$$P_D = P(\bar{y}_{12} \geq Q, \bar{y}_{24} < Q) - (1 - P_{Q-15}^{12}). \qquad (3.2.3)$$

For $P(S_1 \cap S_2^c \cap S_3^c)$, consider the fact that

$$P(S_1 \cap S_2^c \cap S_3^c) = P(S_1 \cap S_{21}^c \cap S_3^c) + P(S_1 \cap S_{21} \cap S_{22}^c \cap S_3^c)$$
$$\geq P(S_1 \cap S_{21}^c \cap S_3^c)$$
$$= P(S_1 \cap S_{21}^c \cap S_{31}^c) + P(S_1 \cap S_{21}^c \cap S_{31} \cap S_{32}^c)$$
$$+ P(S_1 \cap S_{21}^c \cap S_{31} \cap S_{32} \cap S_{33}^c)$$
$$\geq P(S_1 \cap S_{21}^c \cap S_{31}^c) + P(S_1 \cap S_{21}^c \cap S_{31} \cap S_{32}^c)$$
$$= P(S_1 \cap S_{21}^c \cap S_{31}^c) + P(S_1 \cap S_{21}^c \cap S_{31})$$
$$- P(S_1 \cap S_{21}^c \cap S_{31} \cap S_{32})$$
$$= P(S_1 \cap S_{21}^c) - P(S_1 \cap S_{31} \cap S_{32})$$
$$+ P(S_1 \cap S_{21} \cap S_{31} \cap S_{32}).$$

Since

$$P(S_1 \cap S_{21}^c) = P(S_1) - P(S_1 \cap S_{21}) = P_{Q+5}^6 - P_{Q+5}^6 P_{Q-15}^6,$$

$$P(S_1 \cap S_{31} \cap S_{32}) = P\left(\begin{array}{c} y_i \geq Q+5, i = 1, ..., 6 \\ y_i \geq Q-15, i = 7, ..., 24 \end{array} \right)$$

$$+18P\left(\begin{array}{c} y_i \geq Q+5, i = 1, ..., 6 \\ y_i \geq Q-15, i = 7, ..., 23 \\ Q-25 \leq y_{24} < Q-15 \end{array} \right)$$

$$+\binom{18}{2}P\left(\begin{array}{c} y_i \geq Q+5, i = 1, ..., 6 \\ y_i \geq Q-15, i = 7, ..., 22 \\ Q-25 \leq y_i < Q-15, i = 23, 24 \end{array} \right)$$

$$= P_{Q+5}^6 P_{Q-25}^{18} + 18 P_{Q+5}^6 P_{Q-15}^{17}(P_{Q-25} - P_{Q-15})$$
$$+153 P_{Q+5}^6 P_{Q-15}^{16}(P_{Q-25} - P_{Q-15})^2$$

and

$$P(S_1 \cap S_{21} \cap S_{31} \cap S_{32}) = P\left(\begin{array}{c} y_i \geq Q+5, i = 1, ..., 6 \\ y_i \geq Q-15, i = 7, ..., 24 \end{array} \right)$$

$$+12P\left(\begin{array}{c} y_i \geq Q+5, i = 1, ..., 6 \\ y_i \geq Q-15, i = 7, ..., 23 \\ Q-25 \leq y_{24} < Q-15 \end{array} \right)$$

$$+\binom{12}{2}P\left(\begin{array}{c} y_i \geq Q+5, i = 1, ..., 6 \\ y_i \geq Q-15, i = 7, ..., 22 \\ Q-25 \leq y_i < Q-15, i = 23, 24 \end{array} \right)$$

$$= P_{Q+5}^6 P_{Q-15}^{18} + 12 P_{Q+5}^6 P_{Q-15}^{17}(P_{Q-25} - P_{Q-15})$$
$$+66 P_{Q+5}^6 P_{Q-15}^{16}(P_{Q-25} - P_{Q-15})^2,$$

a lower bound for $P(S_1 \cap S_2^c \cap S_3^c)$ is

$$P_E = P_{Q+5}^6 - P_{Q+5}^6 P_{Q-15}^6 - 6P_{Q+5}^6 P_{Q-15}^{17}(P_{Q-25} - P_{Q-15})$$
$$- 87P_{Q+5}^6 P_{Q-15}^{16}(P_{Q-25} - P_{Q-15})^2. \quad (3.2.4)$$

Combining these results, we obtain the following lower bound for P_{DT}:

$$\underline{P_{DT}} = \max(0, P_B) + \max(0, P_C, P_D) + P_E, \quad (3.2.5)$$

where P_B, P_C, P_D and P_E are given by (3.2.1)-(3.2.4), respectively. This lower bound is given in terms of six probabilities P_{Q+5}, P_{Q-15}, P_{Q-25}, $P(\bar{y}_{12} < Q)$, $P(\bar{y}_{24} < Q)$, and $P(\bar{y}_{12} \geq Q, \bar{y}_{24} < Q)$. If y_i is normally distributed with mean μ and variance σ^2, then

$$P_x = 1 - \Phi\left(\frac{x - \mu}{\sigma}\right),$$

$$P(\bar{y}_k < Q) = \Phi\left(\frac{\sqrt{k}(Q - \mu)}{\sigma}\right),$$

and

$$P(\bar{y}_{12} \geq Q, \bar{y}_{24} < Q) = P(\bar{y}_{24} < Q) - P(\bar{y}_{12} < Q, \bar{y}_{24} < Q)$$
$$= \Phi\left(\frac{\sqrt{24}(Q - \mu)}{\sigma}\right) - \Psi(Q - \mu, Q - \mu),$$

where $x = Q + 5$, $Q - 15$, or $Q - 25$, $k = 12$ or 24, Φ is the standard normal distribution function, and Ψ is the bivariate normal distribution with mean 0 and covariance matrix

$$\frac{\sigma^2}{24}\begin{pmatrix} 2 & 1 \\ 1 & 1 \end{pmatrix}.$$

If μ and σ^2 are unknown, they can be estimated using data from previously sampled test results.

It is clear that the lower bound in (3.2.5) is more precise than that given by Bergum (1990) since $\underline{P_{DT}} \geq P_B$. But how accurate is $\underline{P_{DT}}$? A numerical comparison of P_{DT}, $\underline{P_{DT}}$ and Bergum's lower bound P_B is given in Figure 3.2.1 for the case where $Q = 75$ and y_i's are independently distributed as $N(\mu, \sigma^2)$ with some values of μ and σ. The true probability P_{DT} is approximated by Monte Carlo with size $N = 10,000$. It can be seen from Figure 3.2.1 that the lower bound $\underline{P_{DT}}$ is better than Bergum's lower bound and, in fact, $\underline{P_{DT}}$ is a very accurate approximation to P_{DT} when $\sigma \geq 5$.

Note that if the USP/NF dissolution test is modified according to Tsong et al. (1995), i.e., $Q - 15\%$ at stages 2 and 3 of the USP/NF dissolution test is changed to $Q - 5\%$, then the lower bound for the probability of passing the dissolution test is still given by (3.2.5) except that P_{Q-15} should be replaced by P_{Q-5}.

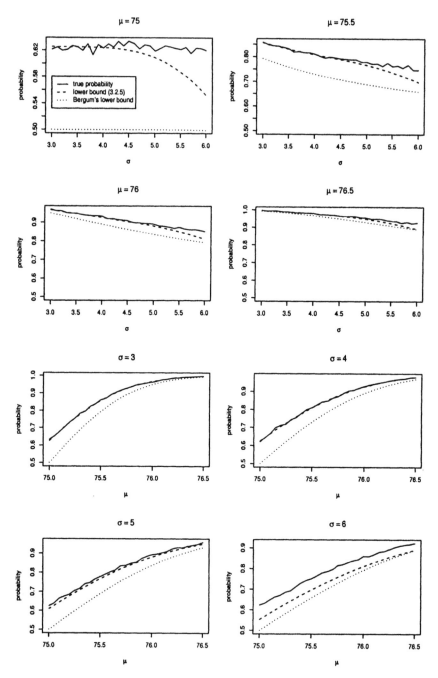

Figure 3.2.1. Probability of Passing the Dissolution
Test and Its Lower Bounds

3.3 Dissolution Profile and Similarity

As discussed in §3.1, dissolution testing may be performed at multiple time points, e.g., at 15, 30, 45, 60, and 120 minutes or until asymptote is reached. For a drug product, the curve of the mean dissolution rate over time is referred to as its *dissolution profile.*

To assess the dissolution profile of a drug product, a model-dependent approach is usually considered. For example, Langenbucher (1972) indicated that the dissolution profile can be approximately by a Weibull distribution after linearlization. Dawoodbhai et al. (1991) considered the so-called Gompertz model to characterize the dissolution profile, while Pena Romero et al. (1991) introduced the use of the logistic curve, which was found useful in the study of water uptake and force development in an optimized prolonged-release formulation. Kervinen and Yliruusi (1993) proposed three control factor models for S-shaped dissolution profile curves to connect the curves with the physical phenomenon of dissolution. Tsong et al. (1995) indicated that we may consider a sigmoid curve or a probit model to describe the dissolution profile.

In practice, drug products are often compared in terms of their dissolution curves. For example, a testing drug product is considered to be similar to a reference drug product if their dissolution profiles are similar in some sense. For drug products with minor postapproval changes, the FDA SUPAC guidances indicate that *in vitro* dissolution testing for profile comparison can be used as a surrogate for *in vivo* bioequivalence testing. Types of changes and levels of changes are listed in Table 3.3.1. It, however, should be noted that dissolution profile comparison is usually performed provided that the acceptance criteria of the USP/NF dissolution test as specified in §3.1 is met for each drug product under comparison.

Since dissolution profiles are curves over time, we introduce the concepts of *local similarity* and *global similarity.* Two dissolution profiles are said to be locally similar at a given time point if their difference or ratio at the given time point is within certain equivalence limits. Two dissolution profiles are considered globally similar if their differences or ratios are within certain equivalence limits across all time points.

The assessment of local similarity or global similarity depends upon the selection of equivalence limits. However, there are no justifiable equivalence limits in the literature or regulatory guidelines. Benet (1992) pointed out that for some drug products with narrow therapeutic index, relatively small changes in systemic concentrations can lead to marked changes in pharmacodynamic response. In practice, since an *in vitro* dissolution testing is usually simple and highly controllable as compared to the *in vivo* bioequivalence testing, which is often more complicated, variable, unpredictable,

Table 3.3.1. Types and Levels of Changes Specified in SUPAC

Type	Change
1	Components and composition
2	Site of manufacture
3	Scale of manufacture (scale up or down)
4	Manufacturing process and equipment

Level	Change
1	Changes that are unlikely to have any detectable impact on formulation quality and performance
2	Moderate changes that could have a significant impact on formulation quality and performance
3	Major changes likely to have a significant impact on formulation quality and performance

Source: SUPAC-IR (1995)

and uncontrollable, Chow and Ki (1997) suggested that the equivalence limits should be narrow enough, e.g., narrower than those for *in vivo* bioequivalence testing, to ensure that the corresponding drug absorption will reach the desired bioavailability. For this purpose, Chow and Ki (1997) proposed the following equivalence limits. Let δ be a meaningful difference of scientific importance in mean dissolution profiles of two drug products under consideration. In practice, δ is usually determined by a pharmaceutical scientist. Suppose that Q is the desired mean dissolution rate of a drug product (standard) as specified in the USP/NF individual monograph. Chow and Ki (1997) considered a drug product to have a similar mean dissolution rate to the standard if its mean dissolution rate falls within $(Q - \delta, Q + \delta)$. For two drug products that are similar to the standard (i.e., both of them passed the USP/NF dissolution test), their mean dissolution rates, denoted by μ_1 and μ_2, at a particular time point are both in the interval $(Q - \delta, Q + \delta)$. At the extreme case where one of μ_1 and μ_2 is $Q - \delta$ and the other one is $Q + \delta$, the ratio μ_1/μ_2 is equal to $\frac{Q-\delta}{Q+\delta}$ or $\frac{Q+\delta}{Q-\delta}$. Thus, Chow and Ki (1997) proposed the equivalence limits (δ_L, δ_U) for similarity between dissolution profiles of two drug products, where

$$\delta_L = \frac{Q - \delta}{Q + \delta} \quad \text{and} \quad \delta_U = \frac{Q + \delta}{Q - \delta}.$$

Since $Q + 5\%$ is used in the USP/NF dissolution test described in §3.1, $\delta = 5\%$ is considered to be a scientific (or chemical) meaningful difference in dissolution testing. When $\delta = 5\%$, the corresponding lower and upper limits for similarity with various Q are

Q	70%	75%	80%	85%	90%	95%
δ_L	86.7%	87.5%	88.2%	88.9%	89.47%	90.00%
δ_U	115.4%	114.3%	113.3%	112.5%	111.76%	111.11%

Note that the lower and upper equivalence limits are not symmetric about 100% and they are narrower than the bioequivalence limits of 80% and 125%. When $Q = 95\%$, the lower and upper limits (i.e., 90% and 111.11%) agree with those for *in vitro* bioequivalence testing for nasal aerosols and sprays drug products as specified by the FDA (FDA, 1999b). Details regarding bioequivalence testing can be found in Chapter 5.

3.4 Methods for Assessing Similarity

Since the dissolution profiles of drug products are unknown, assessing similarity has to be based on data from dissolution testing. In this section we review some statistical methods for assessing the similarity between two drug products. Some recent developments for this problem are introduced in §3.5-3.6.

3.4.1 Model-Dependent Approach

The model-dependent approach introduced in §3.3 can be employed not only to describe dissolution profiles but also to compare the similarity between dissolution profiles.

For comparison of dissolution profiles between a test product and a reference product, Tsong et al. (1995) suggested first modeling the dissolution profile curve based on previously approved batches for the reference drug product and determining the specifications on the parameters of the dissolution profile curve. Then, the dissolution profile curve of the test product is modeled. If the parameters of the test product fall within some predetermined specifications, then we conclude the two drug products have similar dissolution profiles. This approach may sound reasonable. However, some questions remain unsolved, which limits the application of this procedure. These questions include: (i) How do we select an appropriate model for the dissolution profile? (ii) What is the interpretation of the parameters for the selected model? (iii) Does the dissolution profile of the test product follow the same model as that of the reference product?

3.4.2   Model-Independent Approach

Some model-independent approaches such as the analysis of variance, the analysis of covariance, and the split-plot analysis are considered in assessing similarity between two dissolution profiles. However, these methods are not appropriate because dissolution testing results over time are not independent due to the nature of dissolution testing. As an alternative, Tsong, Hammerstrom, and Chen (1997) proposed a multivariate analysis by considering the distance between mean dissolution rates of two drug products at two time points. The idea is to use Hotelling T^2 statistic to construct a 90% confidence region for the difference in dissolution means of two batches of the reference product at the two time points. This confidence region is then used as equivalence criteria for assessment of similarity between dissolution profiles. For a given test product, if the constructed confidence region for the difference in dissolution means between the test product and the reference product at the two time points is within the equivalence region, then we conclude that the two dissolution profiles are similar at the two time points. One disadvantage of Tsong, Hammerstrom, and Chen's method is that it is impossible to visualize the confidence region when there are more than two time points. Another model-independent approach is to consider the method of analysis of variance with repeated measures proposed by Gill (1988). The idea is to consider a nested model with a covariate error structure to account for correlation between the observations (repeated measurements). This model is useful in (i) comparing dissolution rates between drug products at given time points, (ii) detecting time effect within treatment, and (iii) comparing mean dissolution rates change from one time point to another. One disadvantage of Gill's method is that the dissolution profiles can only be compared at each time point when there is a significant treatment-by-time interaction.

3.4.3   The f_2 Similarity Factor

Instead of comparing two dissolution profiles, we may consider a statistic that measures the closeness of two dissolution profiles. Such a statistic is called a *similarity factor*. Two dissolution profiles are considered to be similar if the similarity factor is within some specified equivalence limits. If the similarity factor involves only a single time point, then it is related to the local similarity. On the other hand, if the similarity factor depends on the entire dissolution profile curves, then it is related to the global similarity.

Moore and Flanner (1996) considered a similarity factor that is referred to as the f_2 similarity factor. The f_2 similarity factor can be described as follows. Since the FDA SUPAC guidances require that all profiles be conducted on at least 12 individual dosage units, we assume that at each time point and for each drug product, there are n individual dosage units. Let y_{hti} be the cumulative percent dissolved for dosage unit i at the tth sampling time point for drug product h, where $i = 1, ..., n$, $t = 1, ..., T$, and $h = 1, 2$. Denote the average cumulative percent dissolved at the tth time point for product h as

$$\bar{y}_{ht} = \frac{1}{n} \sum_{i=1}^{n} y_{hti}$$

and the sum of squares of difference in average cumulative percent dissolved between the two drug products over all sampling time points as

$$D = \sum_{t=1}^{T} (\bar{y}_{1t} - \bar{y}_{2t})^2.$$

The f_2 similarity factor proposed by Moore and Flanner (1996) is then defined to be the logarithmic reciprocal square root transformation of one plus the mean squared (the average sum of squares) difference in observed average cumulative percent dissolved between the two products over all sampling time points, i.e.,

$$f_2 = 50 \log_{10} \left(100/\sqrt{1 + D/T} \right) = 100 - 25 \log_{10}(1 + D/T), \qquad (3.4.1)$$

where $\log_{10}$ denotes the logarithm base 10 transformation. Note that f_2 is a strictly decreasing function of D. If there is no difference in average cumulative percent at all sampling time points $(D = 0)$, f_2 reaches its maximum value 100. A large value of f_2 indicates the similarity of the two dissolution profiles. For immediate-release solid dosage forms, the FDA suggests that two dissolution profiles are considered to be similar if the f_2 similarity factor is between 50 and 100 (SUPAC-IR, 1995).

The use of the f_2 factor has been discussed and criticized by many researchers. See, for example, Chow and Liu (1997), Liu, Ma, and Chow (1997), Shah et al. (1998), Tsong et al. (1996), and Ma, Lin, and Liu (1999). Ma et al. (2000) studied the size and power of the f_2 similarity factor for assessment of similarity, based on the method of moments and the method of bootstrap. In what follows, we focus on two main problems in using the f_2 similarity factor for assessing similarity between dissolution profiles of two drug products.

The first problem of using the f_2 similarity factor for assessing similarity is its lack of statistical justification. Since f_2 is a statistic and, thus, a random variable, $P(f_2 > 50)$ may be quite large when the two dissolution profiles are not similar. On the other hand, $P(f_2 > 50)$ can be very small when the two dissolution profiles are actually similar. Suppose that the expected value $E(f_2)$ exists and that we can find a 95% lower confidence bound for $E(f_2)$, which is denoted by $\tilde{f}_2$. Then a reasonable modification to the approach of using f_2 is to replace f_2 by $\tilde{f}_2$, i.e., two dissolution profiles are considered to be similar if $\tilde{f}_2 > 50$. However, Liu, Ma, and Chow (1997) indicated that the distribution of f_2 is very complicated and almost intractable because of the unnecessary logarithmic reciprocal square root transformation, which they believe was just to make the artificial acceptable range from 50 to 100. Since f_2 is a strictly decreasing function of D/T, $f_2 > 50$ if and only if $D/T < 99$. Hence, an alternative way is to consider a 95% upper confidence bound $\tilde{D}/T$ for $E(D)/T$ as a similarity factor, i.e., two dissolution profiles are similar if $\tilde{D}/T < 99$. Note that

$$\frac{E(D)}{T} = \frac{1}{T} \sum_{t=1}^{T} \mu_{Dt}^2 + \frac{1}{nT} \sum_{t=1}^{T} \sigma_{Dt}^2,$$

where $\mu_{Dt} = E(y_{1ti} - y_{2ti})$ is the difference of two dissolution profiles at the tth time point and $\sigma_{Dt}^2 = \text{Var}(y_{1ti} - y_{2ti})$. However, the construction of an upper confidence bound for $E(D)/T$ is still a difficult problem and more research is required.

The second problem of using the f_2 similarity factor for assessing similarity is that the f_2 factor assess neither local similarity nor global similarity, owing to the use of the average of $(\bar{y}_{1t} - \bar{y}_{2t})^2$, $t = 1, ..., T$. To illustrate the problem, let us consider the following example. Suppose that n is large enough so that $D \approx E(D) = \sum_{t=1}^{T} \mu_{Dt}^2$ and that T is an even integer, $\mu_{Dt} = 0$ when $t = 1, ..., T/2$, and $|\mu_{Dt}| = 10$ when $t = T/2 + 1, ..., T$. Since $E(D)/T = 10^2/2 = 50 < 99$, the value of f_2 is larger than 50. On the other hand, the two profiles are not globally similar, if a difference of ± 10 is considered to be large enough for nonsimilarity. At time points $t = T/2 + 1, ..., T$, the two profiles are not locally similar either.

3.5   Chow and Ki's Method

For statistical comparison of dissolution profiles between two drug products, Chow and Ki (1997) considered the ratio of the dissolution results of the ith dosage unit at the tth time point, denoted by

$$R_{ti} = \frac{y_{1ti}}{y_{2ti}}, \tag{3.5.1}$$

which can be viewed as a measure of the relative dissolution rate at the ith dissolution medium (or the ith location) and the tth time point. In the following discussion, R_{ti} can be replaced by the difference $y_{1ti} - y_{2ti}$ or the log-transformation on y_{1ti}/y_{2ti}. Since the dissolution results at the tth time point depend on the results at the previous time point $t - 1$, dissolution results are correlated over time. To account for this correlation, Chow and Ki (1997) considered the following autoregressive time series model for R_{ti}:

$$R_{ti} - \gamma_t = \phi(R_{(t-1)i} - \gamma_{(t-1)}) + \epsilon_{ti},$$
$$i = 1, ..., n, \ t = 2, ..., T, \tag{3.5.2}$$

where $\gamma_t = E(R_{ti})$ is the mean relative dissolution rate at the tth time point, $|\phi| < 1$ is an unknown parameter, and ϵ_{ti}'s are independent and identically normally distributed with mean 0 and variance σ_ϵ^2.

3.5.1 The Case of Constant Mean Relative Dissolution Rate

We consider the case where $\gamma_t = \gamma$ for all t. This occurs when there are only minor changes or modifications of the test formulation (drug product 1) over the reference formulation (drug product 2). When $\gamma_t = \gamma$ for all t, local similarity is the same as global similarity. Chow and Ki (1997) proposed to construct a 95% confidence interval (L, U) for γ and then compare (L, U) with the equivalence limits (δ_L, δ_U) (see §3.3). If (L, U) is within (δ_L, δ_U), then we claim that the two dissolution profiles are similar. Thus, the pair of statistics L and U can be viewed as a similarity factor (§3.4.3).

Under (3.5.2) and the assumption that $\gamma_t = \gamma$,

$$E(R_{ti}) = \gamma \quad \text{and} \quad \text{Var}(R_{ti}) = \sigma_R^2,$$

where

$$\sigma_R^2 = \frac{\sigma_\epsilon^2}{1 - \phi^2}. \tag{3.5.3}$$

Let

$$\hat{\gamma} = \frac{1}{nT} \sum_{t=1}^{T} \sum_{i=1}^{n} R_{ti}. \tag{3.5.4}$$

Then

$$E(\hat{\gamma}) = \gamma$$

and

$$\text{Var}(\hat{\gamma}) = \frac{1}{n} \text{Var}\left(\frac{1}{T} \sum_{t=1}^{T} R_{t1}\right)$$

$$= \frac{\sigma_R^2}{nT}\left(1 + 2\sum_{t=1}^{T} \frac{T-t}{T}\phi^t\right).$$

If σ_R^2 and ϕ are known, then a 95% confidence interval for γ is (L, U) with

$$L = \hat{\gamma} - z_{0.975}\sqrt{\text{Var}(\hat{\gamma})}$$

and

$$U = \hat{\gamma} + z_{0.975}\sqrt{\mathrm{Var}(\hat{\gamma})},$$

where z_a is the $100a$th percentile of the standard normal distribution. When σ_R^2 and ϕ are unknown, we replace σ_R^2 and ϕ in L and U by their estimators

$$\hat{\sigma}_R^2 = \frac{1}{nT-1}\sum_{t=1}^{T}\sum_{i=1}^{n}(R_{ti}-\hat{\gamma})^2$$

and

$$\hat{\phi} = \sum_{t=1}^{T-1}\sum_{i=1}^{n}(R_{ti}-\hat{\gamma})(R_{(t+1)i}-\hat{\gamma})\Big/\sum_{t=1}^{T}\sum_{i=1}^{n}(R_{ti}-\hat{\gamma})^2,$$

respectively, which results an approximate 95% confidence interval (L, U) for γ, since, by the theory of time series (e.g., Fuller, 1996), $\hat{\sigma}_R^2$ and $\hat{\phi}$ are consistent estimators as $nT \to \infty$.

3.5.2 The Random Effects Model Approach

In many practical situations, γ_t varies with t. There are two approaches to model γ_t. One approach, adopted by Chow and Ki (1997), is to model γ_t by a random effects model, i.e., γ_t's are assumed to be independent and normally distributed random variables with mean γ and variance σ_γ^2. The other approach is to model γ_t by a deterministic function such as a polynomial of time. We consider the random effects model approach here. The other approach will be discussed in §3.6.

First, consider the local similarity between two dissolution profiles at the tth time point. Under the random effects model for γ_t, Chow and Ki (1997) proposed to construct an approximate 95% prediction interval for γ_t to assess the local similarity at the tth time point. For a fixed t,

$$R_{ti}|\gamma_t \sim N(\gamma_t, \sigma_R^2),$$

where σ_R^2 is given by (3.5.3), and

$$\bar{R}_t|\gamma_t \sim N(\gamma_t, n^{-1}\sigma_R^2).$$

Hence, unconditionally,

$$\bar{R}_t \sim N(\gamma, n^{-1}\sigma_R^2 + \sigma_\gamma^2),$$

where $\bar{R}_t$ is the average of R_{ti}, $i = 1, ..., n$. Then,

$$\gamma_t|\bar{R}_t \sim N\left(\frac{\sigma_R^2/n}{\sigma_R^2/n + \sigma_\gamma^2}\gamma + \frac{\sigma_\gamma^2}{\sigma_R^2/n + \sigma_\gamma^2}\bar{R}_t, \frac{\sigma_\gamma^2\sigma_R^2}{\sigma_R^2 + n\sigma_\gamma^2}\right).$$

Therefore, when γ, σ_R^2, and σ_γ^2 are known, a 95% prediction interval for γ_t is given by (L_t, U_t) with

$$L_t = \frac{\sigma_R^2/n}{\sigma_R^2/n + \sigma_\gamma^2}\gamma + \frac{\sigma_\gamma^2}{\sigma_R^2/n + \sigma_\gamma^2}\bar{R}_t - z_{0.975}\sqrt{\frac{\sigma_\gamma^2\sigma_R^2}{\sigma_R^2 + n\sigma_\gamma^2}}$$

and

$$U_t = \frac{\sigma_R^2/n}{\sigma_R^2/n + \sigma_\gamma^2}\gamma + \frac{\sigma_\gamma^2}{\sigma_R^2/n + \sigma_\gamma^2}\bar{R}_t + z_{0.975}\sqrt{\frac{\sigma_\gamma^2\sigma_R^2}{\sigma_R^2 + n\sigma_\gamma^2}}.$$

When γ, σ_R^2, and σ_γ^2 are unknown, we replace γ by $\hat{\gamma}$ defined in (3.5.4); replace σ_R^2 by its unbiased estimator

$$\hat{\sigma}_R^2 = \frac{1}{T(n-1)}\sum_{t=1}^{T}\sum_{i=1}^{n}(R_{ti} - \bar{R}_t)^2;$$

replace $\sigma_R^2/n + \sigma_\gamma^2$ by its unbiased estimator

$$s^2 = \frac{1}{T-1}\sum_{t=1}^{T}(\bar{R}_t - \hat{\gamma})^2;$$

and replace σ_γ^2 by

$$\hat{\sigma}_\gamma^2 = \max\{0, s^2 - \hat{\sigma}_R^2/n\}.$$

The resulting prediction limits are

$$L_t = \bar{R}_t - \min\left\{1, \frac{\hat{\sigma}_R^2}{ns^2}\right\}(\bar{R}_t - \hat{\gamma}) - z_{0.975}\frac{\hat{\sigma}_\gamma\hat{\sigma}_R}{s\sqrt{n}}$$

and

$$U_t = \bar{R}_t - \min\left\{1, \frac{\hat{\sigma}_R^2}{ns^2}\right\}(\bar{R}_t - \hat{\gamma}) + z_{0.975}\frac{\hat{\sigma}_\gamma\hat{\sigma}_R}{s\sqrt{n}}.$$

Thus, the two dissolution profiles are claimed to be locally similar at the tth time point if (L_t, U_t) is within (δ_L, δ_U).

Under the random effects model approach, however, it is difficult to assess the global similarity between two dissolution profiles. We consider instead the similarity of the two dissolution profiles at all time points considered in dissolution testing. That is, we construct simultaneous prediction intervals $(\tilde{L}_t, \tilde{U}_t)$, $t = 1, ..., T$, satisfying

$$P\left(\tilde{L}_t < \gamma_t < \tilde{U}_t, \ t = 1, ..., T \middle| \bar{R}_t, t = 1, ..., T\right) \geq 95\%$$

and consider the two dissolution profiles to be global similar when $(\tilde{L}_t, \tilde{U}_t)$ is within (δ_L, δ_U) for $t = 1, ..., T$. Using Bonferroni's method, simultaneous prediction intervals can be constructed using the limits

$$\tilde{L}_t = \bar{R}_t - \min\left\{1, \frac{\hat{\sigma}_R^2}{ns^2}\right\}(\bar{R}_t - \hat{\gamma}) - z_{1-0.025/T}\frac{\hat{\sigma}_\gamma \hat{\sigma}_R}{s\sqrt{n}}$$

and

$$\tilde{U}_t = \bar{R}_t - \min\left\{1, \frac{\hat{\sigma}_R^2}{ns^2}\right\}(\bar{R}_t - \hat{\gamma}) + z_{1-0.025/T}\frac{\hat{\sigma}_\gamma \hat{\sigma}_R}{s\sqrt{n}}.$$

3.6 Chow and Shao's Method

The random effects model approach considered in §3.5.2 has two disadvantages. First, as indicated by the plot of $\bar{R}_t$ in Figure 3.6.1, there are often deterministic/monotone trend in γ_t, $t = 1, ..., T$, which cannot be appropriately described by random effects. Second, it is difficult to use the random effects approach to assess the global similarity between two dissolution profiles.

Consider the following polynomial model for γ_t:

$$\gamma_t = \beta_0 + \beta_1 x_t + \beta_2 x_t^2 + \cdots + \beta_p x_t^p, \tag{3.6.1}$$

where x_t is the value of the tth time point and β_j's are unknown parameters. Also, the variances $\sigma_t^2 = \text{Var}(\epsilon_{ti})$, $t = 1, ..., T$, may depend on t. Let

$$\bar{R} = \begin{pmatrix} \bar{R}_1 \\ \bar{R}_2 \\ \vdots \\ \bar{R}_T \end{pmatrix}, \quad X = \begin{pmatrix} 1 & x_1 & x_1^2 & \cdots & x_1^p \\ 1 & x_2 & x_2^2 & \cdots & x_2^p \\ \vdots & \vdots & \vdots & \ddots & \vdots \\ 1 & x_T & x_T^2 & \cdots & x_T^p \end{pmatrix}, \quad \beta = \begin{pmatrix} \beta_0 \\ \beta_1 \\ \vdots \\ \beta_p \end{pmatrix},$$

and $\bar{R}_t$ be the average of R_{ti}, $i = 1, ..., n$, where R_{ti} is given by (3.5.1)-(3.5.2). Then the ordinary least squares estimator of β is

$$\hat{\beta}_{\text{OLS}} = (X'X)^{-1}X'\bar{R},$$

which is unbiased with

$$\text{Var}(\hat{\beta}_{\text{OLS}}) = n^{-1}(X'X)^{-1}X'V_\epsilon X(X'X)^{-1},$$

where V_ϵ is a $T \times T$ matrix whose element of the tth row and sth column is $\phi^{|t-s|}\sigma_t\sigma_s$. Let

$$\hat{\sigma}_t^2 = \frac{1}{n-1}\sum_{i=1}^{n}(R_{ti} - \bar{R}_t)^2$$

and

$$\hat{\phi} = \sum_{t=1}^{T-1} \sum_{i=1}^{n} z_{ti} z_{(t+1)i} \Big/ \sum_{t=1}^{T} \sum_{i=1}^{n} z_{ti}^2,$$

where

$$z_{ti} = R_{ti} - (1, x_t, ..., x_t^p)\hat{\beta}_{\text{OLS}}.$$

Then, approximately (when nT is large)

$$[n^{-1}(X'X)^{-1}X'\hat{V}_\epsilon X(X'X)^{-1}]^{-1/2}(\hat{\beta}_{\text{OLS}} - \beta) \sim N(0, I_{p+1}),$$

where $\hat{V}_\epsilon$ is V_ϵ with σ_t replaced by $\hat{\sigma}_t$ and ϕ replaced by $\hat{\phi}$, and I_{p+1} is the identity matrix of order $p + 1$. Consequently, an approximate 95% confidence interval for the mean relative dissolution rate at time x (which may be different from any of x_t, $t = 1, ..., T$) is $(L(x), U(x))$ with

$$L(x) = \hat{\beta}_{\text{OLS}}'a(x) - z_{0.975}\sqrt{n^{-1}a(x)'(X'X)^{-1}X'\hat{V}_\epsilon X(X'X)^{-1}a(x)}$$

and

$$U(x) = \hat{\beta}_{\text{OLS}}'a(x) + z_{0.975}\sqrt{n^{-1}a(x)'(X'X)^{-1}X'\hat{V}_\epsilon X(X'X)^{-1}a(x)},$$

where $a(x) = (1, x, ..., x^p)'$. Thus, two dissolution profiles are locally similar at time x if $(L(x), U(x))$ is within (δ_L, δ_U). The pair of $L(x)$ and $U(x)$ is a similarity factor.

To assess the global similarity of two dissolution profiles, we can consider the simultaneous confidence intervals $(\tilde{L}(x), \tilde{U}(x))$, where $\tilde{L}(x)$ and $\tilde{U}(x)$ are the same as $L(x)$ and $U(x)$, respectively, with $z_{0.975}$ replaced by $\sqrt{\chi_{0.975, p+1}^2}$. Thus, two dissolution profiles are globally similar if $(\tilde{L}(x), \tilde{U}(x))$ is within (δ_L, δ_U) for all possible time values x. In this case, the pairs of curves $(\tilde{L}(x)$ and $\tilde{U}(x))$ is a similarity factor.

The ordinary least squares estimator $\hat{\beta}_{\text{OLS}}$ may be improved by the generalized least squares estimator

$$\hat{\beta}_{\text{GLS}} = (X'\hat{V}_\epsilon^{-1}X)^{-1}X'\hat{V}_\epsilon^{-1}\bar{R},$$

which has its asymptotic variance-covariance matrix $n^{-1}(X'V_\epsilon^{-1}X)^{-1}$ (see, e.g., Fuller, 1996, §9.1, and Shao, 1999, §3.5.4). Therefore, the previously described procedures for assessing similarity can be modified by replacing $\hat{\beta}_{\text{OLS}}$ and $(X'X)^{-1}X'\hat{V}_\epsilon X(X'X)^{-1}$ with $\hat{\beta}_{\text{GLS}}$ and $(X'\hat{V}_\epsilon^{-1}X)^{-1}$, respectively, which may result in shorter confidence intervals and, thus, more efficient methods of assessing similarity.

Example 3.6.1. To illustrate the use of the statistical methods in this section and §3.4-3.5, we consider the dissolution data discussed in Tsong et

al. (1996). For illustration purposes, we consider dissolution data from the
new lot as the dissolution data of the test product (y_{1ti}'s) and dissolution
data from lot #1 as the dissolution data of the reference product (y_{2ti}'s).
The dissolution data are listed in Table 3.6.1.

Based on the dissolution data in Table 3.6.1, D and the f_2 similarity
factor defined in (3.4.1) are 193.3 and 63.6, respectively. Since the f_2 factor
is between 50 and 100, the two dissolution profiles are considered to be
similar according to the FDA's criterion of using the f_2 similarity factor.

Consider the ratio of the dissolution data R_{ti} given in (3.5.1) and model
(3.5.2). If we assume that $\gamma_t = \gamma$ for all t, then, according to Chow and Ki
(1997), a 95% confidence interval for γ is (96.5%, 103.1%). Suppose that
the desired mean dissolution rate is $Q = 75\%$. Then the equivalence limits
for similarity are given by $(\delta_L, \delta_U) = (87.5\%, 114.3\%)$ (see §3.3). Since
$(96.5\%, 103.1\%) \subset (87.5\%, 114.3\%)$, we conclude that the two dissolution
profiles are globally similar. However, it can be seen from Figure 3.6.1 that
γ_t varies with t and, in fact, a quadratic relationship between γ_t and the
time (hour) is revealed. Hence, the conclusion based on the assumption of
$\gamma_t = \gamma$ for all t may not be appropriate.

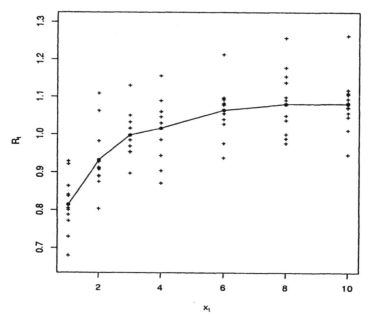

Figure 3.6.1. Dissolution Data and Their Averages
over Locations (Solid Curve)

Table 3.6.1. Dissolution Data (% label claim)

Product	Location	Time (hour)						
		1	2	3	4	6	8	10
Test	1	34	45	61	66	75	85	91
	2	36	51	62	67	83	85	93
	3	37	48	60	69	76	84	91
	4	35	51	63	61	79	82	88
	5	36	49	62	68	79	81	89
	6	37	52	65	73	82	93	95
	7	39	51	61	69	77	85	93
	8	38	49	63	66	79	84	90
	9	35	51	61	67	80	88	96
	10	37	49	61	68	79	91	91
	11	37	51	63	71	83	89	94
	12	37	54	64	70	80	90	93
Reference	1	50	56	68	73	80	86	87
	2	43	48	65	71	77	85	92
	3	44	54	63	67	74	81	82
	4	48	56	64	70	81	84	93
	5	45	56	63	69	76	81	83
	6	46	57	64	67	76	79	85
	7	42	56	62	67	73	81	88
	8	44	54	60	65	72	77	83
	9	38	46	54	58	66	70	76
	10	46	55	63	65	73	80	85
	11	47	55	62	67	76	81	85
	12	48	55	62	66	73	78	85

Table 3.6.2. Analysis of Similarity

Time (hour)	x_t	1	2	3	4	6	8	10
Mean (%)	$\bar{R}_t$	0.81	0.93	1.00	1.02	1.06	1.08	1.08
Lower bound	L_t	78.2	89.3	95.6	97.3	101.9	103.5	103.6
(%)	$\tilde{L}_t$	76.7	87.8	94.1	95.8	100.4	102.0	102.1
	$L(x_t)$	80.0	87.9	93.9	98.4	104.2	105.9	102.4
	$\tilde{L}(x_t)$	77.7	86.1	92.2	96.6	102.1	103.8	99.9
Upper bound	U_t	86.5	97.7	103.9	105.7	110.2	111.8	111.9
(%)	$\tilde{U}_t$	88.0	99.2	105.4	107.2	111.7	113.3	113.4
	$U(x_t)$	88.3	94.4	100.1	105.1	111.6	113.3	111.3
	$\tilde{U}(x_t)$	90.7	96.2	101.8	106.9	113.7	115.4	113.8

The method in §3.5.2 (the random-effect model approach) is applied to this data set and yields prediction bounds L_t and U_t and simultaneous prediction bounds $\tilde{L}_t$ and $\tilde{U}_t$ (see Table 3.6.2). To apply Chow and Shao's method introduced in this section, we choose a quadratic model for γ_t, i.e., $p = 2$ in (3.6.1). The corresponding confidence bounds $L(x_t)$ and $U(x_t)$ and simultaneous confidence bounds $\tilde{L}(x_t)$ and $\tilde{U}(x_t)$ are given in Table 3.6.2. These confidence/prediction bounds are displayed in Figure 3.6.2 for comparison.

Using the equivalence limits $(\delta_L, \delta_U) = (87.5\%, 114.3\%)$, it can be seen from Table 3.6.2 or Figure 3.6.2 that the two dissolution profiles are not globally similar, although they are locally similar when $x_t \geq 2$.

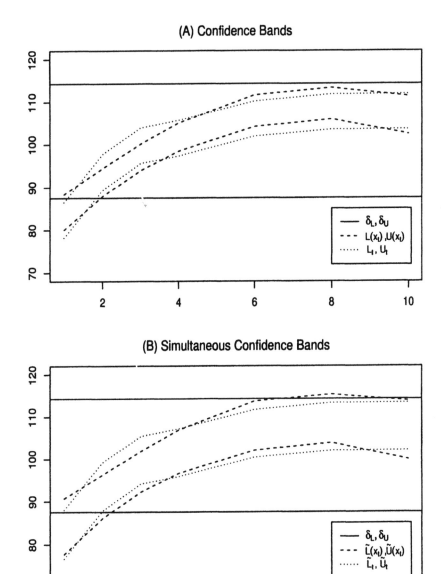

Figure 3.6.2. Confidence and Prediction Bounds

Chapter 4

Stability Analysis

For every drug product in the marketplace, the FDA requires that an expiration dating period (which is usually referred to as shelf-life) be indicated on the immediate container label. The shelf-life of a drug product is defined as the time interval in which the characteristic of the drug product (e.g., potency) remains within the approved USP/NF specification after being manufactured. The FDA has the authority to issue recalls for drug products that fail to meet the USP/NF specifications for the identity, strength, quality, purity, stability, and reproducibility prior to the expiration date.

A drug's shelf-life is usually established through a stability study under the appropriate storage conditions. As indicated in both the FDA stability guideline (FDA, 1987b) and the ICH guideline for stability (ICH, 1993), the purpose of a stability study is not only to characterize the degradation of a drug product, but also to establish a shelf-life applicable to all future batches of the drug product.

Statistical models, designs, and procedures for stability analysis, as described in the FDA stability guideline, are given in §4.1-4.3. Our focus is mainly on the statistical issues that have not been fully documented in the FDA guideline, such as stability study design (§4.1), batch-to-batch variation (§4.2-4.3), two-phase shelf-life estimation (§4.4), stability analysis with discrete responses (§4.5), and shelf-life for drug products with multiple responses and ingredients (§4.6).

4.1 Statistical Model and Design

The primary covariate in stability analysis is the storage time. The FDA and ICH guidelines suggest that stability testing be performed at three-month intervals during the first year, six-month intervals during the second year, and annually thereafter. Since different batches of a drug product may exhibit different degradations, the FDA requires that at least three batches of the drug product be tested for stability analysis. Other covariates, such as package type and strength, may also be included in stability analysis.

We consider the case where the drug characteristic decreases with time. The other case where the drug characteristic increases with time can be treated similarly. For continuous assay results (e.g., potency expressed in percent of label claim), the following linear model is usually considered to describe the degradation in stability analysis:

$$y_{ij} = \beta_i' x_{ij} + e_{ij}, \quad i = 1, ..., k, \ j = 1, ..., n, \qquad (4.1.1)$$

where i is the index for batch, x_{ij} is a $p \times 1$ vector of nonrandom covariates of the form $(1, t_{ij}, w_{ij})'$, $(1, t_{ij}, t_{ij} w_{ij})'$ or $(1, t_{ij}, w_{ij}, t_{ij} w_{ij})'$, t_{ij} is the jth time point for the ith batch, w_{ij} is the jth value of a vector of nonrandom covariates (e.g., package type and strength), β_i is an unknown $p \times 1$ vector of parameters, and e_{ij}'s are independent random errors (in observing y_{ij}'s), which are assumed to be identically distributed as $N(0, \sigma_e^2)$.

When $\beta_i = \beta$ for all i, we say that there is no batch-to-batch variation. In such a case, model (4.1.1) reduces to a fixed effects linear regression model. When β_i's are different, the best way to interpret the batch-to-batch variation is to consider β_i, $i = 1, ..., k$, as a random *sample* from a population of all future batches, which the established shelf-life is to be applied. Throughout this chapter, we assume that β_i's are independent and identically distributed as $N(\beta, \Sigma)$, where β and Σ are respectively the unknown mean vector and covariance matrix of β_i. Consequently, model (4.1.1) becomes a mixed effects linear regression model. The fixed effects linear regression model is a special case of the general mixed effects model. Statistical procedures utilized in these two cases may be different, which is discussed in the later sections of this chapter.

The FDA stability guideline provides some design considerations for stability studies under ambient conditions. These design considerations include batch sampling, container-closure and drug product sampling, and sampling time considerations. An appropriate stability design can help to achieve the objective of a stability study. Basically, a stability design consists of two parts: the selection of design factors (e.g., batch, strength, and package type) and the choice of sampling intervals (e.g., three-month during the first year, six-month during the second year, and yearly thereafter). For the selection of design factors, the stability designs commonly employed are the full factorial design and fractional factorial designs. In the interest of reducing the number of sampling intervals for stability testing, Nordbrock (1992) introduced various choices of subsets of sampling intervals for the intended stability studies for up to four years (see Table 4.1.1). In practice, these subsets can be classified into four groups, namely, the complete group, the $\frac{1}{2}$-group, the $\frac{1}{3}$-group, and the $\frac{2}{3}$-group. For a $\frac{i}{j}$-group, only a fraction ($\frac{i}{j}, i < j$) of the stability tests will be done except for the initial and the last sampling time points. For example, for the $\frac{1}{2}$-group, half of the stability tests will be performed at 0, 3, 9, 18, 36, and 48 months, and the other half will be done at 0, 6, 12, 24, and 48 months. A design of this kind is usually referred to as a one-half design. In his comprehensive review of stability designs, Nordbrock (1992) also provided a summary of some useful reduced stability designs with various choices of subsets of sampling time intervals for long-term stability studies at room temperature (see Table 4.1.2). These stability designs, which are commonly adopted in the pharmaceutical industry, are accepted by the FDA and ICH.

For design selection, Nordbrock (1992) proposed a criterion based on the power for detection of a significant difference between regression slopes (i.e., stability loss over time). For a fixed sample size, the design with the highest power for detection of a significant difference between slopes is the best design. On the other hand, for a given desired power, the design with the smallest sample size is the best design. Alternatively, Chow (1992) and Ju and Chow (1995) proposed to select a design based on the precision of the estimated shelf-life. For a fixed sample size, the design with the best precision for shelf-life estimation is the best design. For a given desired precision for shelf-life estimation, the design with the smallest sample size is the best design.

Since long-term stability testing requires a drug product be tested at more sampling time intervals, the cost of the stability studies could be substantial. As a result, it is of interest to adopt a design where only a fraction of the total number of samples are tested, but still maintain the validity,

Table 4.1.1. Subsets of Sampling Time Intervals

Subset	Selected time intervals (in month)									Group
T_1	0	3	6	9	12	18	24	36	48	Complete
T_2	0	3		9		18		36	48	$\frac{1}{2}$
T_3	0		6		12		24		48	$\frac{1}{2}$
T_5	0	3			12			36	48	$\frac{1}{3}$
T_6	0		6			18			48	$\frac{1}{3}$
T_7	0			9			24		48	$\frac{1}{3}$
T_8	0	3		9	12		24	36	48	$\frac{2}{3}$
T_9	0	3	6		12	18		36	48	$\frac{2}{3}$
T_{10}	0		6	9		18	24		48	$\frac{2}{3}$

Table 4.1.2. Stability Designs

Design description	Sample time intervals	Number of assays[†]
Complete	all tested using T_1	$9kab$
Complete-$\frac{2}{3}$	$\frac{1}{3}$ tested using T_8	$20kab/3^*$
	$\frac{1}{3}$ tested using T_9	
	$\frac{1}{3}$ tested using T_{10}	
Complete-$\frac{1}{2}$	$\frac{1}{2}$ tested using T_2	$11kab/2^*$
	$\frac{1}{2}$ tested using T_3	
Complete-$\frac{1}{3}$	$\frac{1}{3}$ tested using T_5	$13kab/3^*$
	$\frac{1}{3}$ tested using T_6	
	$\frac{1}{3}$ tested using T_7	
Fractional	all tested using T_1	$6kab$
Two strengths per batch	all tested using T_1	$18ka$
Two packages per strength	all tested using T_1	$18kb$
Fractional-$\frac{1}{2}$	$\frac{1}{2}$ tested using T_2	$11kab/3^*$
	$\frac{1}{2}$ tested using T_3	
Two strength per batch-$\frac{1}{2}$	$\frac{1}{2}$ tested using T_2	$11ka$
	$\frac{1}{2}$ tested using T_3	
Two packages per strength-$\frac{1}{2}$	$\frac{1}{2}$ tested using T_2	$11kb$
	$\frac{1}{2}$ tested using T_3	

[†] a = the number of packages, b = the number of strengths
 k = the number of batches

[*] integer part plus 1 if this number is not an integer

accuracy, and reliability of the estimated shelf-life. For this consideration, matrixing and bracketing designs have become increasingly popular in drug research and development for stability. As indicated in the ICH guideline for stability, a bracketing design is defined as the design of a stability schedule, so that at any time point, only the samples on the extremes, for example, of container size and/or dosage strengths, are tested (Helboe, 1992; ICH, 1993). A matrixing design is a design where only a fraction of the total number of samples are tested at any specified sampling point (Helboe, 1992; ICH, 1993; Nordbrock, 2000). Alternatively, Chow (1992) and Chow and Liu (1995) define any subset of a full factorial design as a matrixing design. Some statistical justification for use of matrixing and bracketing designs can be found in Lin (1994) and Nordbrock (2000).

Lin (1994) indicated that a matrixing design may be applicable to strength if there are no changes in the proportion of active ingredients, container size, and immediate sampling time points. The application of a matrixing design to situations, such as closure systems, the orientation of container during storage, packaging form, manufacturing process, and batch size, should be evaluated carefully. It is discouraged to apply a matrixing design to sampling times at two endpoints (i.e., the initial and the last) and at any time points beyond the desired expiration date. If the drug product is sensitive to temperature, humidity, and light, the matrixing design should be avoided.

4.2 Testing for Batch-to-Batch Variation

If the batch-to-batch variability is small, it would be advantageous to combine the data from different batches for an overall shelf-life estimation with high precision. However, combining the data from different batches should be supported by a preliminary test of batch similarity. The FDA guideline recommends a preliminary test for batch-to-batch variation be performed at the significance level of 0.25 (Bancroft, 1964), though it has been criticized by many researchers (see, e.g., Ruberg and Stegeman, 1991; Chow and Liu, 1995).

Under model (4.1.1), testing for batch-to-batch variation is equivalent to testing whether $\Sigma = 0$, i.e., the distribution of β_i is degenerated at β. In the following, we describe a test procedure proposed by Shao and Chow (1994). Other procedures of testing for batch-to-batch variation can be found in the literature, for example, Chow and Shao (1989) and Murphy and Weisman (1990).

Let $Y_i = (y_{i1}, ..., y_{in})'$ be the vector of assay results from the ith batch and $X_i = (x_{i1}', ..., x_{in}')'$, $i = 1, ..., k$. First, consider the case where $X_i = X$ for all i. Under model (4.1.1), the ordinary least squares estimator of $\beta = E(\beta_i)$ is $(X'X)^{-1}X'\bar{Y}$, where $\bar{Y}$ is the average of Y_i's. Let SSR be the sum of squared residuals,

$$S = \sum_{i=1}^{k}(Y_i - \bar{Y})(Y_i - \bar{Y})',$$

and

$$\text{SE} = k\bar{Y}'[I_n - X(X'X)^{-1}X']\bar{Y},$$

where I_n is the $n \times n$ identity matrix. Shao and Chow's test procedure is motivated by the decomposition

$$\text{SSR} = \text{tr}(S) + \text{SE},$$

where $\text{tr}(S)$ is the trace of the matrix S. A direct calculation shows that

1. $E(\text{SE}) = \sigma_e^2$ and SE/σ_e^2 has the chi-square distribution with $n - p$ degrees of freedom.

2. S has a Wishart distribution and $E[\text{tr}(S)] = (k-1)[\text{tr}(X\Sigma X') + n\sigma_e^2]$.

3. The statistics SE and S are independent.

4. Under the hypothesis that $\Sigma = 0$, $\text{tr}(S)/\sigma_e^2$ has the chi-square distribution with $n(k-1)$ degrees of freedom.

Thus, a p-value for testing the hypothesis of $\Sigma = 0$ is given by

$$1 - F\left(\frac{(n-p)\text{tr}(S)}{n(k-1)\text{SE}}\right), \qquad (4.2.1)$$

where F is the distribution function of the F-distribution with degrees of freedom $n(k-1)$ and $n - p$.

When some X_i's are different, the previous procedure can still be applied by replacing X with the average of X_i's. The p-value given in (4.2.1) is not exact but approximately correct when either n is large or σ_e is small (small error asymptotics). Note that stability studies are often conducted under well-controlled conditions so that the error variance σ_e^2 is small. More discussion about testing for batch-to-batch variation can be found in §4.5.3.

Example 4.2.1. A stability study was conducted on a 300mg tablet of a drug product. The tablets from five batches were stored at room temperature in two types of containers (high-density polyethylene bottle and blister package). The tablets were tested for potency at 0, 3, 6, 9, 12, and 18 months. Using the assay results listed in Table 4.2.1 and model (4.1.1) with $x_{ij} = (1, t_j, t_j w_j)$ ($w_j = 0$ for bottle container and $w_j = 1$ for blister package), we obtain that $\text{tr}(S) = 88.396$ and $\text{SE} = 4.376$. Thus, the p-value computed according to (4.2.1) is

$$1 - F(3.367) = 0.028,$$

which is much less than 0.25. Thus, we can conclude that there is a significant batch-to-batch variation in this case.

4.3 Shelf-Life Estimation

4.3.1 Fixed-Batches Approach

For a single batch, the FDA stability guideline indicates that an acceptable approach for drug characteristics that are expected to decrease in potency with time is to determine the time at which the 95% one-sided lower confi-

Table 4.2.1. Assay Results (% of Claim) in Example 4.2.1

Package	Batch						
		0	3	6	9	12	18
Bottle	1	104.8	102.5	101.5	102.4	99.4	96.5
	2	103.9	101.9	103.2	99.6	100.2	98.8
	3	103.5	102.1	101.9	100.3	99.2	101.0
	4	101.5	100.3	101.1	100.6	100.7	98.4
	5	106.1	104.3	101.5	101.1	99.4	98.2
Blister	1	102.0	101.6	100.9	101.1	101.7	97.1
	2	104.7	101.3	103.8	99.8	98.9	97.1
	3	102.5	102.3	100.0	101.7	99.0	100.9
	4	100.1	101.8	101.4	99.9	99.2	97.4
	5	105.2	104.1	102.4	100.2	99.6	97.5

Source: Shao and Chow (1994, *Biometrics*, Vol. 50, p. 761)

dence bound for the mean degradation curve intersects the acceptable lower product specification limit as specified in the USP/NF (FDA, 1987b). For multiple batches, if a preliminary test for batch-to-batch variation is not significant at the 0.25 level, then all batches are considered from the same population of production batches with a common degradation pattern, and a single estimated shelf-life can be obtained by combining data from the different batches. If we adopt the test procedure as described in §4.2, then no batch-to-batch variation is concluded when the p-value in (4.2.1) is larger than 0.25.

When there is no batch-to-batch variation, model (4.1.1) reduces to

$$y_{ij} = \beta' x_{ij} + e_{ij}, \quad i = 1, ..., k, \ j = 1, ..., n.$$

Using the ordinary least squares method, we obtain the following 95% lower confidence bound for $\beta' x(t)$:

$$L(t) = \hat{\beta}' x(t) - t_{0.95;nk-p}\sqrt{\frac{x(t)'(X_1'X_1 + \cdots + X_k'X_k)^{-1}x(t)\text{SSR}}{nk-p}}, \quad (4.3.1)$$

where $x(t)$ is x_{ij} with t_{ij} replaced by t and w_{ij} (package type or strength) fixed at a particular value, $\hat{\beta}$ is the ordinary least squares estimator of β, $X_i = (x_{i1}, ..., x_{in})'$, SSR is the sum of squared residuals, and $t_{0.95;nk-p}$ is the 95th percentile of the t-distribution with $nk - p$ degrees of freedom. According to the FDA stability guideline (FDA, 1987b), the estimated shelf-life can be determined as

$$\hat{t}^* = \inf\{t : L(t) \leq \eta\}, \quad (4.3.2)$$

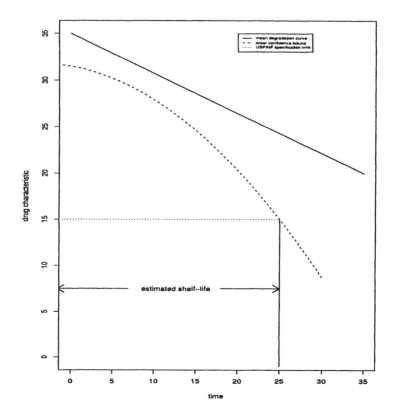

Figure 4.3.1. Shelf-Life Estimation

where η is the given lower specification limit. If $L(t)$ is decreasing in t, $\hat{t}^*$ is the solution of $\eta = L(t)$, i.e., $\eta = L(\hat{t}^*)$ (see Figure 4.3.1). Since $\beta'x(t)$ is the average drug characteristic at time t, the true shelf-life is

$$t^* = \inf\{t : \beta'x(t) \leq \eta\}.$$

Note that t^* is nonrandom but unknown. The estimated shelf-life $\hat{t}^*$ in (4.3.2) is actually a 95% lower confidence bound for t^*, since

$$P\left(\hat{t}^* > t^*\right) \leq P\left(L(t^*) > \eta\right) = P\left(L(t^*) > \beta'x(t^*)\right) = 0.05.$$

Note that $\hat{t}^*$ may be much larger than the study range, the maximum of t_{ij}'s in the study. The reliability of $\hat{t}^*$ depends on the validity of the statistical model for t-values beyond the study range. In practice, an estimated shelf-life of more than 6 months beyond the study range may not be reliable.

When a preliminary test for batch-to-batch variation is significant, the FDA suggests that the minimum of the individual estimated shelf-lives obtained from individual batches be considered as the estimated shelf-life of the drug product. The minimum approach for determination of shelf-life, however, has received a considerable amount of criticism because it lacks statistical justification (Chow and Shao, 1991) and suffers from some shortcomings (Ruberg and Stegeman, 1991; Ruberg and Hsu, 1992). As an alternative, Ruberg and Hsu (1992) proposed an approach using the concept of multiple comparison to derive some criteria for pooling batches with the worst batches. The idea is to pool the batches that have slopes similar to the worst degradation rate with respect to a predetermined equivalence limit. Although the fixed-batches approach may ensure that the estimated shelf-life is applicable to the k batches of the drug product under study, it does not provide a valid estimated shelf-life applicable to all future batches that may have different degradation curves from any of the k batches under study.

4.3.2 Random-Batches Approach

As indicated in the FDA stability guideline, the batches used in stability studies for the establishment of drug shelf-life should constitute a random sample from the population of future production batches. In addition, a single estimated shelf-life should be applicable to all future batches. As a result, statistical methods based on the mixed effects model seem more appropriate. In recent years, several methods for determining a drug's shelf-life with random batches have been considered. See, for example, Chow and Shao (1991), Murphy and Weisman (1990), Chow (1992), Shao and Chow (1994), and Shao and Chen (1997). We now describe the procedure proposed by Shao and Chow (1994) and Shao and Chen (1997), which is based on model (4.1.1) with $\Sigma \neq 0$.

Let $\beta'_{\text{future}}x(t)$ be the mean degradation curve at time t for a future batch of the drug product. Given β_{future}, the shelf-life for this batch is

$$t^*_{\text{future}} = \inf\{t : \beta'_{\text{future}}x(t) \leq \eta\}.$$

Since β_{future} should be considered as a random vector having the same distribution as β_i in model (4.1.1), the shelf-life t^*_{future} is an unknown random quantity with distribution

$$F_{\text{shelf}}(t) = P\left(\beta'_{\text{future}}x(t) \leq \eta\right) = \Phi\left(\frac{\eta - \beta'x(t)}{\sqrt{x(t)'\Sigma x(t)}}\right),$$

where $\beta = E(\beta_{\text{future}})$, $\Sigma = \text{Var}(\beta_{\text{future}})$, and Φ is the standard normal distribution. Therefore, it makes more sense to consider a 95% lower prediction bound for t^*_{future}, instead of a lower confidence bound, as the estimated shelf-life.

Let $Y_i = (y_{i1}, ..., y_{in})'$ and $\hat{\beta}_i = (X_i'X_i)^{-1}X_i'Y_i$. Conditioning on β_i, $\hat{\beta}_i \sim N(\beta_i, \sigma_e^2(X_i'X_i)^{-1})$. Since $\beta_i \sim N(\beta, \Sigma)$, the unconditional distribution of $\hat{\beta}_i$ is $N(\beta, \Sigma + \sigma_e^2(X_i'X_i)^{-1})$. Define

$$L(t) = x(t)'\hat{\beta} - \rho_{0.95}(k)\sqrt{v(t)/k}, \qquad (4.3.3)$$

where $\hat{\beta}$ is the average of $\hat{\beta}_i$'s,

$$v(t) = x(t)' \left[\frac{1}{k-1} \sum_{i=1}^{k}(\hat{\beta}_i - \hat{\beta})(\hat{\beta}_i - \hat{\beta})' \right] x(t),$$

$\rho_a(k)$ satisfies

$$\int_0^1 P\{T_k(u) \le \rho_a(k)\}\, du = a,$$

and $T_k(u)$ denotes a random variable having the noncentral t-distribution with $k-1$ degrees of freedom and $\sqrt{k}\Phi^{-1}(1-u)$ as the noncentrality parameter. Values of $\rho_a(k)$ for $a = 0.99, 0.95, 0.90$ and $k = 3, 4, ..., 20$ are listed in Table 4.3.1.

Assume that n is large or σ_e is small. Then $[\hat{\beta}'x(t) - \eta]/\sqrt{v(t)/k}$ approximately has the noncentral t-distribution with $k-1$ degrees of freedom and the noncentrality parameter $[\beta'x(t) - \eta]/\sqrt{x(t)'\Sigma x(t)/k}$, since

$$E[v(t)] = x(t)'\Sigma x(t) + \frac{\sigma_e^2}{k} \sum_{i=1}^{k} x(t)'(X_i'X_i)^{-1}x(t)$$

$$\approx x(t)'\Sigma x(t)$$

when n is large or σ_e^2 is small. Let $\xi_u = F^{-1}_{\text{shelf}}(u)$. Then

$$u = F_{\text{shelf}}(\xi_u) = \Phi\left(\frac{\eta - \beta'x(\xi_u)}{\sqrt{x(\xi_u)'\Sigma x(\xi_u)}} \right)$$

and, thus, the noncentrality parameter of the random variable $[\hat{\beta}'x(\xi_u) - \eta]/\sqrt{v(\xi_u)/k}$ is

$$\sqrt{k}\Phi^{-1}(1-u) = \frac{\beta'x(\xi_u) - \eta}{\sqrt{x(\xi_u)'\Sigma x(\xi_u)/k}}.$$

Define

$$\hat{t}^* = \inf\{t : L(t) \le \eta\}, \qquad (4.3.4)$$

Table 4.3.1. Values of $\rho_a(k)$

k	a 0.99	0.95	0.90
3	13.929	5.840	3.771
4	10.153	5.262	3.662
5	9.178	5.222	3.756
6	8.903	5.331	3.905
7	8.889	5.496	4.072
8	8.994	5.684	4.245
9	9.160	5.881	4.417
10	9.358	6.080	4.587
11	9.574	6.279	4.753
12	9.800	6.475	4.916
13	10.031	6.669	5.074
14	10.265	6.859	5.229
15	10.498	7.045	5.380
16	10.730	7.228	5.527
17	10.961	7.407	5.671
18	11.189	7.583	5.812
19	11.417	7.755	5.950
20	11.637	7.924	6.084

where $L(t)$ is given by (4.3.3). Then

$$
P\left(t^*_{\text{future}} < \hat{t}^*\right) = \int_0^\infty P_Y\left(t < \hat{t}^*\right) dF_{\text{shelf}}(t)
$$

$$
= \int_0^\infty P_Y\left\{L(t) > \eta\right\} dF_{\text{shelf}}(t)
$$

$$
= \int_0^1 P_Y\left\{L(\xi_u) > \eta\right\} du
$$

$$
= \int_0^1 P\left\{\frac{\hat{\beta}' x(\xi_u) - \eta}{\sqrt{v(\xi_u)/k}} > \rho_{0.95}(k)\right\} du
$$

$$
\approx \int_0^1 P\left\{T_k(u) > \rho_{0.95}(k)\right\} du
$$

$$
= 0.05,
$$

where P_Y denotes the probability related to $Y = (Y_1, ..., Y_k)$ and P is the joint probability related to Y and β_{future}. This means that $\hat{t}^*$ defined by

(4.3.4) is an approximate 95% lower prediction bound for t^*_{future} and, thus, can be used as an estimated shelf-life for all future batches of the drug product. Note that $\hat{t}^*$ in (4.3.4) has the same form as that of $\hat{t}^*$ in the case of no batch-to-batch variation (§4.3.1, Figure 4.3.1), except that $L(t)$ in (4.3.1) is replaced by a more conservative bound to incorporate the batch-to-batch variability.

Example 4.3.1. To illustrate the shelf-life estimation procedure, we use the stability data in Example 4.2.1 (Table 4.2.1). We consider model (4.1.1) with $x'_{ij} = (1, t_j, t_j w_j)$, where $w_j = 0$ for the bottle container and 1 for the blister package. Values of $L(t)$ given by (4.3.3) are listed in Table 4.3.2. For $\eta = 90\%$, the estimated shelf-life $\hat{t}^*$ defined by (4.3.4) is 27 months for bottle container and 26 months for blister package.

Table 4.3.2. Values of $L(t)$ in (4.3.3)

t (in months)	Bottle container	Blister package
18	95.642	95.208
19	95.037	94.626
20	94.430	94.040
21	93.822	93.450
22	93.210	92.859
23	92.596	92.264
24	91.985	91.670
25	91.371	91.072
26	90.754	90.474
27	90.145	89.884
28	89.537	89.304

4.3.3 Discussion

Since the estimated shelf-life in §4.3.1 or §4.3.2 is a lower confidence or prediction bound, it generally underestimates the true shelf-life and, thus, is a conservative estimator. Theoretical and empirical properties of shelf-life estimators can be found in the statistical literature. For example, Sun et al. (1999) studied the distributional properties of the shelf-life estimator proposed by Shao and Chow (1994); Ho, Liu and Chow (1992) examined, by simulation, the bias and mean squared error of shelf-life estimators; and Shao and Chow (2001a) obtained some formulas for the asymptotic bias and mean squared error of shelf-life estimators. These results may have an impact on the selection of appropriate stability study designs.

4.4 Two-Phase Shelf-Life

Unlike most drug products, some drug products must be stored at certain temperatures, such as -20^0C (frozen temperature), 5^0C (refrigerator temperature), and 25^0C (room temperature), in order to maintain their stability until use (Mellon, 1991). Drug products of this kind are usually referred to as frozen drug products. A shelf-life statement for frozen drug products usually consists of multiple phases with different storage temperatures. For example, a commonly adopted shelf-life statement for frozen products could be 24 months at -20^0C followed by 2 weeks at 5^0C. As a result, the drug's shelf-life is determined based on a two-phase stability study. The first phase of the stability study is to determine the drug's shelf-life under a frozen storage condition such as -20^0C, while the second phase of the stability study is to estimate the drug's shelf-life under a refrigerated condition. The first phase of the stability study is usually referred to as the *frozen study*, and the second phase of the stability study is known as the *thawed study*. The frozen study is usually conducted similarly to a regular long-term stability study, except that the drug is stored in frozen conditions. In other words, stability testing will be normally conducted at 3-month intervals during the first year, 6-month intervals during the second year, and annually thereafter. Stability testing for the thawed study is conducted following the stability testing for the frozen study. It may be performed at 1-week (or 1-day) intervals, for up to several weeks.

Mellon (1991) suggested that stability data from the frozen study and a thawed study be analyzed separately to obtain a combined shelf-life for the drug product. However, his method does not account for the fact that the stability at the second phase (thawed study) may depend upon the stability at the first phase (frozen study), i.e., an estimated shelf-life from a thawed study following 3-months of frozen storage may be longer than that of one following 6-months of frozen storage. Shao and Chow (2001b) proposed a method for the determination of drug shelf-lives for the two-phases using a two phase linear regression based on the statistical principle described in both the FDA and ICH stability guidelines.

For simplicity's sake, in this section we will assume that the time interval is the only covariate and that there is no batch-to-batch variation. Results for general situations can be obtained by combining the results in this section and those in §4.3.

4.4.1 A Two-Phase Linear Regression Model

For the first phase of the stability study, we have data

$$y_{ij} = \alpha + \beta t_j + e_{ij}, \quad i = 1, ..., k, \ j = 1, ..., n, \qquad (4.4.1)$$

where y_{ij} is the assay result from the ith batch at time t_j, α and β are unknown parameters, and e_{ij}'s are independent random errors that are identically distributed as $N(0, \sigma_e^2)$. Note that this is a special case of model (4.1.1). Since there is no batch-to-batch variation, α and β do not depend on i. Hence, data from different batches at each time point can be treated as replicates.

At time t_j, second-phase stability data are collected at time intervals t_{jh}, $h = 1, ..., m \geq 2$. The total number of data for the second phase is knm. Data from the two phases are independent. Typically, $t_{jh} = t_j + s_h$, where s_h is time in the second phase and $s_h = 1, 2, 3$ days (or weeks), etc.

Since the degradation lines for the two phases intersect, the intercept of the second phase degradation line at time t is $\alpha + \beta t$. Let $\gamma(t)$ be the slope of the second phase degradation line at time t. Then, at time t_j, we have second-phase stability data

$$y_{ijh} = \alpha + \beta t_j + \gamma(t_j)s_h + e_{ijh}, \quad i = 1, ..., k, \ h = 1, ..., m,$$

where $j = 1, ..., n$ and e_{ijh}'s are independent random errors identically distributed as $N(0, \sigma_{e2}^2)$.

It is assumed that $\gamma(t)$ is a polynomial in t with unknown coefficients, i.e.,

$$\gamma(t) = \sum_{l=0}^{L} \gamma_l t^l \qquad (4.4.2)$$

where γ_l's are unknown parameters and $L + 1 < km$ and $L < n$. Typically, $L \leq 2$. When $L = 0$, $\gamma(t) = \gamma_0$ is a common slope model. When $L = 1$, $\gamma(t) = \gamma_0 + \gamma_1 t$ is a linear trend model, while when $L = 2$, $\gamma(t) = \gamma_0 + \gamma_1 t + \gamma_2 t^2$ is a quadratic trend model.

4.4.2   The Second-Phase Shelf-Life

The first-phase shelf-life can be estimated based on the first-phase data $\{y_{ij}\}$ and the method in §4.3. We now consider the second-phase shelf-life under assumption (4.4.2). Since the slope of the second-phase degradation line may vary with t, we estimate the slope at time t_j using the second-phase data at t_j:

$$b_j = \frac{\sum_{i=1}^{k} \sum_{h=1}^{m} (s_h - \bar{s})y_{ijh}}{k \sum_{h=1}^{m} (s_h - \bar{s})^2},$$

where $\bar{s}$ is the average of s_h's. Since $L < n$, the unknown parameters γ_l in (4.4.2) can be estimated by the least squares estimators under the following "model":

$$b_j = \sum_{l=0}^{L} \gamma_l t_j^l + \text{error},$$

i.e., the parameter vector $(\gamma_0, \gamma_1, ..., \gamma_L)'$ can be estimated by

$$(W'W)^{-1}W'b, \qquad (4.4.3)$$

where $b = (b_1, ..., b_n)'$, $W' = [g(t_1), ..., g(t_n)]$, and $g(t) = (1, t, ..., t^L)'$. Consequently, the slope $\gamma(t)$ can be estimated by

$$\hat{\gamma}(t) = g(t)'(W'W)^{-1}W'b.$$

The covariance matrix of $(W'W)^{-1}W'b$ is

$$V = \frac{\sigma_{e2}^2}{k\sum_{h=1}^{m}(s_h - \bar{s})^2}(W'W)^{-1},$$

where the unknown variance σ_{e2}^2 can be estimated by

$$\hat{\sigma}_{e2}^2 = \frac{1}{knm - n(L+2)}\sum_{i=1}^{k}\sum_{j=1}^{n}\sum_{h=1}^{m}(y_{ijh} - \bar{y}_j - b_i(s_h - \bar{s}))^2,$$

and $\bar{y}_j$ is the average of y_{ijh}'s with a fixed j. Let $\hat{V}$ be the same as V but with σ_{e2}^2 replaced by $\hat{\sigma}_{e2}^2$. Then $(W'W)^{-1}W'b$ and its estimated covariance matrix $\hat{V}$ can be used to form approximate t-tests to select a polynomial model in (4.4.2).

The variance of $\hat{\gamma}(t)$ can be estimated by $g(t)'\hat{V}g(t)$. For fixed t and s, let

$$v(t, s) = v(t) + g(t)'\hat{V}g(t)s^2 \qquad (4.4.4)$$

and

$$L(t, s) = \hat{\alpha} + \hat{\beta}t + \hat{\gamma}(t)s - t_{0.95;kn+knm-2-n(L+2)}\sqrt{v(t, s)}, \qquad (4.4.5)$$

where $\hat{\alpha}$ and $\hat{\beta}$ are the least square estimators of α and β in (4.4.1) based on the data from the first phase. For any fixed t less than the first-phase true shelf-life, i.e., t satisfying $\alpha + \beta t > \eta$, the second-phase shelf-life can be estimated as

$$\hat{s}^*(t) = \inf\{s \geq 0 : L(t, s) \leq \eta\}$$

(if $L(t, s) < \eta$ for all s, then $\hat{s}^*(t) = 0$), where η is the given lower limit for the drug characteristic. That is, if the drug product is taken out of the first-phase storage condition at time t, then the estimated second-phase shelf-life is $\hat{s}^*(t)$. The justification for $\hat{s}^*(t)$ is that for any t satisfying $\alpha + \beta t > \eta$,

$$P\{\hat{s}^*(t) \leq \text{the true second-phase shelf-life }\} \approx 95\%$$

for large sample sizes or small error variances.

In practice, the time at which the drug product is taken out of the first-phase storage condition may be unknown. In such a case, we may apply the following method to assess the second-phase shelf-life. Select a set of time intervals $t_v < \hat{t}^*$, $v = 1, ..., J$, where $\hat{t}^*$ is the estimated first-phase shelf-life, and construct a table (or a figure) for $(t_v, \hat{s}^*(t_v))$, $v = 1, ..., J$ (see, for example, Table 4.4.2). If a drug product is taken out of the first-phase storage condition at time t_0 which is between t_v and t_{v+1}, then its second-phase shelf-life is $\hat{s}^*(t_{v+1})$.

Example 4.4.1. A pharmaceutical company wishes to establish a shelf-life for a drug product at a frozen condition of -20^0C followed by a shelf-life at a refrigerated condition of 5^0C. During the frozen phase, the product stored at -20^0C was tested at 0, 3, 6, 9, 12, and 18 months. At each sampling time point of the frozen phase, the product was tested at 1, 2, 3, and 5 weeks at the refrigerated condition of 5^0C. Three batches of the drug product were used at each sampling time point ($k = 3$). Assay results in the percent of labeled concentration (g/50 ml) are given in Table 4.4.1. The p-values from the F-tests of batch-to-batch variation for the two phases of data are larger than 0.25, and, thus, we combined three batches in the analysis.

Assay results in Table 4.4.1 indicate that the degradation of the drug product at the refrigerated phase is faster at later sampling time points of the frozen phase. Assuming the linear trend model $\gamma(t) = \gamma_0 + \gamma_1 t$ (model (4.4.2) with $L = 1$) and using formula (4.4.3), we obtain estimates $\hat{\gamma}_0 = -0.2025$ and $\hat{\gamma}_1 = -0.0031$ with estimated standard errors of 0.0037 and 0.0004, respectively. Hence, the hypothesis that $\gamma_1 = 0$ (which leads to the common slope model $\gamma(t) = \gamma_0$) is rejected based on an approximate t-test with the significance level ≤ 0.0001.

Table 4.4.2 lists the lower confidence bounds $L(t)$ and $L(t,s)$, where $L(t)$ is obtained by using (4.3.2) and the first-phase data, and $L(t,s)$ is computed by using (4.4.5) and the second-phase data. For comparison, the results are given under both common slope and linear trend models. The acceptable lower product specification limit in this example is $\eta = 90$. Thus, the first-phase (frozen) shelf-life for this drug product is 32 months.

The results for $L(t,s)$ in Table 4.4.2 are given at s such that $L(t,s) > 90$ whereas $L(t,s+1) < 90$. Thus, s values listed in Table 4.4.2 are the second-phase (refrigerated) shelf-lives for various t values. For example, if the drug product is taken out of the frozen storage condition at month 10, then its refrigerated shelf-life is 29 days under the common slope model or 28 days under the linear trend model.

If we are unable to determine which of the two models (common slope and linear trend) is significantly better than the other, then we could adopt a conservative approach by selecting the shorter of the shelf-lives computed under the two models. Note that a higher degree polynomial model does not always produce shorter shelf-lives at the second phase. In the example, the linear trend model produced shorter second-phase shelf-lives in later months, but longer second-phase shelf-lives in early months. This is because under the common slope model, the estimated common slope is the average of the five estimated slopes (in different months) that become increasingly with time (t), since $\hat{\gamma}_1 < 0$.

Table 4.4.1. Stability Data in Example 4.4.1

Time		Stability Data	
t (month)	s (day)	Frozen condition	Refrigerated condition
0		100.0, 100.1, 100.1	
3		99.2, 99.0, 99.1	
	7		97.7, 97.4, 97.4
	14		96.5, 96.2, 95.9
	21		94.8, 94.5, 94.6
	35		91.7, 91.8, 91.4
6		98.2, 98.2, 98.1	
	7		96.7, 96.5, 96.7
	14		95.4, 95.2, 95.1
	21		93.6, 93.5, 93.6
	35		90.3, 90.6, 90.5
9		97.5, 97.4, 97.5	
	7		95.9, 95.6, 95.7
	14		94.5, 94.3, 94.1
	21		92.7, 92.5, 92.5
	35		89.3, 89.5, 89.3
12		96.4, 96.5, 96.5	
	7		94.5, 94.7, 94.8
	14		92.8, 93.3, 93.4
	21		91.3, 91.4, 91.5
	35		88.2, 88.2, 87.9
18		94.4, 94.6, 94.5	
	7		92.6, 92.6, 92.4
	14		91.0, 91.1, 90.6
	21		88.9, 89.0, 89.0
	35		85.1, 85.6, 85.6

Table 4.4.2. Lower Confidence Bounds and Estimated
Shelf-Lives in Example 4.4.1

Month t	$L(t)$	Common slope model		Linear trend model	
		Day s	$L(t,s)$	Day s	$L(t,s)$
1	99.70	40	90.14	42	90.21
2	99.41	39	90.05	41	90.08
3	99.11	38	90.21	39	90.19
4	98.82	37	90.15	38	90.06
5	98.52	36	90.09	36	90.15
6	98.22	35	90.02	35	90.01
7	97.93	33	90.19	33	90.10
8	97.63	32	90.13	31	90.19
9	97.34	31	90.06	30	90.03
10	97.02	29	90.23	28	90.12
11	96.72	28	90.17	26	90.21
12	96.42	27	90.10	25	90.05
13	96.11	26	90.04	23	90.16
14	95.81	24	90.20	22	90.01
15	95.50	23	90.14	20	90.14
16	95.20	22	90.07	19	90.01
17	94.89	20	90.23	17	90.17
18	94.59	19	90.16	16	90.06
19	94.28	18	90.09	14	90.25
20	93.97	17	90.02	13	90.17
21	93.67	15	90.18	12	90.09
22	93.36	14	90.11	11	90.03
23	93.05	13	90.04	9	90.28
24	92.75	11	90.20	8	90.24
25	92.44	10	90.13	7	90.20
26	92.13	9	90.05	6	90.18
27	91.82	7	90.21	5	90.16
28	91.52	6	90.14	4	90.15
29	91.21	5	90.06	3	90.15
30	90.90	3	90.22	2	90.15
31	90.60	2	90.14	1	90.15
32	90.30	1	90.07	0	90.30
33	89.98	–	–	–	–

4.4.3   Discussion

In practice, the assumption of simple linear regression in the second phase of a stability study may not be appropriate. For example, there may be an acceleration in decay with s in the second phase. The method in §4.4.2 can be easily extended to the case where polynomial regression models are considered in the second phase. For example, suppose that in the second phase,

$$y_{ijh} = \alpha + \beta t_j + \gamma(t_j)s_h + \rho(t_j)s_h^2 + e_{ijh},$$

where both $\gamma(t)$ and $\rho(t)$ are polynomials. At month t_j, let b_j and c_j be the least squares estimates of the coefficients of the linear and quadratic terms in the second-phase quadratic model. Then the estimators of $\gamma(t)$ and $\rho(t)$ can be obtained using

$$b_j = \gamma(t_j) + \text{error}$$

and

$$c_j = \rho(t_j) + \text{error}.$$

Usual model diagnostic methods may be applied to select an adequate model.

The selection of sampling time points at the second-phase stability study depends on how fast the degradation would be. It may be a good idea to have shorter time intervals for the second phase in later months; for example, we may test the drug product more frequently in later weeks. For a fixed total sample size, it is of interest to examine the relative efficiency for the estimation of shelf-lives using either more sampling time points in the first phase and less sampling time points in the second phase or less sampling time points in the first phase and more sampling time points in the second phase. The allocation of sampling time points at each phase then becomes an interesting research topic for two-phase shelf-life estimation. In addition, since the degradation at the second phase is highly correlated with the degradation at the first phase, it may be of interest to examine such correlation for future design planning.

For the method in §4.4.2, equal assay variabilities for the second phase data at different t_j are assumed. If this assumption is not true, the variance estimator $\hat{V}$ in (4.4.4) should be modified; see, for example, Shao and Chow (2001b).

Finally, the method in §4.4.1-4.4.2 can be extended to the case of multiple-phase shelf-life estimation in a straightforward manner.

4.5   Discrete Responses

In stability studies, drug characteristics, such as the hardness and color, often result in discrete responses. For solid oral dosage forms such as tablets and capsules, the 1987 FDA stability guideline indicates the following characteristics should be studied in stability studies:

> Tablets: A stability study should include tests for the following characteristics of the tablet: appearance, friability, hardness, color, odor, moisture, strength, and dissolution.

> Capsules: A stability study should include tests for the following characteristics: strength, moisture, color, appearance, shape brittleness, and dissolution.

Information on the stability based on discrete responses is useful for quality assurance of the drug product prior to the expiration date established based on the primary continuous response such as the strength (potency). For establishment of drug shelf-life based on discrete responses, however, there is little discussion in the FDA stability guideline. In this section, we introduce some methods for analysis of discrete stability data proposed in Chow and Shao (2001a).

4.5.1   The Case of No Batch-to-Batch Variation

When there is no batch-to-batch variation, we assume that binary responses y_{ij}'s are independent and follow the logistic regression model

$$
\begin{aligned}
E(y_{ij}) &= \psi(\beta' x_{ij}), & i &= 1, ..., k, \\
\mathrm{Var}(y_{ij}) &= \tau(\beta' x_{ij}), & j &= 1, ..., n_i,
\end{aligned}
\tag{4.5.1}
$$

where $\psi(z) = e^z/(1 + e^z)$, $\tau(z) = \psi(z)[1 - \psi(z)]$, x_{ij}'s are the same as those in (4.1.1), and β is a vector of unknown parameters. Let $x(t)$ be x_{ij} with t_{ij} replaced by t and w_{ij} fixed at a particular value. Since $\psi(z)$ is a strictly increasing function of z, the true shelf-life t^* satisfies $\beta' x(t^*) = \psi^{-1}(\eta)$, where η is an approved specification limit.

Under model (4.5.1), $\hat{\beta}$, the maximum likelihood estimator of β, is the solution of the equation

$$
\sum_{i=1}^{k} \sum_{j=1}^{n_i} x_{ij}[y_{ij} - \psi(\beta' x_{ij})] = 0.
$$

When $\sum_i n_i$ is large, $\hat{\beta} - \beta$ is approximately distributed as $N(0, V)$, where

$$
V = \left[\sum_{i=1}^{k} \sum_{j=1}^{n_i} x_{ij} x_{ij}' \tau(\beta' x_{ij}) \right]^{-1};
$$

see, for example, Shao (1999, §4.4-4.5). Consequently, an approximate 95% lower confidence bound for $\beta'x(t)$ is

$$L(t) = \hat{\beta}'x(t) - z_{0.95}\sqrt{x(t)'\hat{V}x(t)},$$

where $\hat{V}$ is V with β replaced by $\hat{\beta}$ and z_a is the $100a$th standard normal percentile. An estimated shelf-life is then $\hat{t}^* = \inf\{t : L(t) \leq \psi^{-1}(\eta)\}$.

Unlike the case for continuous responses, a large number of observations (a large $\sum_i n_i$) is required for discrete y_{ij}'s, in order to apply the asymptotic results for $\hat{\beta}$.

4.5.2 The Case of Random Batches

When there is batch-to-batch variation, we consider the following mixed effects model

$$\begin{aligned}
E(y_{ij}|\beta_i) &= \psi(\beta_i'x_{ij}), & i &= 1, ..., k, \\
\text{Var}(y_{ij}|\beta_i) &= \tau(\beta_i'x_{ij}), & j &= 1, ..., n_i, \quad (4.5.2)
\end{aligned}$$

β_i's are independently distributed as $N(\beta, \Sigma)$,

where ψ and τ are the same as those in (4.5.1) and $E(y_{ij}|\beta_i)$ and $\text{Var}(y_{ij}|\beta_i)$ are respectively the conditional expectation and variance of y_{ij}, given β_i.

Let $\psi(\beta_{\text{future}}'x(t))$ be the mean degradation curve at time t for a future batch of the drug product. The shelf-life for this batch is

$$t_{\text{future}}^* = \inf\{t : \beta_{\text{future}}'x(t) \leq \psi^{-1}(\eta)\},$$

which is a random variable since β_{future} is random (see §4.3.2). Consequently, a shelf-life estimator should be a 95% lower prediction bound for t_{future}^*.

Since β_i's are unobserved random effects, the prediction bound has to be obtained based on the marginal model specified by

$$E(y_{ij}) = E[E(y_{ij}|\beta_i)] = E[\psi(\beta_i'x_{ij})]$$

and

$$\begin{aligned}
\text{Var}(y_{ij}) &= \text{Var}[E(y_{ij}|\beta_i)] + E[\text{Var}(y_{ij}|\beta_i)] \\
&= \text{Var}[\psi(\beta_i'x_{ij})] + E[\tau(\beta_i'x_{ij})].
\end{aligned}$$

For a nonlinear function ψ, however, neither $E(y_{ij})$ nor $\text{Var}(y_{ij})$ is an explicit function of $\beta'x_{ij}$, and, hence, an efficient estimator of β, such as the maximum likelihood estimator, is difficult to compute.

We introduce here a method that is easy to compute (Chow and Shao, 2001b). Assume that n_i's are large so that we can fit the logistic regression model for each fixed batch. For each fixed i, let $\hat{\beta}_i$ be a solution of the equation

$$\sum_{j=1}^{n_i} x_{ij}[y_{ij} - \psi(\beta' x_{ij})] = 0,$$

i.e., $\hat{\beta}_i$ is the maximum likelihood estimator of β_i based on the data in the ith batch, given β_i. For large n_i, $\hat{\beta}_i$ is approximately and conditionally distributed as $N(\beta_i, V_i(\beta_i))$, where

$$V_i(\beta_i) = \left[\sum_{j=1}^{n_i} x_{ij} x'_{ij} \tau(\beta'_i x_{ij})\right]^{-1}.$$

Unconditionally, $\hat{\beta}_i$ is approximately distributed as $N(\beta, D_i)$, where

$$\begin{aligned} D_i &= E[\mathrm{Var}(\hat{\beta}_i|\beta_i)] + \mathrm{Var}[E(\hat{\beta}_i|\beta_i)] \\ &= E[V_i(\beta_i)] + \mathrm{Var}(\beta_i) \\ &= E[V_i(\beta_i)] + \Sigma. \end{aligned}$$

Consequently, we may apply the method described in §4.3.2. Let $\hat{\beta}$ be the average of $\hat{\beta}_i$'s and

$$v(t) = \frac{1}{k-1} \sum_{i=1}^{k} x(t)'(\hat{\beta}_i - \hat{\beta})(\hat{\beta}_i - \hat{\beta})' x(t).$$

Then $[\hat{\beta}' x(t) - \psi^{-1}(\eta)]/\sqrt{v(t)/k}$ is approximately distributed as the non-central t-distribution with $k-1$ degrees of freedom and the non-centrality parameter $[\beta' x(t) - \psi^{-1}(\eta)]/\sqrt{x(t)' \Sigma x(t)}$. Following the derivation in §4.3.2, we obtain the following approximate 95% lower prediction bound for t^*_{future}:

$$\hat{t}^* = \inf\{t : L(t) \le \psi^{-1}(\eta)\},$$

where $L(t) = \hat{\beta}' x(t) - \rho_{0.95}(k)\sqrt{v(t)/k}$ and the value of $\rho_{0.95}(k)$ is given in Table 4.3.1.

4.5.3 Testing for Batch-to-Batch Variation

A test for batch-to-batch variation may be performed to determine which of the methods in §4.5.1 and §4.5.2 should be used. We introduce the tests for batch-to-batch variation proposed in Chow and Shao (2001b). Note that testing for batch-to-batch variation is equivalent to testing the hypotheses

$$H_0 : \Sigma = 0 \quad \text{versus} \quad H_1 : \Sigma \ne 0.$$

First, consider the case where $x_{ij} = x_j$ and $n_i = n$ for all i (i.e., the stability designs for all batches are the same). From the result in §4.5.2, under H_0, approximately

$$[V_0(\hat{\beta})]^{-1/2}(\hat{\beta}_i - \beta) \sim N(0, I_p),$$

where I_p is the identity matrix of order p and

$$V_0(\beta) = \left[\sum_{j=1}^{n} x_j x_j' \tau(\beta' x_j) \right]^{-1}.$$

Since $\hat{\beta}_i$'s are independent, approximately

$$T_0 = \sum_{i=1}^{k} (\hat{\beta}_i - \hat{\beta})'[V_0(\hat{\beta})]^{-1}(\hat{\beta}_i - \hat{\beta}) \sim \chi^2_{p(k-1)}$$

under H_0, where χ^2_r denotes the chi-square distribution with r degrees of freedom. Under H_1, since $\text{Var}(\hat{\beta}_i) = \Sigma + E[V_i(\beta_i)]$, $E(T_0)$ is much larger than $p(k-1)$, which is $E(T_0)$ under H_0. Therefore, a large value of T_0 indicates that H_1 is true. The proposed p-value for testing batch-to-batch variation is then

$$1 - \chi^2_{p(k-1)}(T_0).$$

According to the FDA guideline (for continuous responses), to obtain an estimated shelf-life, we may apply the method in §4.5.1 when the p-value is larger than or equal to 0.25 and apply the method in §4.5.2 when the p-value is smaller than 0.25.

Next, consider the general case where x_{ij}'s depend on i. Let $c = (c_1, ..., c_k)$ be a constant vector satisfying $\sum_{i=1}^{k} c_i = 0$. From the result in §4.5.2, under H_0, approximately

$$\left[\sum_{i=1}^{k} c_i V_i(\hat{\beta}) \right]^{-1/2} \sum_{i=1}^{k} c_i \hat{\beta}_i \sim N(0, I_p),$$

where

$$V_i(\beta) = \left[\sum_{j=1}^{n_i} x_{ij} x_{ij}' \tau(\beta' x_{ij}) \right]^{-1}.$$

Then, approximately

$$T = \sum_{i=1}^{k} c_i \hat{\beta}_i' \left[\sum_{i=1}^{k} c_i V_i(\hat{\beta}) \right]^{-1} \sum_{i=1}^{k} c_i \hat{\beta}_i \sim \chi^2_p$$

Table 4.5.1. Test Results for Odor Intensity

Package	Batch	Replicate	0	3	6	9	12	18	24	30	36
			\multicolumn{9}{c}{Sampling time (month)}
Bottle	1	1	0	0	0	0	0	1	0	0	0
		2	0	0	0	0	0	0	0	0	1
		3	0	0	0	0	0	0	0	0	1
		4	0	0	0	0	0	0	0	0	0
		5	0	0	0	0	0	0	0	0	0
	2	1	0	0	0	0	0	0	0	0	1
		2	0	0	0	0	0	0	0	0	0
		3	0	0	0	0	1	0	0	0	0
		4	0	0	0	0	0	0	0	0	1
		5	0	0	0	0	0	0	0	0	0
	3	1	0	0	0	0	0	0	0	0	1
		2	0	0	0	0	0	0	0	0	0
		3	0	0	0	0	0	0	1	0	1
		4	0	0	0	0	0	0	0	0	0
		5	0	0	0	0	0	0	0	0	0
Blister	1	1	0	0	0	0	0	0	0	1	0
		2	0	0	0	0	0	0	0	0	0
		3	0	0	0	0	0	0	0	0	0
		4	0	0	0	0	0	0	0	0	0
		5	0	0	0	0	0	0	0	0	1
	2	1	0	0	0	0	0	0	0	1	0
		2	0	0	0	0	0	0	0	0	0
		3	0	0	0	0	0	0	0	0	1
		4	0	0	0	0	0	0	0	0	0
		5	0	0	0	0	0	0	0	0	0
	3	1	0	0	0	0	0	0	1	0	0
		2	0	0	0	0	0	0	0	0	0
		3	0	0	0	0	0	0	0	0	1
		4	0	0	0	0	0	0	0	0	1
		5	0	0	0	0	0	0	0	0	0

under H_0. Our proposed p-value for testing batch-to-batch variation is then

$$1 - \chi_p^2(T).$$

The constant vector c can be chosen as follows. If $k = 3$, we may choose $c = (1, 1, -2)$. If k is even, we may choose $c = (1, -1, 1, -1, ..., 1, -1)$. If k is odd and $k \geq 5$, we may choose $c = (1, 1, -2, 1, -1, ..., 1, -1)$.

4.5.4 An Example

A stability study was conducted on tablets of a drug product to establish a shelf-life of the drug product. Tablets from three batches were stored at room temperature (25^OC) in two different types of containers (bottle and blister package). In addition to the potency test, the tablets were also tested for odor at 0, 3, 6, 9, 12, 18, 24, 30, and 36 months. At each time point, five independent assessments were performed. The results of the odor intensity were expressed as either "acceptable" (denoted by 0) or "not acceptable" (denoted by 1). Table 4.5.1 displays the data from odor intensity test.

With $x_j' = (1, t_j, w_j t_j)$, where w_j is the indicator for bottle or blister package, the statistic T_0 given in §4.5.3 is equal to 0.5035 based on the data in Table 1, which results in a p-value of 0.9978, i.e., the batch-to-batch variation is not significant (§4.5.3). Thus, the shelf-life estimation procedure in §4.5.1 should be applied by combining data in different batches. The confidence bound $L(t)$ was plotted (over t) in Figure 4.5.1. The two horizontal lines in Figure 4.5.1 correspond to $\psi^{-1}(\eta)$ with $\eta = 80\%$ and 90%, respectively. For a given η, the intersect of the horizontal line and $L(t)$ gives the shelf-life of the drug product. For $\eta = 90\%$, it can be seen from Figure 4.5.1 that the estimated shelf-life is about 21 months for bottle container and 22 months for blister package.

4.5.5 Ordinal Responses

We consider the situation where y_{ij} is an ordinal response with more than two categories. We introduce the following three approaches in Chow and Shao (2001b).

Generalized Linear Models

Suppose that a parametric model (conditional the covariate) can be obtained for the response y_{ij}. For example, y_{ij} follows a binomial distribution or a (truncated) Poisson distribution, given x_{ij}. Then, model (4.5.1) (which is a generalized linear model) still holds with a proper modification of the variance function τ. For example, if y_{ij} is binomial taking

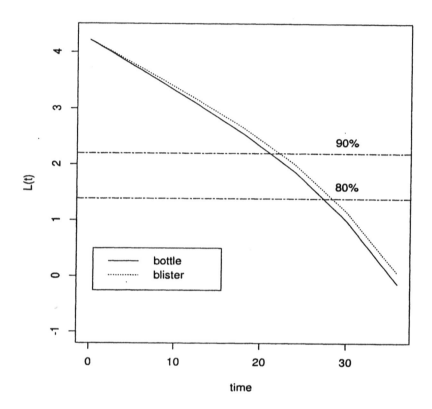

Figure 4.5.1. $L(t)$ Without Batch-to-Batch Variation

values $0, 1, ..., m$, then $\tau(z) = m\psi(z)[1 - \psi(z)]$. Consequently, the results in §4.5.1-4.5.3 can still be applied with the modification of the function τ. Under this approach, it is assumed that the mean of the discrete response is an appropriate summary measure for the stability analysis.

Threshold Approach (Multivariate Generalized Models)

Suppose that the ordinal response y is a categorized version of a latent continuous variable U. For example, if y is a grouped continuous response, then U may be the unobserved underlying continuous variable. Suppose that the relationship between y and U is determined by

$$y = r \quad \text{if and only if} \quad \theta_r < U \le \theta_{r+1}, \quad r = 0, 1, ..., m,$$

where $\theta_0 = -\infty$, $\theta_m = \infty$, and θ_r, $r = 1, ..., m-1$, are unknown parameters. Assume further that the latent variable U and the covariate x follow a linear regression model

$$U = -\beta' x + \epsilon,$$

where ϵ is a random error with distribution function F. Then,

$$P(y \le r|x) = F(\theta_{r+1} + \beta' x), \quad r = 0, 1, ..., m.$$

This is referred to as the threshold approach Fahrmeir and Tutz (1994). If $F(z) = 1/(1 + e^{-z/\sigma})$ (the logistic distribution with mean 0 and variance $\sigma^2 \pi^2/3$), then

$$P(y \le r|x) = \frac{e^{(\theta_{r+1}+\beta' x)/\sigma}}{1 + e^{(\theta_{r+1}+\beta' x)/\sigma}} = \psi(\tilde{\theta}_{r+1} + \tilde{\beta}' x),$$

where $\tilde{\theta}_r = \theta_r/\sigma$ and $\tilde{\beta} = \beta/\sigma$.

Consider the case of no batch-to-batch variation. Suppose that the shelf-life of the drug product is defined to be the time interval that the mean of U remains above the specification $\psi^{-1}(\eta)$. Let $y_{ij}^{(r)} = I(y_{ij} \le r)$, where $I(\cdot)$ is the indicator function. Then, an extension of model (4.5.1) is

$$\begin{aligned} E(y_{ij}^{(r)}) &= \psi(\tilde{\beta}' x_{ij}), & i &= 1, ..., k, \\ \mathrm{Var}(y_{ij}^{(r)}) &= \tau(\tilde{\beta}' x_{ij}), & j &= 1, ..., n_i, \end{aligned} \quad r = 0, 1, ..., m-1. \quad (4.5.3)$$

Since $y_{ij}^{(r)}$, $r = 0, 1, ..., m$, are dependent, model (4.5.3) is a multivariate generalized linear model. Maximum likelihood estimation can be carried out as described in Section 3.4 of Fahrmeir and Tutz (1994). Let $L(t)$ be an approximate 95% lower confidence bound for $\tilde{\beta}' x(t)$ based on the maximum likelihood estimation. Then the estimated shelf-life can still be defined as $\hat{t}^* = \inf\{t : L(t) \le \psi^{-1}(\eta)\}$. A combination of this approach and the method in §4.5.2 can be used to handle the case where random batch-to-batch variation is present.

Binary Approach

The threshold approach involves some complicated computation, since a multivariate generalized linear model has to be fitted. A simple but not very efficient approach is to binarize the ordinal responses. Let r_0 is a fixed threshold and define $\tilde{y}_{ij} = 0$ if $y_{ij} \le r_0$ and 1 otherwise. Note that if the ordinal response y follows the model described in the threshold approach, then

$$P(y \le r_0|x) = F(\theta_{r_0+1} + \beta' x) = \psi(\tilde{\theta}_{r_0+1} + \tilde{\beta}' x)$$

and, hence, model (4.5.1) holds for the summary data set $\{\tilde{y}_{ij}\}$. Thus, we can apply the methods described in §4.5.1-4.5.3.

4.6   Multiple Components/Ingredients

For drug products with a single active ingredient, stability data may contain multiple responses. Some responses are continuous (e.g., potency), while the others are discrete (e.g., hardness). We refer to stability analysis of this kind as shelf-life estimation with multiple responses. On the other hand, for drug products with multiple active ingredients, stability data for each active ingredient are necessarily collected for evaluation of an overall shelf-life of the drug product. We refer to stability analysis of this kind as shelf-life estimation with multiple ingredients.

4.6.1   Shelf-Life Estimation with Multiple Responses

For the study of drug stability, the FDA guideline requires that all drug characteristics be evaluated. A naive approach is to establish a shelf-life for each drug characteristic separately and then consider the minimum of the individual estimated shelf-lives as the single estimated shelf-life for the drug product. This method, however, lacks of statistical justification. Let $\hat{t}_l^*$ be the estimated shelf-life for the lth drug characteristic (obtained using the method in §4.3.1, §4.3.2, §4.5.1, or §4.5.2), $l = 1, ..., m$. Then

$$P\left(\hat{t}_l^* \leq t_l^*\right) \geq 0.95, \quad l = 1, ..., m, \tag{4.6.1}$$

where t_l^* is the true shelf-life for the lth drug characteristic. However, if we define the overall true drug shelf-life to be $t^* = \min_{l \leq m} t_l^*$, the minimum of individual shelf-lives, then (4.6.1) does not ensure that

$$P\left(\min_{l \leq m} \hat{t}_l^* \leq t^*\right) \geq 0.95.$$

A simple modification is to replace $\hat{t}_1^*, ..., \hat{t}_m^*$, which are individual lower confidence bounds, by a set of simultaneous lower confidence bounds for $t_1^*, ..., t_m^*$. The simplest way to obtain simultaneous confidence bounds is the Bonferroni method; see, for example, Shao (1999, §7.5). Let $\tilde{t}_l^*$ be the same as $\hat{t}_l^*$ but with confidence level $1 - 0.05/m$ instead of $1 - 0.05 = 0.95$, $l = 1, ..., m$. Then we can use $\min_{l \leq m} \tilde{t}_l^*$ as the estimated overall shelf-life, since

$$P\left(\min_{l \leq m} \tilde{t}_l^* \leq t^*\right) \geq P\left(\tilde{t}_l^* \leq t_l^*, l = 1, ..., m\right)$$

$$\geq 1 - \sum_{l=1}^m P\left(\tilde{t}_l^* > t_l^*\right)$$

$$\geq 1 - \sum_{l=1}^m \frac{0.05}{m}$$

$$= 0.95.$$

4.6.2 Shelf-Life Estimation with Multiple Ingredients

In most cases, each drug product contains a single active ingredient. An estimated shelf-life is obtained based on one or several characteristics of the active ingredient. However, some drug products may contain more than one active ingredient (Pong, 2001). For example, Premarin (conjugated estrogens, USP) is known to contain more than three active ingredients, including estrone, equilin, and 17α-dihydroequilin. The specification limits for different active ingredients may be different. Other examples include combinational drug products, such as traditional Chinese herbal medicines. One may still apply the simultaneous confidence bounds approach in §4.6.1 to obtain an overall estimated shelf-life. However, the resulting shelf-life may be too conservative to be of practical interest, since the potential ingredient-to-ingredient or drug-to-drug interaction is not taken into consideration. For example, the true shelf-life may not be $\min_{l \le m} t_l^*$, but equal to the time interval that the mean curve of $f(y_{ij}^{(1)}, ..., y_{ij}^{(m)})$ remains within $f(\eta_1, ..., \eta_m)$, where $y_{ij}^{(l)}$ is the characteristic of the lth ingredient of the drug product at time t_{ij}, η_l is the USP/NF specification for the lth ingredient, and f is a function that relates the impact of all ingredients. The problem can be easily solved if the function f is known, i.e., one can obtain an estimated shelf-life based on data $z_{ij} = f(y_{ij}^{(1)}, ..., y_{ij}^{(m)})$. In the case of unknown f, we may consider an approach that uses factor analysis in multivariate analysis.

For simplicity, we consider the case where there is no batch-to-batch variation. Suppose that there are m active ingredients or components and each of them follows model (4.1.1), i.e.,

$$E(y_{ij}^{(l)}) = x_{ij}'\beta^{(l)}, \quad i = 1, ..., k, \ j = 1, ..., n, \ l = 1, ..., m.$$

Let $y_{ij} = (y_{ij}^{(1)}, ..., y_{ij}^{(m)})'$. Assume that for any i and j,

$$y_{ij} - E(y_{ij}) = LF + \varepsilon, \tag{4.6.2}$$

where L is an $m \times q$ nonrandom unknown matrix of full rank, F and ε are unobserved independent random vectors of dimensions $q \times 1$ and $m \times 1$, respectively, F is distributed as $N(0, I_q)$, ε is distributed as $N(0, \Psi)$, and Ψ is an unknown diagonal matrix. Model (4.6.2) with the assumptions on F and ε is the so-called orthogonal factor model (Johnson and Wichern, 1998).

Normally q is a predetermined integer and is much smaller than m (e.g., $q = 1$ or 2). If (4.6.2) holds, then

$$(L'L)^{-1}L'[y_{ij} - E(y_{ij})] = F + (L'L)^{-1}L'\varepsilon. \tag{4.6.3}$$

If we ignore the error part $(L'L)^{-1}L'\varepsilon$, then (4.6.3) indicates that the components of y_{ij} can be grouped into q groups that are represented by q independent components of F. Hence, an overall estimated shelf-life can be obtained by applying the method in §4.3.1 to stability data

$$(\hat{L}'\hat{L})^{-1}\hat{L}'y_{ij},$$

where $\hat{L}$ is an estimator of L. If $q > 1$, the approach of simultaneous confidence bounds can be applied.

There are two commonly used approaches for estimating L. The first approach is to apply the method of principal components. The lth column of L is estimated by $\lambda_l L_l$, where λ_l is the lth eigenvalue of the sample covariance matrix based on data

$$(y_{ij}^{(1)} - x_{ij}'\hat{\beta}^{(1)}, ..., y_{ij}^{(m)} - x_{ij}'\hat{\beta}^{(m)}), \quad i = 1, ..., k, j = 1, ..., n, \qquad (4.6.4)$$

L_l is the corresponding eigenvector, and $\hat{\beta}^{(l)}$ is the least squares estimator of $\beta^{(l)}$ for the lth ingredient. The second method is the maximum likelihood method under model (4.6.2) by treating values in (4.6.4) as the observed data. The maximum likelihood estimator of L can be computed numerically, using an existing computer program (Johnson and Wichern, 1998).

Model (4.6.2) is essential in applying the factor analysis method. Further research for this problem is needed, including the validation of model (4.6.2), the determination of q (the number of important factors), and the estimation methodology for L.

Chapter 5

Bioavailability and Bioequivalence

When a brand-name drug is going off patent, the innovator drug company will usually develop a new formulation to extend its exclusivity in the marketplace. At the same time, generic drug companies may file abbreviated new drug applications (ANDA) for generic drug approval. An approved generic drug can be used as a substitute for the brand-name drug. In 1984, the FDA was authorized to approve generic drugs through *bioavailability* and *bioequivalence* studies under the Drug Price and Patent Term Restoration Act. As defined in 21 CFR 320.1, bioavailability refers to the rate and extent to which the active ingredient or active moiety is absorbed from a drug product and becomes available at the site of action. *In vivo* bioequivalence testing is usually considered as a surrogate for clinical evaluation of drug products based on the *Fundamental Bioequivalence Assumption* that when two formulations of the same drug product or two drug products (e.g., a brand-name drug and its generic copy) are equivalent in bioavailability, they will reach the same therapeutic effect or they are therapeutically equivalent (Chow and Liu, 1999a). Pharmacokinetic (PK) responses such as area under the blood or plasma concentration-time curve (AUC) and maximum concentration (C_{max}) are usually considered the primary measures for bioavailability. *In vivo* bioequivalence testing is commonly conducted with a crossover design on healthy volunteers to assess bioavailability through PK responses. The PK responses are then analyzed with appropriate statistical method to determine whether bioequivalence criterion is met according to the regulatory requirement for bioequivalence review. Throughout this chapter, the brand-name drug is referred to as the reference product (formulation) whereas its new dosage form or generic

107

copy is called a test product (formulation).

In this chapter, some concepts related to *in vivo* bioequivalence and FDA's regulations are described (§5.1). Statistical design and model for *in vivo* bioequivalence studies are introduced in §5.2, followed by a review of the statistical methods currently adopted by the FDA (§5.3). Recent developments for *in vivo* bioequivalence, such as statistical designs and methods other than those in the FDA guidances, are introduced in §5.4-5.5. Recent development for *in vitro* bioequivalence testing for nasal aerosols and sprays products is discussed in §5.6. Sample size determination for bioequivalence testing is considered in §5.7.

5.1 Average, Population, and Individual Bioequivalence

In 1992, the FDA published its first guidance on statistical procedures for *in vivo* bioequivalence studies (FDA, 1992). The 1992 FDA guidance requires that the evidence of bioequivalence in average bioavailability in PK responses between the two drug products be provided. Let y_R and y_T denote PK responses (or log-PK responses if appropriate) of the reference and test formulations, respectively, and let $\delta = E(y_T) - E(y_R)$. Under the 1992 FDA guidance, two formulations are said to be bioequivalent if δ falls in the interval (δ_L, δ_U) with 90% assurance, where δ_L and δ_U are given limits specified in the FDA guidance. For example, if $(\hat{\delta}_L, \hat{\delta}_U)$ is a 90% confidence interval for δ based on PK responses, then bioequivalence is claimed if $\delta_L \leq \hat{\delta}_L$ and $\delta_U \geq \hat{\delta}_U$, i.e., the 90% confidence interval for δ is entirely within the interval (δ_L, δ_U). Since only the averages $E(y_T)$ and $E(y_R)$ are concerned in this method, this type of bioequivalence is usually referred to as *average bioequivalence* (ABE). In 2000, the FDA issued a guidance on general considerations of bioavailability and bioequivalence studies for orally administered drug products, which replaces the 1992 FDA guidance (FDA, 2000a). Statistical design and analysis for assessment of ABE as described in the 2000 FDA guidance are the same as those given in the 1992 FDA guidance.

The ABE approach for bioequivalence, however, has limitations for addressing drug interchangeability, since it focuses only on the comparison of population averages between the test and reference formulations (Chen, 1997). Drug interchangeability can be classified as either drug prescribability or drug switchability. Drug prescribability is referred to as the physician's choice for prescribing an appropriate drug for his/her new patients among the drug products available, while drug switchability is related to the switch from a drug product to an alternative drug product within the same patient whose concentration of the drug product has been titrated to a steady, efficacious, and safe level. To assess drug prescribability and switchability, *population bioequivalence* (PBE) and *individual bioequivalence* (IBE) are proposed, respectively (see Anderson and Hauck, 1990; Esinhart and Chinchilli, 1994; Sheiner, 1992; Schall and Luus, 1993; Chow and Liu, 1995; and Chen, 1997). The concepts of PBE and IBE are described in two FDA draft guidances (FDA, 1997a, 1999a) and a recently published FDA guidance for industry (FDA, 2001). Let y_T be the PK response from the test formulation, y_R and y'_R be two identically distributed PK responses from the reference formulation, and

$$
\theta = \begin{cases}
\dfrac{E(y_R - y_T)^2 - E(y_R - y'_R)^2}{E(y_R - y'_R)^2/2} & \text{if } E(y_R - y'_R)^2/2 \geq \sigma_0^2 \\[3mm]
\dfrac{E(y_R - y_T)^2 - E(y_R - y'_R)^2}{\sigma_0^2} & \text{if } E(y_R - y'_R)^2/2 < \sigma_0^2,
\end{cases}
\tag{5.1.1}
$$

where σ_0^2 is a given constant specified in the 2001 FDA guidance. If y_R, y'_R and y_T are independent observations from different subjects, then the two formulations are population bioequivalent (PBE) when $\theta < \theta_{PBE}$, where θ_{PBE} is an equivalence limit for assessment of PBE as specified in the 2001 FDA guidance. If y_R, y'_R and y_T are from the same subject ($E(y_R - y'_R)^2/2$ is then the within-subject variance), then the two formulations are individual bioequivalent (IBE) when $\theta < \theta_{IBE}$, where θ_{IBE} is an equivalence limit for IBE as specified in the 2001 FDA guidance. Note that θ in (5.1.1) is a measure of the relative difference between the mean squared errors of $y_R - y_T$ and $y_R - y'_R$. When y_R, y'_R and y_T are from the same individual, it measures the drug switchability within the same individual. On the other hand, it measures drug prescribability when y_R, y'_R and y_T are from different subjects. Thus, IBE addresses drug switchability, whereas PBE addresses drug prescribability. According to the 2001 FDA guidance, IBE or PBE can be claimed if a 95% upper confidence bound for θ is smaller than θ_{IBE} or θ_{PBE}, provided that the observed ratio of geometric means is within the limits of 80% and 125%.

Note that each of the three types of bioequivalence criteria is based on a single function of moments of the PK responses, instead of their entire distributions. Although the IBE and PBE approaches focus on the second-order moments whereas the ABE approach focuses on the first-order moments, it is generally not true that IBE (or PBE) implies ABE. Statistical procedures for testing IBE or PBE is considerably more complicated than that for testing ABE. Searching for a better bioequivalence criterion is still an interesting research topic in the area of bioavailability and bioequivalence. For example, Schall (1995) considered a probability-based (instead of moment-based) bioequivalence criterion; Liu and Chow (1992a) proposed to assess bioequivalence using two functions of moments, where one function contains the means and the other involves variances of the PK responses.

5.2   Statistical Design and Model

For *in vivo* bioequivalence testing, crossover designs (see Jones and Kenward, 1989; Chow and Liu, 1999a) are usually considered. For ABE, a standard two-sequence, two-period (2×2) crossover design is recommended by the FDA guidances (FDA, 1992; FDA, 2000a). This design can also be employed for assessment of PBE. In a standard 2×2 crossover design, subjects are randomly assigned to one of the two sequences of formulations. In the first sequence, n_1 subjects receive treatments in the order of TR (T = test formulation, R = reference formulation) at two different dosing periods, whereas in the second sequence, n_2 subjects receive treatments in the order of RT at two different dosing periods. A sufficient length of washout between dosing periods is usually applied to wear off the possible residual effect that may be carried over from one dosing period to the next dosing period. Let y_{ijk} be the original or the log-transformation of the PK response of interest from the ith subject in the kth sequence at the jth dosing period. The following statistical model is considered:

$$y_{ijk} = \mu + F_l + P_j + Q_k + S_{ikl} + e_{ijk}, \tag{5.2.1}$$

where μ is the overall mean; P_j is the fixed effect of the jth period ($j = 1, 2$, and $P_1 + P_2 = 0$); Q_k is the fixed effect of the kth sequence ($k = 1, 2$, and $Q_1 + Q_2 = 0$); F_l is the fixed effect of the lth formulation (when $j = k$, $l = T$; when $j \neq k$, $l = R$; $F_T + F_R = 0$); S_{ikl} is the random effect of the ith subject in the kth sequence under formulation l and (S_{ikT}, S_{ikR}), $i = 1, ..., n_k$, $k = 1, 2$, are independent and identically distributed bivariate normal random vectors with mean 0 and an unknown covariance matrix

$$\begin{pmatrix} \sigma_{BT}^2 & \rho\sigma_{BT}\sigma_{BR} \\ \rho\sigma_{BT}\sigma_{BR} & \sigma_{BR}^2 \end{pmatrix};$$

e_{ijk}'s are independent random errors distributed as $N(0, \sigma_{Wl}^2)$; and S_{ikl}'s and e_{ijk}'s are mutually independent. Note that σ_{BT}^2 and σ_{BR}^2 are between-subject variances and σ_{WT}^2 and σ_{WR}^2 are within-subject variances, and that $\sigma_{TT}^2 = \sigma_{BT}^2 + \sigma_{WT}^2$ and $\sigma_{TR}^2 = \sigma_{BR}^2 + \sigma_{WR}^2$ are the total variances for the test and reference formulations, respectively. Under model (5.2.1), the ABE parameter δ defined in §5.1 is equal to $\delta = F_T - F_R$, whereas the parameter θ in (5.1.1) for PBE is equal to

$$\theta = \frac{\delta^2 + \sigma_{TT}^2 - \sigma_{TR}^2}{\max\{\sigma_0^2, \sigma_{TR}^2\}}. \tag{5.2.2}$$

For IBE, however, the standard 2×2 crossover design is not useful because each subject only receives each formulation once. Thus, it is not possible to obtain unbiased estimators of within-subject variances. To obtain unbiased estimators of the within-subject variances, FDA (2001) suggested that the following 2×4 crossover design be used. In the first sequence, n_1 subjects receive treatments at four periods in the order of TRTR (or TRRT), while in the second sequence, n_2 subjects receive treatments at four periods in the order of RTRT (or RTTR). Let y_{ijk} be the observed response (or log-response) of the ith subject in the kth sequence at jth period, where $i = 1, ..., n_k$, $j = 1, ..., 4$, $k = 1, 2$. The following statistical model is assumed:

$$y_{ijk} = \mu + F_l + W_{ljk} + S_{ikl} + e_{ijk}, \qquad (5.2.3)$$

where μ is the overall mean; F_l is the fixed effect of the lth formulation ($l = T, R$ and $F_T + F_R = 0$); W_{ljk}'s are fixed period, sequence, and interaction effects ($\sum_k \bar{W}_{lk} = 0$, where $\bar{W}_{lk}$ is the average of W_{ljk}'s with fixed (l, k), $l = T, R$); and S_{ikl}'s and e_{ijk}'s are similarly defined as those in (5.2.1). If we define $W_{ljk} = P_j + Q_k$ in (5.2.1), then model (5.2.1) has the same form as that in (5.2.3). Under model (5.2.3), θ in (5.1.1) for IBE is equal to

$$\theta = \frac{\delta^2 + \sigma_D^2 + \sigma_{WT}^2 - \sigma_{WR}^2}{\max\{\sigma_0^2, \sigma_{WR}^2\}}, \qquad (5.2.4)$$

which is a nonlinear function of $\delta = F_T - F_R$ and variance components, where

$$\sigma_D^2 = \sigma_{BT}^2 + \sigma_{BR}^2 - 2\rho\sigma_{BT}\sigma_{BR}$$

is the variance of $S_{ikT} - S_{ikR}$, which is referred to as the variance due to the subject-by-formulation interaction.

5.3 Statistical Tests Suggested by the FDA

In this section, we review statistical testing procedures for ABE, IBE, and PBE as described in the FDA guidances (FDA, 2000a; FDA, 2001).

5.3.1 Testing for ABE

ABE is usually assessed based on PK responses from the standard 2×2 crossover design described in §5.2. According to the 2000 FDA guidance, ABE is claimed if the following null hypothesis H_0 is rejected at the 5% level of significance:

$$H_0 : \delta \leq \delta_L \text{ or } \delta \geq \delta_U \quad \text{versus} \quad H_1 : \delta_L < \delta < \delta_U, \qquad (5.3.1)$$

where $\delta = F_T - F_R$ and δ_L and δ_U are given bioequivalence limits. Under model (5.2.1),

$$\hat{\delta} = \frac{\bar{y}_{11} - \bar{y}_{12} - \bar{y}_{21} + \bar{y}_{22}}{2} \quad \sim \quad N\left(\delta, \ \frac{\sigma_{1,1}^2}{4}\left(\frac{1}{n_1} + \frac{1}{n_2}\right)\right), \qquad (5.3.2)$$

where $\bar{y}_{jk}$ is the sample mean of the observations in the kth sequence at the jth period and $\sigma_{1,1}^2$ is

$$\sigma_{a,b}^2 = \sigma_D^2 + a\sigma_{WT}^2 + b\sigma_{WR}^2 \qquad (5.3.3)$$

with $a = 1$ and $b = 1$. Let

$$\hat{\sigma}_{1,1}^2 = \frac{1}{n_1 + n_2 - 2}\sum_{k=1}^{2}\sum_{i=1}^{n_k}(y_{i1k} - y_{i2k} - \bar{y}_{1k} + \bar{y}_{2k})^2. \qquad (5.3.4)$$

Then $\hat{\sigma}_{1,1}^2$ is independent of $\hat{\delta}$ and

$$(n_1 + n_2 - 2)\hat{\sigma}_{1,1}^2 \quad \sim \quad \sigma_{1,1}^2\chi_{n_1+n_2-2}^2,$$

where χ_r^2 is the chi-square distribution with r degrees of freedom. Thus, the limits of a 90% confidence interval for δ are given by

$$\hat{\delta}_{\pm} = \hat{\delta} \pm t_{0.95;n_1+n_2-2}\frac{\hat{\sigma}_{1,1}}{2}\sqrt{\frac{1}{n_1} + \frac{1}{n_2}},$$

where $t_{0.95;r}$ is the 95th quantile of the t-distribution with r degrees of freedom. According to the 2000 FDA guidance, ABE can be claimed if and only if the 90% confidence interval falls within $(-\delta_L, \delta_U)$, i.e., $\delta_L < \hat{\delta}_- < \hat{\delta}_+ < \delta_U$. Note that this is based on the two one-sided tests procedure proposed by Schuirmann (1987). The idea of Schuirmann's two one-sided tests is to decompose H_0 in (5.3.1) into the following two one-sided hypotheses:

$$H_{01} : \delta \leq \delta_L \quad \text{and} \quad H_{02} : \delta \geq \delta_U.$$

Apparently, both H_{01} and H_{02} are rejected at the 5% significance level if and only if $\delta_L < \hat{\delta}_- < \hat{\delta}_+ < \delta_U$. Schuirmann's two one-sided tests procedure is a test of size 5% (Berger and Hsu, 1996, Theorem 2). Further discussion about the procedure of two one-sided tests is given in §8.2.2.

Example 5.3.1. The log-transformed PK responses listed in Table 5.3.1 are from a 2×2 crossover design for bioequivalence testing between a test formulation and a reference formulation. Using the method previously described, we obtain the following 90% confidence interval for δ: $(-0.0342, 0.0949)$. From FDA (2000a), $\delta_L = -0.223$ and $\delta_U = 0.223$, which corresponds to $(80\%, 125\%)$ in the original scale. Thus, we can claim ABE between the two formulations.

Table 5.3.1. Log-PK Responses from a 2×2 Crossover Design

Sequence 1		Sequence 2	
Period 1	Period 2	Period 1	Period 2
4.9622	4.7198	4.6001	4.6721
4.7994	4.7665	4.4820	4.6282
4.6686	4.5408	4.6419	4.7608
4.6045	4.7574	4.8766	4.4202
4.6134	4.3737	4.7865	4.6704
4.7692	4.5999	4.4985	5.0941
4.5495	4.9195	4.7723	4.5420
4.9369	4.6509	4.6581	4.4687
4.8391	4.5823	4.7311	4.4645
4.7146	4.4432	4.7698	4.8313
4.6918	4.8072	4.5879	4.5909
4.6751	4.5374	4.3235	4.8580

5.3.2 Testing for IBE

According to the 2001 FDA guidance, IBE can be assessed based on data
from a 2×4 crossover design as described in §5.2. IBE is claimed if the
following null hypothesis H_0 is rejected at the 5% level of significance provided that the observed ratio of geometric means is within the limits of
80% and 125%.

$$H_0 : \theta \geq \theta_{IBE} \quad \text{versus} \quad H_1 : \theta < \theta_{IBE}, \qquad (5.3.5)$$

where θ is given in (5.2.4) and θ_{IBE} is the IBE limit specified in the 2001
FDA guidance.

Since θ is a nonlinear function of δ and variance components, an exact
confidence bound for θ does not exist. FDA (1997a) considered a nonparametric bootstrap percentile method, which leads to many discussions (e.g.,
Schall and Luus, 1993; Chow, 1999; Shao, Chow, and Wang, 2000; and
Shao, Kübler, and Pigeot, 2000). The procedure recommended in the 1999
FDA draft guidance and the 2001 FDA guidance is based on the following
idea (Hyslop, Hsuan, and Holder, 2000).

Note that hypotheses given in (5.3.5) are equivalent to

$$H_0 : \gamma \geq 0 \quad \text{versus} \quad H_1 : \gamma < 0, \qquad (5.3.6)$$

where

$$\gamma = \delta^2 + \sigma_D^2 + \sigma_{WT}^2 - \sigma_{WR}^2 - \theta_{IBE} \max\{\sigma_0^2, \sigma_{WR}^2\}.$$

Therefore, it suffices to find a 95% upper confidence bound $\hat{\gamma}_U$ for γ. IBE is concluded if $\hat{\gamma}_U < 0$. Since γ is the sum of δ^2 and some variance components, the idea in Howe (1974), Graybill and Wang (1980), and Ting et al. (1990) can be applied; that is, if $\gamma = \gamma_1 + \cdots + \gamma_r - \gamma_{r+1} - \cdots - \gamma_m$, where γ_j's are positive parameters, then an approximate upper confidence bound is

$$\hat{\gamma}_1 + \cdots + \hat{\gamma}_r - \hat{\gamma}_{r+1} - \cdots - \hat{\gamma}_m + \sqrt{(\tilde{\gamma}_1 - \hat{\gamma}_1)^2 + \cdots + (\tilde{\gamma}_m - \hat{\gamma}_m)^2},$$

where $\hat{\gamma}_j$ is an estimator of γ_j, $\tilde{\gamma}_j$ is a 95% upper confidence bound for γ_j when $j = 1, ..., r$, $\tilde{\gamma}_j$ is a 95% lower confidence bound for γ_j when $j = r+1, ..., m$, and $\hat{\gamma}_j$'s are independent.

Hyslop, Hsuan, and Holder (2000) considered the following decomposition of γ:

$$\gamma = \delta^2 + \sigma_{0.5,0.5}^2 + 0.5\sigma_{WT}^2 - 1.5\sigma_{WR}^2 - \theta_{IBE}\max\{\sigma_0^2, \sigma_{WR}^2\}, \qquad (5.3.7)$$

where $\sigma_{0.5,0.5}^2 = \sigma_D^2 + 0.5\sigma_{WT}^2 + 0.5\sigma_{WR}^2$ is the special case of $\sigma_{a,b}^2$ given by (5.3.3) with $a = b = 0.5$. The reason to decompose γ in this way is because independent unbiased estimators of δ, $\sigma_{0.5,0.5}^2$, σ_{WT}^2 and σ_{WR}^2 can be derived under the 2×4 crossover design. For subject i in sequence k, let x_{ilk} and z_{ilk} be the average and the difference, respectively, of two observations from formulation l, and let $\bar{x}_{lk}$ and $\bar{z}_{lk}$ be respectively the sample mean based on x_{ilk}'s and z_{ilk}'s. Under model (5.2.3), an unbiased estimator of δ is

$$\hat{\delta} = \frac{\bar{x}_{T1} - \bar{x}_{R1} + \bar{x}_{T2} - \bar{x}_{R2}}{2} \sim N\left(\delta, \frac{\sigma_{0.5,0.5}^2}{4}\left(\frac{1}{n_1} + \frac{1}{n_2}\right)\right); \qquad (5.3.8)$$

an unbiased estimator of $\sigma_{0.5,0.5}^2$ is

$$\hat{\sigma}_{0.5,0.5}^2 = \frac{(n_1 - 1)s_{d1}^2 + (n_2 - 1)s_{d2}^2}{n_1 + n_2 - 2} \sim \frac{\sigma_{0.5,0.5}^2 \chi_{n_1+n_2-2}^2}{n_1 + n_2 - 2}, \qquad (5.3.9)$$

where s_{dk}^2 is the sample variance based on $x_{iTk} - x_{iRk}$, $i = 1, ..., n_k$; an unbiased estimator of σ_{WT}^2 is

$$\hat{\sigma}_{WT}^2 = \frac{(n_1 - 1)s_{T1}^2 + (n_2 - 1)s_{T2}^2}{2(n_1 + n_2 - 2)} \sim \frac{\sigma_{WT}^2 \chi_{n_1+n_2-2}^2}{n_1 + n_2 - 2},$$

where s_{Tk}^2 is the sample variance based on z_{iTk}, $i = 1, ..., n_k$; and an unbiased estimator of σ_{WR}^2 is

$$\hat{\sigma}_{WR}^2 = \frac{(n_1 - 1)s_{R1}^2 + (n_2 - 1)s_{R2}^2}{2(n_1 + n_2 - 2)} \sim \frac{\sigma_{WR}^2 \chi_{n_1+n_2-2}^2}{n_1 + n_2 - 2},$$

where s_{Rk}^2 is the sample variance based on z_{iRk}, $i = 1, ..., n_k$. Furthermore, estimators $\hat{\delta}$, $\hat{\sigma}_{0.5,0.5}^2$, $\hat{\sigma}_{WT}^2$ and $\hat{\sigma}_{WR}^2$ are independent.

Assume that $\sigma_{WR}^2 \geq \sigma_0^2$, γ in (5.3.7) reduces to

$$\gamma = \delta^2 + \sigma_{0.5,0.5}^2 + 0.5\sigma_{WT}^2 - (1.5 + \theta_{IBE})\sigma_{WR}^2.$$

Following the idea in Howe (1974) and Graybill and Wang (1980), Hyslop, Hsuan, and Holder (2000) obtained the following approximate 95% upper confidence bound for γ:

$$\hat{\gamma}_U = \hat{\delta}^2 + \hat{\sigma}_{0.5,0.5}^2 + 0.5\hat{\sigma}_{WT}^2 - (1.5 + \theta_{IBE})\hat{\sigma}_{WR}^2 + \sqrt{U}, \qquad (5.3.10)$$

where U is the sum of the following four quantities:

$$\left[\left(|\hat{\delta}| + t_{0.95;n_1+n_2-2} \frac{\hat{\sigma}_{0.5,0.5}}{2} \sqrt{\frac{1}{n_1} + \frac{1}{n_2}} \right)^2 - \hat{\delta}^2 \right]^2,$$

$$\hat{\sigma}_{0.5,0.5}^4 \left(\frac{n_1 + n_2 - 2}{\chi_{0.05;n_1+n_2-2}^2} - 1 \right)^2,$$

$$0.5^2 \hat{\sigma}_{WT}^4 \left(\frac{n_1 + n_2 - 2}{\chi_{0.05;n_1+n_2-2}^2} - 1 \right)^2,$$

and

$$(1.5 + \theta_{IBE})^2 \hat{\sigma}_{WR}^4 \left(\frac{n_1 + n_2 - 2}{\chi_{0.95;n_1+n_2-2}^2} - 1 \right)^2, \qquad (5.3.11)$$

and $\chi_{a;r}^2$ is the $100a$th percentile of the chi-square distribution with r degrees of freedom.

If it is known that $\sigma_0^2 > \sigma_{WR}^2$, then, by (5.3.7),

$$\gamma = \delta^2 + \sigma_{0.5,0.5}^2 + 0.5\sigma_{WT}^2 - 1.5\sigma_{WR}^2 - \theta_{IBE}\sigma_0^2.$$

An approximate 95% upper confidence bound for γ is

$$\hat{\gamma}_U = \hat{\delta}^2 + \hat{\sigma}_{0.5,0.5}^2 + 0.5\hat{\sigma}_{WT}^2 - 1.5\hat{\sigma}_{WR}^2 - \theta_{IBE}\sigma_0^2 + \sqrt{U_0}, \qquad (5.3.12)$$

where U_0 is the same as U except that the quantity in (5.3.11) should be replaced by

$$1.5^2 \hat{\sigma}_{WR}^4 \left(\frac{n_1 + n_2 - 2}{\chi_{0.95;n_1+n_2-2}^2} - 1 \right)^2. \qquad (5.3.13)$$

The confidence bound $\hat{\gamma}_U$ in (5.3.10) is referred to as the confidence bound under the reference-scaled criterion, whereas $\hat{\gamma}_U$ in (5.3.12) is referred to as the confidence bound under the constant-scaled criterion. In practice, whether $\sigma_{WR}^2 \geq \sigma_0^2$ is usually unknown. Hyslop, Hsuan, and Holder (2000) recommend using the reference-scaled criterion or the constant-scaled criterion according to $\hat{\sigma}_{WR}^2 \geq \sigma_0^2$ or $\hat{\sigma}_{WR}^2 < \sigma_0^2$, which is referred to as the estimation method. Intuitively, the estimation method works well if the true value of σ_{WR}^2 is not close to σ_0^2. Alternatively, we may test the hypothesis of $\sigma_{WR}^2 \geq \sigma_0^2$ versus $\sigma_{WR}^2 < \sigma_0^2$ to decide which confidence bound should be used; i.e., if

$$\hat{\sigma}_{WR}^2(n_1 + n_2 - 2) \geq \sigma_0^2 \chi_{0.05;n_1+n_2-2}^2,$$

then $\hat{\gamma}_U$ in (5.3.10) should be used; otherwise $\hat{\gamma}_U$ in (5.3.12) should be used. This is referred to as the test method and is more conservative than the estimation method. The estimation method and the test method were compared in a simulation study in Chow, Shao, and Wang (2002). It was found that when $\sigma_{WR}^2 > \sigma_0^2$, the two methods produce almost the same results; when $\sigma_{WR}^2 \approx \sigma_0^2$; the test method performs better; and when $\sigma_{WR}^2 < \sigma_0^2$, the estimation method is better and the test method is too conservative unless the sample size $n_k \geq 35$.

5.3.3   Testing for PBE

At the first glance, testing for PBE seems to be similar to testing for IBE. In view of (5.2.2), PBE can be claimed if the null hypothesis in

$$H_0 : \lambda \geq 0 \quad \text{versus} \quad H_1 : \lambda < 0$$

is rejected at the 5% significance level provided that the observed ratio of geometric means is within the limits of 80% and 125%, where

$$\lambda = \delta^2 + \sigma_{TT}^2 - \sigma_{TR}^2 - \theta_{PBE} \max\{\sigma_0^2, \sigma_{TR}^2\} \tag{5.3.14}$$

and θ_{PBE} is a constant specified in FDA (2001).

Under the 2×4 crossover design, the 2001 FDA guidance describes a test procedure for PBE using the same method introduced in §5.3.2. First, λ is decomposed into a linear function of δ^2, σ_{TT}^2, and $(1 + \theta_{PBE})\sigma_{TR}^2$ (or σ_{TR}^2 when $\sigma_{TR}^2 < \sigma_0^2$). Then, the method described in §5.3.2 is applied with the following estimators of δ, σ_{TT}^2, and σ_{TR}^2: the estimator of δ is $\hat{\delta}$ given in (5.3.8) and the estimator of σ_{Tl}^2 is

$$\hat{\sigma}_{Tl}^2 = \frac{1}{n_1 + n_2 - 2} \sum_{k=1}^{2} \sum_{i=1}^{n_k} [(x_{ilk} - \bar{x}_{lk})^2 + (z_{ilk} - \bar{z}_{lk})^2/4],$$

where $l = T, R$, and x_{ilk}, z_{ilk}, $\bar{x}_{lk}$, and $\bar{z}_{lk}$ are the same as those in §5.3.2.

However, we note that this test recommended by FDA (2001) is inappropriate due to the violation of the primary assumption of independence among the estimated components in the decomposition of λ. That is, $\hat{\delta}$, $\hat{\sigma}_{TT}^2$, and $\hat{\sigma}_{TR}^2$ are not mutually independent. In fact, Chow, Shao, and Wang (2001b) showed that

$$\text{Cov}(\hat{\sigma}_{TT}^2, \hat{\sigma}_{TR}^2) = 2\rho^2 \sigma_{BT}^2 \sigma_{BR}^2 / (n_1 + n_2 - 2),$$

although $\hat{\delta}$ is independent of $(\hat{\sigma}_{TT}^2, \hat{\sigma}_{TR}^2)$.

What is the effect of the use of FDA's procedure? To address this question, consider the asymptotic size of FDA's test procedure assuming that $n_1 = n_2 = n$ and n is large. Note that the size of a PBE test is the largest possible probability of concluding PBE when two products are in fact not PBE. Chow, Shao, and Wang (2001b) showed that, as $n \to \infty$, the asymptotic size of FDA's test procedure is given by

$$\Phi\left(\frac{z_{0.05}}{\sqrt{1 - 2a\rho^2 \sigma_{BT}^2 \sigma_{BR}^2 / \sigma_\lambda^2}}\right),$$

where Φ is the standard normal distribution function, $z_{0.05}$ is the 5th percentile of the standard normal distribution,

$$\sigma_\lambda^2 = 2\delta^2(\sigma_D^2 + 0.5\sigma_{WT}^2 + 0.5\sigma_{WR}^2) + 0.25\sigma_{WT}^4 + 0.25a^2\sigma_{WR}^4$$
$$+ (\sigma_{BT}^2 + 0.5\sigma_{WT}^2)^2 + a^2(\sigma_{BR}^2 + 0.5\sigma_{WR}^2)^2,$$

$a = 1 + \theta_{BE}$ if $\sigma_{TR}^2 \geq \sigma_0^2$, and $a = 1$ if $\sigma_{TR}^2 < \sigma_0^2$. This indicates that the asymptotic size of FDA's test for PBE is always less than the nominal level 5% unless $\rho = 0$ (which is impractical). Note that if the size of a PBE test is less than the nominal level 5%, it means that this test is too conservative and has unnecessarily low power (the probability of correctly concluding that the two products are PBE).

Statistical tests for PBE whose asymptotic sizes are exactly equal to 5% are given in §5.5.

5.4 Alternative Designs for IBE

Although the 2×2 crossover design and the 2×4 crossover design have the same number of subjects, the 2×4 crossover design yields four observations, instead of two, from each subject. This may increase the overall cost substantially. As an alternative to the 2×4 crossover design, the 2001 FDA guidance also recommends a 2×3 crossover design, in which n_1 subjects in sequence 1 receive treatments at three periods in the order of TRT (or RTT), while n_2 subjects in sequence 2 receive treatments at three periods in the order of RTR (or TRR). In §5.4.1 we derive the test procedure for IBE under this design. A different 2×3 design and the related test procedure are introduced in §5.4.2.

5.4.1   The 2×3 Crossover Design

Statistical model for the 2×3 crossover design with two sequences TRT and RTR (or RTT and TRR) is given by (5.2.3). The test procedure described in §5.3.2, however, needs to be modified. Let x_{ilk}, z_{ilk}, $\bar{x}_{lk}$, $\bar{z}_{lk}$, s_{dk}^2, s_{Tk}^2, and s_{Rk}^2 be the same as those defined in §5.3.2 (when there is only one observation under formulation l for a fixed (i,k), x_{ilk} is the same as the original y-value and z_{ilk} is defined to be 0). Then, an unbiased estimator of δ is

$$\hat{\delta} = \frac{\bar{x}_{T1} - \bar{x}_{R1} + \bar{x}_{T2} - \bar{x}_{R2}}{2} \sim N\left(\delta, \frac{\sigma_{0.5,1}^2}{4n_1} + \frac{\sigma_{1,0.5}^2}{4n_2}\right),$$

where $\sigma_{a,b}^2$ is given by (5.3.3); an unbiased estimator of $\sigma_{0.5,1}^2$ is

$$\hat{\sigma}_{0.5,1}^2 = s_{d1}^2 \sim \frac{\sigma_{0.5,1}^2 \chi_{n_1-1}^2}{n_1 - 1};$$

an unbiased estimator of $\sigma_{1,0.5}^2$ is

$$\hat{\sigma}_{1,0.5}^2 = s_{d2}^2 \sim \frac{\sigma_{1,0.5}^2 \chi_{n_2-1}^2}{n_2 - 1};$$

an unbiased estimator of σ_{WT}^2 is

$$\hat{\sigma}_{WT}^2 = s_{T1}^2/2 \sim \frac{\sigma_{WT}^2 \chi_{n_1-1}^2}{n_1 - 1};$$

and an unbiased estimator of σ_{WR}^2 is

$$\hat{\sigma}_{WR}^2 = s_{R2}^2/2 \sim \frac{\sigma_{WR}^2 \chi_{n_2-1}^2}{n_2 - 1}.$$

Furthermore, estimators $\hat{\delta}$, $\hat{\sigma}_{0.5,1}^2$, $\hat{\sigma}_{1,0.5}^2$, $\hat{\sigma}_{WT}^2$ and $\hat{\sigma}_{WR}^2$ are independent. The independence of $\hat{\delta}$ and $\hat{\sigma}_{WT}^2$ follows from the fact that

$$\mathrm{Cov}(z_{i11}, z_{i21}) = \mathrm{Cov}(e_{i11} + e_{i31} - 2e_{i21}, e_{i11} - e_{i31}) = 0.$$

Independence of other estimators can be shown similarly. Consequently, we consider to decompose γ in (5.3.7) as follows:

$$\gamma = \delta^2 + 0.5(\sigma_{0.5,1}^2 + \sigma_{1,0.5}^2) + 0.25\sigma_{WT}^2 - 1.75\sigma_{WR}^2 - \theta_{IBE}\max\{\sigma_0^2, \sigma_{WR}^2\}. \tag{5.4.1}$$

This leads to the following approximate 95% upper confidence bound $\hat{\gamma}_U$ for γ. When $\sigma^2_{WR} \geq \sigma^2_0$,

$$\hat{\gamma}_U = \hat{\delta}^2 + 0.5(\hat{\sigma}^2_{0.5,1} + \hat{\sigma}^2_{1,0.5}) + 0.25\hat{\sigma}^2_{WT} - (1.75 + \theta_{IBE})\hat{\sigma}^2_{WR} + \sqrt{U},$$

where U is the sum of the following five quantities:

$$\left[\left(|\hat{\delta}| + t_{0.95;n_1+n_2-2}\sqrt{\frac{\hat{\sigma}^2_{0.5,1}}{4n_1} + \frac{\hat{\sigma}^2_{1,0.5}}{4n_2}}\right)^2 - \hat{\delta}^2\right]^2,$$

$$0.5^2\hat{\sigma}^4_{0.5,1}\left(\frac{n_1-1}{\chi^2_{0.05;n_1-1}} - 1\right)^2,$$

$$0.5^2\hat{\sigma}^4_{1,0.5}\left(\frac{n_2-1}{\chi^2_{0.05;n_2-1}} - 1\right)^2,$$

$$0.25^2\hat{\sigma}^4_{WT}\left(\frac{n_1-1}{\chi^2_{0.05;n_1-1}} - 1\right)^2,$$

and

$$(1.75 + \theta_{IBE})^2\hat{\sigma}^4_{WR}\left(\frac{n_2-1}{\chi^2_{0.95;n_2-1}} - 1\right)^2. \qquad (5.4.2)$$

When $\sigma^2_{WR} < \sigma^2_0$,

$$\hat{\gamma}_U = \hat{\delta}^2 + 0.5(\hat{\sigma}^2_{0.5,1} + \hat{\sigma}^2_{1,0.5}) + 0.25\hat{\sigma}^2_{WT} - 1.75\hat{\sigma}^2_{WR} - \theta_{IBE}\sigma^2_0 + \sqrt{U_0},$$

where U_0 is the same as U except that the quantity in (5.4.2) should be replaced by

$$1.75^2\hat{\sigma}^4_{WR}\left(\frac{n_2-1}{\chi^2_{0.95;n_2-1}} - 1\right)^2.$$

When it is unknown whether $\sigma^2_{WR} \geq \sigma^2_0$, the methods discussed in the end of §5.3.2 can be applied to decide which bound should be used.

5.4.2   The 2×3 Extra-Reference Design

Although the 2×3 crossover design requires one fewer observation from each subject than the 2×4 crossover design, it has two disadvantages. First, the differences $x_{iT1} - x_{iR1}$ and $x_{iT2} - x_{iR2}$ from two sequences have different variances $\sigma^2_{0.5,1}$ and $\sigma^2_{1,0.5}$, respectively. This not only results in an extra approximation in the confidence bound for δ^2, but also requires a decomposition of γ into five, instead of four components. As a result, one more confidence bound needs to be constructed. Second, confidence bounds for variance components of $\sigma_{0.5,1}^2$, $\sigma_{1,0.5}^2$, σ_{WT}^2, and σ_{WR}^2 are constructed using chi-square distributions with $n_1 - 1$ or $n_2 - 1$ degrees of freedom, instead of $n_1 + n_2 - 2$ as in the case of the 2×4 crossover design. Consequently, the power for IBE testing based on the 2×3 crossover design is low.

Is there a design having the same number of observations as the 2×3 crossover design but providing a more efficient test procedure for IBE? From (5.3.2), under the 2×2 crossover design, δ and $\sigma_{1,1}^2$ can be independently and unbiasedly estimated by $\hat{\delta}$ in (5.3.2) and $\hat{\sigma}_{1,1}^2$ in (5.3.4), respectively. Note that γ can be decomposed into

$$\gamma = \delta^2 + \sigma_{1,1}^2 - 2\sigma_{WR}^2 - \theta_{IBE} \max\{\sigma_0^2, \sigma_{WR}^2\}.$$

Hence, if we can obtain an unbiased estimator of σ_{WR}^2 independent of the estimators of δ and $\sigma_{1,1}^2$, then a confidence bound for γ can be derived using the same idea in §5.3.2. The simplest way for obtaining an unbiased estimator of σ_{WR}^2 independent of the estimators of δ and $\sigma_{1,1}^2$ is to add an independent third sequence to the 2×2 crossover design, where n_3 subjects in sequence 3 receive two R treatments at two dosing periods. However, to have nearly the same number of observations as that in the 2×3 crossover design, n_3 has to be nearly $(n_1+n_2)/2$. Hence, the degrees of freedom of the chi-square distribution in the confidence bound for σ_{WR}^2 is still much smaller than $n_1 + n_2 - 2$. Alternatively, we may add a third period to the 2×2 crossover design, where subjects in both sequences receive R treatment, i.e., subjects in sequence 1 receive treatments in the order of TRR and subjects in sequence 2 receive treatments in the order of RTR. This design was considered in Schall and Luus (1993) and referred to as the 2×3 *extra-reference* design by Chow, Shao, and Wang (2002). The statistical model under this design is still given by (5.2.3). Chow, Shao, and Wang (2002) showed how to find an unbiased estimator of σ_{WR}^2 independent of the unbiased estimator of δ and its variance estimator. Under the same notation as that in §5.3.2, an unbiased estimator of δ is

$$\hat{\delta} = \frac{\bar{x}_{T1} - \bar{x}_{R1} + \bar{x}_{T2} - \bar{x}_{R2}}{2} \sim N\left(\delta, \frac{\sigma_{1,0.5}^2}{4}\left(\frac{1}{n_1} + \frac{1}{n_2}\right)\right),$$

where $\sigma_{a,b}^2$ is given by (5.3.3); an unbiased estimator of $\sigma_{1,0.5}^2$ is

$$\hat{\sigma}_{1,0.5}^2 = \frac{(n_1 - 1)s_{d1}^2 + (n_2 - 1)s_{d2}^2}{n_1 + n_2 - 2} \sim \frac{\sigma_{1,0.5}^2 \chi_{n_1+n_2-2}^2}{n_1 + n_2 - 1};$$

an unbiased estimator of σ_{WR}^2 is

$$\hat{\sigma}_{WR}^2 = \frac{(n_1 - 1)s_{R1}^2 + (n_2 - 1)s_{R2}^2}{2(n_1 + n_2 - 2)} \sim \frac{\sigma_{WR}^2 \chi_{n_1+n_2-2}^2}{n_1 + n_2 - 2};$$

and estimators $\hat{\delta}$, $\hat{\sigma}_{1,0.5}^2$, and $\hat{\sigma}_{WR}^2$ are independent, since $x_{iT1} - x_{iR1}, x_{iT2} - x_{iR2}, z_{iR1}$, and z_{iR2} are independent.

Chow, Shao, and Wang (2002) considered the following decomposition

$$\gamma = \delta^2 + \sigma_{1,0.5}^2 - 1.5\sigma_{WR}^2 - \theta_{IBE}\max\{\sigma_0^2, \sigma_{WR}^2\} \qquad (5.4.3)$$

and obtained the following approximate 95% upper confidence bound for γ. When $\sigma_{WR}^2 \geq \sigma_0^2$,

$$\hat{\gamma}_U = \hat{\delta}^2 + \hat{\sigma}_{1,0.5}^2 - (1.5 + \theta_{IBE})\hat{\sigma}_{WR}^2 + \sqrt{U},$$

where U is the sum of the following three quantities:

$$\left[\left(|\hat{\delta}| + t_{0.95;n_1+n_2-2}\frac{\hat{\sigma}_{1,0.5}}{2}\sqrt{\frac{1}{n_1} + \frac{1}{n_2}}\right)^2 - \hat{\delta}^2\right]^2,$$

$$\hat{\sigma}_{1,0.5}^4\left(\frac{n_1 + n_2 - 2}{\chi_{0.05;n_1+n_2-2}^2} - 1\right)^2,$$

and

$$(1.5 + \theta_{IBE})^2\hat{\sigma}_{WR}^4\left(\frac{n_1 + n_2 - 2}{\chi_{0.95;n_1+n_2-2}^2} - 1\right)^2. \qquad (5.4.4)$$

When $\sigma_{WR}^2 < \sigma_0^2$,

$$\hat{\gamma}_U = \hat{\delta}^2 + \hat{\sigma}_{1,0.5}^2 - 1.5\hat{\sigma}_{WR}^2 - \theta_{IBE}\sigma_0^2 + \sqrt{U_0},$$

where U_0 is the same as U except that the quantity in (5.4.4) should be replaced by

$$1.5^2\hat{\sigma}_{WR}^4\left(\frac{n_1 + n_2 - 2}{\chi_{0.95;n_1+n_2-2}^2} - 1\right)^2.$$

Again, the methods discussed in the end of §5.3.2 can be applied to decide which bound should be used.

5.4.3 Comparisons

It can be seen from the previous discussion that different designs require different decompositions of the parameter γ, which is a key to the construction of the confidence bound $\hat{\gamma}_U$. A summary of these decompositions is given in Table 5.4.1.

Table 5.4.1. Comparisons of Three Designs for Assessment of IBE

Design	Decomposition	l	df	Variance of $2\hat{\delta}$
2×4 crossover	Formula (5.3.7)	4	$n_1 + n_2 - 2$	$\sigma_{0.5,0.5}^2(n_1^{-1} + n_2^{-1})$
2×3 crossover	Formula (5.4.1)	5	$n_k - 1$	$\sigma_{0.5,1}^2 n_1^{-1} + \sigma_{1,0.5}^2 n_2^{-1}$
Extra-reference	Formula (5.4.3)	3	$n_1 + n_2 - 2$	$\sigma_{1,0.5}^2(n_1^{-1} + n_2^{-1})$

l = the number of components to be estimated in the decomposition.
df = degrees of freedom for variance component estimators.

In terms of the number of components required to be estimated (the smaller the better) and the degrees of freedom for variance component estimators (the larger the better), the 2×3 crossover design is the worst and the 2×3 extra-reference design is the best. In terms of the estimation of δ, the 2×3 crossover design is better than the 2×3 extra-reference design if and only if $\sigma_{1,0.5}^2 > \sigma_{0.5,1}^2$, which is the same as $\sigma_{WT}^2 > \sigma_{WR}^2$, i.e., the test formulation is more variable than the reference formulation. In terms of the estimation of δ, the 2×4 crossover design is the best, since $\sigma_{0.5,0.5}^2$ is smaller than both $\sigma_{0.5,1}^2$ and $\sigma_{1,0.5}^2$. But this comparison is somewhat unfair because 2×3 designs require only 75% of the observations in the 2×4 crossover design. If $4n_1/3$ and $4n_2/3$ are integers and are used as sample sizes in the two sequences of the 2×3 extra-reference design so that the total number of observations is the same as that of the 2×4 crossover design having sample sizes n_1 and n_2, the 2×3 extra-reference design is more efficient than the 2×4 crossover design when σ_{WR}^2 or σ_D^2 is large. This is because (i) the degrees of freedom for the confidence bound of σ_{WR}^2 is $4(n_1 + n_2)/3 - 2$ for the 2×3 extra-reference design and, thus, the gain in having a large degrees of freedom is more when σ_{WR}^2 is larger; (ii) the variance of $\hat{\delta}$ under the 2×4 crossover design over the variance of $\hat{\delta}$ under the 2×3 extra-reference design is $4\sigma_{0.5,0.5}^2/3\sigma_{1,0.5}^2$, which is larger than one if and only if $\sigma_D^2 + 0.5\sigma_{WR}^2 > \sigma_{WT}^2$.

Therefore, the conclusion of the comparison is that the 2×3 crossover design is not as good as the other two types of designs and the 2×3 extra-reference design is comparable to or even better than the 2×4 crossover design. These conclusions are supported by empirical results on the type I error probability and power of the IBE tests based on these three types of designs (Chow, Shao, and Wang, 2002). As an example, Figure 5.4.1 plots the power of the IBE tests (using the estimation method) versus γ when the sample size $n_1 = n_2$ is 15 for the 2×4 crossover design and 20 for the 2×3 designs. Note that a 2×4 design with 15 subjects per sequence has the same total number of observations as that of a 2×3 design with 20 subjects per sequence. It can be seen from Figure 5.4.1 that in terms of the power, the IBE test based on the 2×3 extra-reference design is comparable to or even better than that based on the 2×4 crossover design.

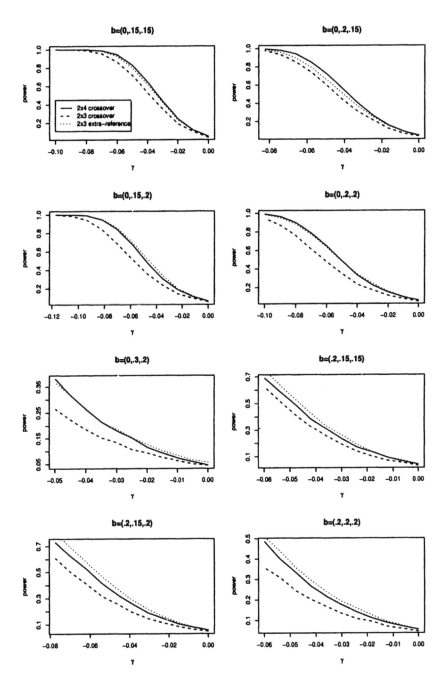

Figure 5.4.1. Power of IBE Tests Versus γ ($n_1 = n_2 = 15$ for 2×4 design and $n_1 = n_2 = 20$ for 2×3 designs); b=$(\sigma_D, \sigma_{WT}, \sigma_{WR})$

5.5 Tests for PBE

For PBE testing, the 2001 FDA guidance does not specify any statistical procedures under a design other than the 2×4 crossover design. Actually, PBE can be assessed under a standard 2×2 crossover design, a 2×3 crossover design, and other higher-order crossover designs. Under the recommended 2×4 crossover design, as shown in §5.3.3, the test procedure given in the 2001 FDA guidance is inappropriate due to the violation of the primary assumption of independence among the estimators of the decomposed components. In what follows, statistical testing procedures under 2×2, 2×3, and 2×4 crossover designs are described using an alternative approach proposed by Chow, Shao, and Wang (2001b), which is based on the method of moments and linearization.

5.5.1 The 2×2 Crossover Design

Under the 2×2 crossover design described in §5.2, an unbiased estimator of δ is $\hat{\delta}$ given in (5.3.2). Commonly used unbiased estimators of σ_{TT}^2 and σ_{TR}^2 are respectively

$$
\hat{\sigma}_{TT}^2 = \frac{1}{n_1 + n_2 - 2} \left[\sum_{i=1}^{n_1} (y_{i11} - \bar{y}_{11})^2 + \sum_{i=1}^{n_2} (y_{i22} - \bar{y}_{22})^2 \right]
$$

$$
\sim \frac{\sigma_{TT}^2 \chi_{n_1+n_2-2}^2}{n_1 + n_2 - 2}
$$

and

$$
\hat{\sigma}_{TR}^2 = \frac{1}{n_1 + n_2 - 2} \left[\sum_{i=1}^{n_1} (y_{i21} - \bar{y}_{21})^2 + \sum_{i=1}^{n_2} (y_{i12} - \bar{y}_{12})^2 \right]
$$

$$
\sim \frac{\sigma_{TR}^2 \chi_{n_1+n_2-2}^2}{n_1 + n_2 - 2}.
$$

It was shown in Chow, Shao, and Wang (2001b) that $\hat{\delta}$ and $(\hat{\sigma}_{TT}^2, \hat{\sigma}_{TR}^2)$ are independent, but $\hat{\sigma}_{TT}^2$ and $\hat{\sigma}_{TR}^2$ are not independent (see §5.3.3).

Applying linearization to the moment estimator

$$
\hat{\lambda} = \hat{\delta}^2 + \hat{\sigma}_{TT}^2 - \hat{\sigma}_{TR}^2 - \theta_{PBE} \max\{\sigma_0^2, \hat{\sigma}_{TR}^2\},
$$

Chow, Shao, and Wang (2001b) obtained the following approximate 95% upper confidence bound for λ. When $\sigma_{TR}^2 \geq \sigma_0^2$,

$$
\hat{\lambda}_U = \hat{\delta}^2 + \hat{\sigma}_{TT}^2 - (1 + \theta_{PBE})\hat{\sigma}_{TR}^2 + t_{0.95;n_1+n_2-2}\sqrt{V}, \qquad (5.5.1)
$$

where V is an estimated variance of $\hat{\delta}^2 + \hat{\sigma}_{TT}^2 - (1 + \theta_{PBE})\hat{\sigma}_{TR}^2$ of the form

$$V = \left(2\hat{\delta}, 1, -(1 + \theta_{PBE})\right) C \left(2\hat{\delta}, 1, -(1 + \theta_{PBE})\right)',$$

and C is an estimated variance-covariance matrix of $(\hat{\delta}, \hat{\sigma}_{TT}^2, \hat{\sigma}_{TR}^2)$. Since $\hat{\delta}$ and $(\hat{\sigma}_{TT}^2, \hat{\sigma}_{TR}^2)$ are independent,

$$C = \begin{pmatrix} \frac{\hat{\sigma}_{1,1}^2}{4}\left(\frac{1}{n_1} + \frac{1}{n_2}\right) & (0,0) \\ (0,0)' & \frac{(n_1-1)C_1}{(n_1+n_2-2)^2} + \frac{(n_2-1)C_2}{(n_1+n_2-2)^2} \end{pmatrix}, \qquad (5.5.2)$$

where $\hat{\sigma}_{1,1}^2$ is defined by (5.3.4), C_1 is the sample covariance matrix of $((y_{i11} - \bar{y}_{11})^2, (y_{i21} - \bar{y}_{21})^2)$, $i = 1, ..., n_1$, and C_2 is the sample covariance matrix of $((y_{i22} - \bar{y}_{22})^2, (y_{i12} - \bar{y}_{12})^2)$, $i = 1, ..., n_2$.

When $\sigma_{TR}^2 < \sigma_0^2$, the upper confidence bound for λ should be modified to

$$\hat{\lambda}_U = \hat{\delta}^2 + \hat{\sigma}_{TT}^2 - \hat{\sigma}_{TR}^2 - \theta_{PBE}\sigma_0^2 + t_{0.95;n_1+n_2-2}\sqrt{V_0}, \qquad (5.5.3)$$

where

$$V_0 = \left(2\hat{\delta}, 1, -1\right) C \left(2\hat{\delta}, 1, -1\right)'.$$

The estimation or test method for IBE described in §5.3.2 can be applied to decide whether the reference-scaled bound $\hat{\lambda}_U$ in (5.5.1) or the constant-scaled bound $\hat{\lambda}_U$ in (5.5.3) should be used.

In theory, the PBE test based on the method of moments and linearization is asymptotically of the nominal size 5% (as $n_1 \to \infty$ and $n_2 \to \infty$), although it is not as good as those in §5.3-5.4 for the assessment of IBE. Thus, empirical studies should be conducted to examine the performance of the PBE test. Chow, Shao, and Wang (2001b) studied by simulation the type I error probability and the power of the PBE test. Some of their results on the type I error are reported in Table 5.5.1, where $\theta_{PBE} = 1.74$ according to the 2001 FDA guidance, $\sigma_0 = 0.2$, and the test method is applied to decide whether the reference-scaled or the constant-scaled bound should be used. It can be seen that in most cases the type I error probability of the PBE test is under the nominal value 5% and is closer to the nominal value when $n = n_1 = n_2$ is large. Selected simulation results on the power of the PBE test are shown in Figure 5.5.1.

Quiroz et al. (2000) proposed another test for assessment of PBE based on the method by Gui et al. (1995) under the 2×2 crossover design. However, their test is not of size 5% even in the asymptotic sense. Asymptotically more accurate tests for PBE can be derived by using, for example, the Edgeworth expansion and the bootstrap.

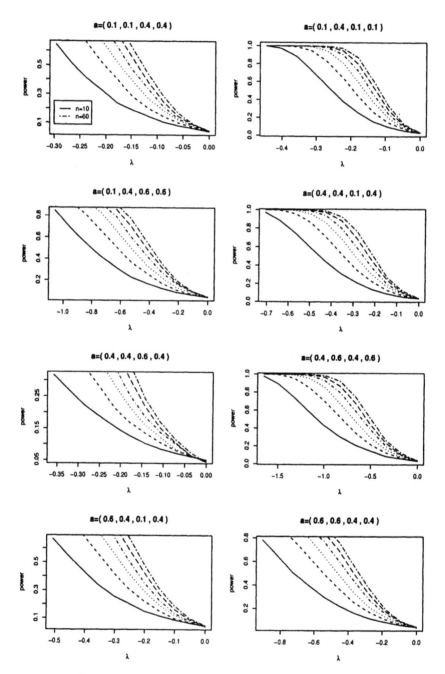

Figure 5.5.1. Power of the PBE Test Versus λ; $\rho = 0.75$,
a=$(\sigma_{BT}, \sigma_{BR}, \sigma_{WT}, \sigma_{WR})$

Table 5.5.1. Type I Error Probability of the PBE Test

$\lambda = 0, \rho = .75$ σ_{BT}, σ_{BR}	n	σ_{WT}, σ_{WR}					
		.1,.1	.1,.4	.4,.4	.4,.6	.6,.4	.6,.6
.1,.1	10	.0406	.0325	.0406	.0360	.0527	.0465
	20	.0508	.0322	.0434	.0365	.0477	.0426
	30	.0583	.0346	.0427	.0426	.0454	.0464
	40	.0576	.0368	.0410	.0389	.0463	.0443
	50	.0601	.0390	.0464	.0404	.0489	.0401
	60	.0556	.0412	.0458	.0430	.0508	.0453
.1,.4	10	.0301	.0306	.0393	.0319	.0419	.0403
	20	.0304	.0331	.0367	.0376	.0416	.0391
	30	.0335	.0357	.0374	.0355	.0445	.0395
	40	.0355	.0324	.0405	.0360	.0400	.0442
	50	.0352	.0367	.0362	.0434	.0415	.0398
	60	.0346	.0364	.0391	.0369	.0431	.0439
.4,.4	10	.0343	.0361	.0408	.0372	.0507	.0401
	20	.0353	.0361	.0355	.0368	.0465	.0413
	30	.0350	.0345	.0339	.0382	.0442	.0449
	40	.0360	.0367	.0389	.0388	.0441	.0429
	50	.0387	.0371	.0408	.0359	.0447	.0409
	60	.0393	.0390	.0425	.0376	.0444	.0431
.4,.6	10	.0312	.0337	.0367	.0313	.0420	.0420
	20	.0320	.0320	.0353	.0347	.0401	.0383
	30	.0306	.0335	.0358	.0386	.0402	.0372
	40	.0335	.0341	.0358	.0344	.0440	.0404
	50	.0317	.0366	.0385	.0399	.0384	.0379
	60	.0366	.0389	.0355	.0364	.0445	.0425
.6,.4	10	.0524	.0406	.0499	.0413	.0584	.0434
	20	.0507	.0427	.0418	.0386	.0502	.0447
	30	.0507	.0353	.0473	.0399	.0493	.0454
	40	.0462	.0419	.0433	.0407	.0475	.0452
	50	.0470	.0405	.0441	.0413	.0436	.0416
	60	.0443	.0445	.0468	.0419	.0452	.0427
.6,.6	10	.0313	.0366	.0408	.0382	.0472	.0412
	20	.0345	.0369	.0388	.0334	.0410	.0419
	30	.0382	.0350	.0396	.0362	.0447	.0381
	40	.0357	.0334	.0335	.0380	.0424	.0419
	50	.0404	.0347	.0414	.0388	.0414	.0415
	60	.0402	.0372	.0418	.0372	.0440	.0430

Example 5.5.1. A 2×2 crossover study was conducted to compare a liquid HSA-free formulation (test formulation) and a standard reconstituted powder formulation (reference formulation) of a drug product intended for treating multiple sclerosis patients. Forty healthy volunteers ($n_1 = n_2 = 20$) were randomly assigned to receive one of the two formulations on Day 1 and Day 14, respectively, after a washout period of 13 days. Blood samples were taken over a 7-day period following each treatment. That is, blood samples were drawn between 5 to 15 minutes predose, at 2, 4, 6, 9, 12, 18, and 21 hours postdose, and at 24, 30, 36, 48, 72, 96, and 168 hours postdose. Serum human interferon-beta concentrations were determined by means of a validated assay.

Pharmacokinetic responses, log-transformed area under the curve from 0 to 168 hours (AUC) and peak concentration ($C_{\max}$) are listed in Table 5.5.2. Statistics for the PBE test are provided in Table 5.5.3, for $\theta_{PBE} = 1.125$ (the most conservative PBE bound) and $\theta_{PBE} = 1.74$ as suggested by FDA (2001). In any case, $\hat{\lambda}_U < 0$. Furthermore, the observed ratios of geometric means are $e^{\hat{\delta}} = 1.205$ for AUC and 1.202 for $C_{\max}$, which are within the limits of 80% and 125%. Hence, PBE can be claimed in terms of either AUC or $C_{\max}$.

It is interesting to compare the PBE analysis with the ABE analysis. According to the result in §5.3.1, ABE can be claimed if and only if the 90% confidence interval $(\hat{\delta}_-, \hat{\delta}_+)$ is within $(-0.223, 0.223)$. Statistics for ABE testing based on data in Table 5.5.2 are included in Table 5.5.3. It turns out that for both AUC and $C_{\max}$, ABE cannot be claimed.

Note that the ABE approach is not suitable for assessment of bioequivalence for highly variable drug products (i.e., the intrasubject CV is greater than 30%). The ABE approach also penalizes the test product that has smaller variability as compared to the reference product, which is the case for this example (Table 5.5.3). As indicated in this example, the PBE analysis provides a more reliable assessment of bioequivalence.

5.5.2 The 2×4 Crossover Design

When the study also considers IBE, the design has to be a higher-order crossover design. If the 2×4 crossover design described in §5.2 is used, a test procedure for PBE can be obtained by using the same idea as that in §5.5.1 but more data to increase accuracy.

Let $\hat{\delta}$, $\hat{\sigma}^2_{0.5,0.5}$, $\hat{\sigma}^2_{WT}$, and $\hat{\sigma}^2_{WR}$ be the same as those defined in §5.3.2, and let $\hat{\sigma}^2_{TT}$ and $\hat{\sigma}^2_{TR}$ be the same as those defined in §5.3.3. Chow, Shao, and Wang (2001b) derived a test for PBE by using $\hat{\lambda}_U$ in (5.5.1) or (5.5.3)

Table 5.5.2. Log-PK Responses

Sequence	Period 1			Period 2		
	Formulation	AUC	C_{max}	Formulation	AUC	C_{max}
1	Liquid	8.09	5.08	Standard	7.75	4.38
2	Standard	6.91	4.04	Liquid	7.97	4.08
1	Liquid	7.87	4.58	Standard	9.92	5.77
2	Standard	8.34	4.38	Liquid	7.28	4.38
1	Liquid	7.70	4.38	Standard	7.33	4.38
2	Standard	7.58	3.71	Liquid	7.70	4.02
1	Liquid	7.99	5.08	Standard	7.43	5.08
2	Standard	7.55	4.70	Liquid	8.28	5.08
2	Standard	8.37	4.38	Liquid	8.03	4.38
1	Liquid	8.84	5.08	Standard	8.65	4.38
2	Standard	7.75	4.38	Liquid	7.48	4.38
1	Liquid	7.78	3.68	Standard	6.27	3.69
2	Standard	7.54	4.38	Liquid	7.87	4.38
1	Liquid	7.61	4.02	Standard	6.91	3.69
2	Standard	7.32	3.69	Liquid	7.95	4.13
1	Liquid	8.21	5.08	Standard	7.90	4.55
2	Standard	8.03	4.38	Liquid	8.44	5.08
1	Liquid	9.50	5.63	Standard	10.8	6.40
2	Standard	8.35	5.08	Liquid	8.54	5.38
2	Standard	8.17	4.38	Liquid	8.25	4.38
1	Liquid	8.52	4.38	Standard	8.10	5.08
2	Standard	8.98	5.25	Liquid	9.56	5.62
1	Liquid	8.93	5.08	Standard	8.93	5.08
2	Standard	7.82	4.58	Liquid	7.83	4.38
1	Liquid	9.10	5.08	Standard	10.1	5.77
1	Liquid	9.34	5.25	Standard	8.69	4.87
2	Standard	7.70	4.38	Liquid	8.29	5.08
1	Liquid	8.61	5.44	Standard	8.70	5.08
2	Standard	7.92	4.61	Liquid	7.14	3.69
2	Standard	8.70	5.25	Liquid	8.71	5.08
1	Liquid	8.05	5.08	Standard	8.20	5.08
1	Liquid	8.22	5.08	Standard	7.86	4.70
2	Standard	7.89	4.38	Liquid	8.17	5.08
2	Standard	7.19	3.69	Liquid	7.63	4.38
1	Liquid	8.69	5.08	Standard	8.32	4.38
1	Liquid	9.33	5.08	Standard	8.47	4.70
2	Standard	7.82	4.38	Liquid	8.18	5.08
1	Liquid	9.11	5.08	Standard	8.15	4.23
1	Liquid	6.19	4.38	Standard	5.78	3.00
2	Standard	7.71	4.38	Liquid	8.39	4.38

Table 5.5.3. Statistics for the PBE and ABE Tests
Based on Data in Table 5.5.2

Variable	$\hat{\delta}$	$\hat{\sigma}_{1,1}^2$	$\hat{\sigma}_{TT}^2$	$\hat{\sigma}_{TR}^2$	The PBE Test $\hat{\lambda}_U^*$	The PBE Test $\hat{\lambda}_U^{**}$	The ABE Test $(\hat{\delta}_-, \hat{\delta}_+)$
AUC	.1868	.4615	.4528	.8539	-.5788	-.7374	(.0057, .3678)
Cmax	.1843	.4101	.2510	.3998	-.2040	-.2820	(.0430, .3255)

$\hat{\lambda}_U^* = \hat{\lambda}_U$ with $\theta_{PBE} = 1.125$
$\hat{\lambda}_U^{**} = \hat{\lambda}_U$ with $\theta_{PBE} = 1.74$

with the new defined $\hat{\delta}$ and $\hat{\sigma}_{Tl}^2$, $l = T, R$, and

$$C = \begin{pmatrix} \frac{\hat{\sigma}_{0.5,0.5}^2}{4}\left(\frac{1}{n_1}+\frac{1}{n_2}\right) & (0,0) \\ (0,0)' & \frac{(n_1-1)C_1}{(n_1+n_2-2)^2} + \frac{(n_2-1)C_2}{(n_1+n_2-2)^2} + \frac{C_0}{2(n_1+n_2-2)} \end{pmatrix},$$

where $\hat{\sigma}_{0.5,0.5}^2$ is defined by (5.3.9), C_1 and C_2 are the same as those in §5.5.1 but with y replaced by x and

$$C_0 = \begin{pmatrix} \hat{\sigma}_{WT}^4 & 0 \\ 0 & \hat{\sigma}_{WR}^4 \end{pmatrix}.$$

Note that Chow, Shao, and Wang's test is different from the one recommended in FDA (2001) (see §5.3.3). Theoretically, the asymptotic size of Chow, Shao, and Wang's test is exactly the same as the nominal level 5%, whereas the asymptotic size of FDA's test is smaller than 5% (see §5.3.3) and is inappropriate. Chow, Shao, and Wang (2001b) studied and compared empirically these two PBE tests. Data were generated according to the standard 2×4 crossover design with normally distributed random subject effects and within-subject errors. Values of the parameters δ, σ_{BT}, σ_{BR}, σ_{WT}, σ_{WR}, and ρ are given in Tables 5.5.4 and 5.5.5. The value of θ_{PBE} is 1.74.

The type I error probability, i.e., the probability of concluding PBE when the two products are in fact not PBE, for FDA's test and Chow, Shao, and Wang's test are listed in Table 5.5.4. At the 5% nominal level, the method by Chow, Shao, and Wang appears to perform better than that of FDA's test. The performance of FDA's test becomes worse when ρ becomes larger or the between subject variances are larger than within subject variances.

Statistically speaking, a relatively conservative test usually results in a relatively low power (the probability of concluding PBE when two products are indeed PBE). The results in Table 5.5.5 are the values of the power of

Table 5.5.4. Type I Error Probability of PBE Tests Under 2 × 4
Crossover Design (10,000 Simulations)

σ_{BT}	σ_{BR}	σ_{WT}	σ_{WR}	δ	n	$\rho = .75$ CSW	$\rho = .75$ FDA	$\rho = 1.00$ CSW	$\rho = 1.00$ FDA
.4	.4	.1	.1	.4373	2	.0335	.0143	.0255	.0000
					30	.0347	.0170	.0296	.0000
					40	.0367	.0172	.0306	.0000
.4	.4	.2	.1	.4016	20	.0401	.0169	.0309	.0001
					30	.0390	.0198	.0335	.0005
					40	.0387	.0175	.0310	.0002
.4	.4	.3	.3	.5303	20	.0388	.0268	.0336	.0143
					30	.0408	.0303	.0354	.0144
					40	.0385	.0307	.0382	.0144
.4	.6	.2	.1	.7657	20	.0311	.0303	.0257	.0135
					30	.0312	.0276	.0246	.0123
					40	.0326	.0301	.0293	.0160
.4	.6	.3	.3	.8404	20	.0296	.0322	.0274	.0205
					30	.0362	.0355	.0348	.0257
					40	.0341	.0347	.0282	.0209
.6	.4	.1	.2	.2345	20	.0509	.0116	.0530	.0000
					30	.0526	.0114	.0486	.0000
					40	.0526	.0120	.0491	.0000
.6	.4	.3	.3	.2850	20	.0524	.0170	.0518	.0031
					30	.0503	.0179	.0470	.0028
					40	.0532	.0207	.0484	.0030
.6	.6	.1	.1	.6452	20	.0365	.0138	.0259	.0000
					30	.0344	.0135	.0278	.0000
					40	.0345	.0143	.0284	.0000
.6	.6	.1	.2	.6928	20	.0321	.0168	.0263	.0000
					30	.0339	.0169	.0273	.0000
					40	.0378	.0188	.0296	.0000
.6	.6	.2	.1	.6215	20	.0344	.0122	.0256	.0000
					30	.0342	.0152	.0302	.0000
					40	.0370	.0167	.0332	.0000
.6	.6	.3	.3	.7115	20	.0373	.0223	.0332	.0022
					30	.0383	.0225	.0346	.0038
					40	.0414	.0268	.0328	.0029

FDA: FDA's PBE test.

CSW: The PBE test proposed by Chow, Shao, and Wang (2001b).

Table 5.5.5. Power of PBE Tests Under 2×4 Crossover Design with $n = 20$ (10,000 Simulations)

σ_{BT}	σ_{BR}	σ_{WT}	σ_{WR}	δ	$\rho = .75$		$\rho = 1.00$	
					CSW	FDA	CSW	FDA
.4	.4	.1	.1	.1956	.7539	.5747	.9977	.7853
				.1383	.8747	.7191	1.000	.9561
				0	.9461	.8330	1.000	.9998
.4	.4	.2	.1	.1796	.5738	.3819	.9180	.3542
				.1270	.6977	.4982	.9751	.5469
				0	.8110	.6075	.9970	.7411
.4	.4	.3	.3	.2372	.7440	.6568	.8848	.7300
				.1677	.8578	.7790	.9623	.8672
				0	.9443	.8888	.9918	.9468
.4	.6	.2	.1	.2421	.9933	.9909	1.000	1.000
				0	.9998	.9997	1.000	1.000
.4	.6	.3	.3	.2658	.9941	.9947	.9997	.9997
				0	1.000	.9998	1.000	1.000
.6	.4	.1	.2	.1049	.1319	.0331	.2701	.0006
				.0742	.1482	.0377	.3211	.0007
				0	.1674	.0402	.3692	.0011
.6	.4	.3	.3	.1275	.1491	.0554	.2072	.0204
				.0901	.1661	.0673	.2347	.0249
				0	.1892	.0755	.2760	.0309
.6	.6	.1	.1	.2040	.8732	.7070	.9999	.9844
				0	.9468	.8252	1.000	.9999
.6	.6	.1	.2	.2191	.9249	.8119	1.000	.9916
				0	.9753	.9054	1.000	.9997
.6	.6	.2	.1	.1965	.7977	.5979	.9994	.8000
				0	.8937	.7253	1.000	.9553
.6	.6	.3	.3	.2250	.8747	.7558	.9931	.8892
				0	.9471	.8646	.9997	.9670

FDA: FDA's PBE test.

CSW: The PBE test proposed by Chow, Shao, and Wang (2001b).

FDA's and Chow, Shao, and Wang's tests when $n = 20$. It can be seen that Chow, Shao, and Wang's test is always more powerful than FDA's test.

5.5.3 The 2×3 Designs

Consider first the 2×3 crossover design described in §5.4.1. Let $\hat{\delta}$, $\hat{\sigma}^2_{1,0.5}$, $\hat{\sigma}^2_{0.5,1}$, $\hat{\sigma}^2_{WT}$, and $\hat{\sigma}^2_{WR}$ be the same as those in §5.4.1, and let $\tilde{\sigma}^2_{TT}$ and $\tilde{\sigma}^2_{TR}$ be the same as those in §5.5.2. Then, an unbiased estimator of σ^2_{Tl} is $\hat{\sigma}^2_{Tl} = \tilde{\sigma}^2_{Tl} + 0.5\hat{\sigma}^2_{Wl}$. Chow, Shao, and Wang's test for PBE can be obtained by using $\hat{\lambda}_U$ in (5.5.1) or (5.5.3) with the new defined $\hat{\delta}$ and $\hat{\sigma}^2_{Tl}$, $l = T, R$, and

$$
C = \begin{pmatrix} \frac{\hat{\sigma}^2_{0.5,1}}{4n_1} + \frac{\hat{\sigma}^2_{1,0.5}}{4n_2} & (0,0) \\ (0,0)' & \frac{(n_1-1)C_1}{(n_1+n_2-2)^2} + \frac{(n_2-1)C_2}{(n_1+n_2-2)^2} + \frac{C_0}{2(n_1+n_2-2)} \end{pmatrix},
$$

where C_1 and C_2 are the same as those in §5.5.2, and

$$
C_0 = \frac{1}{n_1 + n_2 - 2} \begin{pmatrix} (n_1 - 1)\hat{\sigma}^4_{WT} & 0 \\ 0 & (n_2 - 1)\hat{\sigma}^4_{WR} \end{pmatrix}.
$$

Consider next the 2×3 extra-reference design described in §5.4.2. Let $\hat{\delta}$, $\hat{\sigma}^2_{1,0.5}$, and $\hat{\sigma}^2_{WR}$ be the same as those in §5.4.2, let $\hat{\sigma}^2_{TR}$ and $\tilde{\sigma}^2_{TT}$ be the same as that in §5.5.2, and let $\hat{\sigma}^2_{TT} = \tilde{\sigma}^2_{TT}$. Then, a test for PBE can be obtained by using $\hat{\lambda}_U$ in (5.5.1) or (5.5.3) with the the new defined $\hat{\delta}$ and $\hat{\sigma}^2_{Tl}$, $l = T, R$, and

$$
C = \begin{pmatrix} \frac{\hat{\sigma}^2_{1,0.5}}{4}\left(\frac{1}{n_1} + \frac{1}{n_2}\right) & (0,0) \\ (0,0)' & \frac{(n_1-1)C_1}{(n_1+n_2-2)^2} + \frac{(n_2-1)C_2}{(n_1+n_2-2)^2} + \frac{C_0}{2(n_1+n_2-2)} \end{pmatrix},
$$

where C_1 and C_2 are the same as those in §5.5.2 and

$$
C_0 = \begin{pmatrix} 0 & 0 \\ 0 & \hat{\sigma}^4_{WR} \end{pmatrix}.
$$

5.6 In Vitro Bioequivalence

In the previous sections we considered *in vivo* bioequivalence based on bioavailability that is usually assessed through the measures of the rate and extent to which the drug product is absorbed into the bloodstream of human subjects. For some locally acting drug products such as nasal aerosols (e.g., metered-dose inhalers) and nasal sprays (e.g., metered-dose spray pumps) that are not intended to be absorbed into the bloodstream, bioavailability may be assessed by measurements intended to reflect the rate and extent to which the active ingredient or active moiety becomes available at the site of action. For these local delivery drug products, the FDA indicates that bioequivalence may be assessed, with suitable justification, by *in vitro* bioequivalence studies alone (21 CFR 320.24). Although it is recognized that *in vitro* methods are less variable, easier to control, and more likely to detect differences between products if they exist, the clinical relevance of the *in vitro* tests or the magnitude of the differences in the tests are not clearly established until recently a draft guidance on bioavailability and bioequivalence studies for nasal aerosols and nasal sprays for local action was issued by the FDA (FDA, 1999b). In this section we introduce FDA's regulations for *in vitro* bioequivalence studies and the related statistical methods.

5.6.1   Six Tests in the FDA Guidance

For local delivery drug products such as nasal aerosols and nasal sprays, as indicated in the 1999 FDA draft guidance, bioavailability can be determined by several factors, including release of drug substance from the drug product and availability to local sites of action. Release of drug substance from the drug product is characterized by distribution patterns and droplet or drug particle size within the nose that are dependent upon substance, formulation, and device characteristics. As a result, the FDA suggests that *in vitro* bioequivalence for locally acting drugs delivered by nasal aerosol and nasal spray be assessed by the following six tests:

Test	Description
1	Dose or spray content uniformity through container life
2	Droplet and drug particle size distribution
3	Spray pattern
4	Plume geometry
5	Priming and repriming
6	Tail-off profile

For *in vitro* bioequivalence assessment, the FDA requires that dose or spray content uniformity data be determined on primed units at the beginning of unit life (i.e., the first actuation(s) following the labeled number of priming actuations), at the middle of unit life (i.e., the actuation(s) corresponding to 50% of the labeled number of full medication doses), and at the end of unit life (i.e., the actuation(s) corresponding to the label claim number of full medication doses) for nasal aerosols, and at beginning and end of unit life for nasal sprays. Mean dose or spray content uniformity and variability in content uniformity should be determined based on within and between canister or bottle data as well as between batch (lot) data.

Droplet size distribution measurements are critical to delivery of drug to the nose, which could affect the efficiency of the nasal absorption (Chein, 1992). The FDA requires that studies of droplet size distribution and particle size distribution be performed by validated methods such as laser diffraction method for droplet size distribution and multistage cascade impactor (CI) or multistage liquid impriger (MSLI) for particle size distribution. The guidance suggests that the droplet size distribution data (D_{50}) and span (($D_{90}-D_{10}$)/D_{50}) should be analyzed according to the method of comparison for nonprofile analysis, while the cascade impaction data should be analyzed using the method of comparison for profile analysis as specified in the FDA draft guidance (see §5.6.2).

The purpose of the spray pattern test is to characterize the angle at which the spray is emitted from the pump/actuator system (Adams, Singh, and Williams, 1998). Various factors can affect the spray pattern, including the size and shape of the actuator orifice, the design of the actuator, the size of the metering chamber, the size of the stem orifice of the nozzle, and nature of the formulation. Spray pattern characterizes the spray following impaction on an appropriate target. It provides information about the shape and density of the plume following actuation. FDA requires that spray pattern determined on single actuations at three appropriate distances (e.g., 2, 4, and 6 cm) from the actuator to the target (e.g., a thin-layer chromatography plate) at the beginning and end of unit life. The spray pattern image can then be visualized using some developing agents. The spray pattern results include the widest (D_{max}) and shortest (D_{min}) diameters, and the ovality ration (D_{max}/D_{min}). FDA suggests that the spray pattern data be analyzed according to the method of comparison for nonprofile analysis as specified in the draft guidance.

The purpose of the plume geometry test is to visually record the behavior characteristics of the drug formulation plume emitted from the pump/actuator system (Eck et al., 1998). High-speed video photography is usually used to film the plume geometry of a spray. A video camera is positioned level to the spray unit and to one side to capture two side image of the plume at 90 degrees to each other. The plume geometry data, which include plume length, plume width and plume angle can then be analyzed according to the method of comparison for nonprofile analysis as described in the FDA draft guidance. Note that spray pattern and plume geometry are recommended to assist in establishing functional equivalence of products as a result of differences in the device components of the test and reference products. Comparable spray pattern and plume geometry data for the test and reference products in conjunction with other *in vitro* tests ensure equivalent drug deposition patterns, resulting in equivalent delivery of drug to nasal sites of action and equivalent systemic exposure or absorption.

Since the metered-dose pump must be primed prior to initial use, the priming study is to determine the minimum number of actuations required before the metered pump will deliver the labeled dose of drug. The FDA requires that the priming data be analyzed using the method of comparison for nonprofile analysis as specified in the draft guidance. When stored for a time period of nonuse, the metered-dose pump may lose prime. In this case, the repriming study is necessarily performed to determine the minimum number of actuations required delivering the labeled dose of drug after a time period of nonuse. The repriming data should be analyzed similarly. Priming and repriming tests provide information to ensure delivery of the labeled dose of drug, and hence are part of the *in vitro* bioequivalence assessment.

Tail-off profile characterizes the decrease in emitted dose following delivery of the labeled number of actuations (i.e., from end of unit life to product exhaustion). For bioequivalence assessment, comparative tail-off profiles are required to ensue similarity in drug delivery as the product near exhaustion. The tail-off profile data should be analyzed according to the method of comparison for nonprofile analysis as suggested by the FDA.

5.6.2   Nonprofile Analysis

Statistical methods for assessment of *in vitro* bioequivalence testing for nasal aerosols and sprays can be classified as the nonprofile analysis and the profile analysis. The nonprofile analysis applies to tests for dose or spray content uniformity through container life, droplet size distribution, spray pattern, and priming and repriming. The FDA adopts the criterion and limit of the PBE for assessment of *in vitro* bioequivalence in the nonprofile analysis. Let y_T, y_R, and y_R' be independent *in vitro* bioavailabilities, where y_T is from the test formulation and y_R and y_R' are from the reference formulation. Then the two formulations are *in vitro* bioequivalent if $\theta < \theta_{BE}$, where

$$\theta = \frac{E(y_R - y_T)^2 - E(y_R - y_R')^2}{\max\{\sigma_0^2, E(y_R - y_R')^2/2\}} \qquad (5.6.1)$$

and σ_0^2 and θ_{BE} are the same as those in the PBE study. Similar to the PBE, *in vitro* bioequivalence can be claimed if the hypothesis that $\theta \geq \theta_{BE}$ is rejected at the 5% level of significance provided that the observed ratio of geometric means is within the limits of 90% and 111%.

Suppose that m_T and m_R canisters (or bottles) from respectively the test and the reference products are randomly selected and one observation from each canister is obtained. The data can be described by the following model:

$$y_{jk} = \mu_k + \varepsilon_{jk}, \quad j = 1, ..., m_k, \tag{5.6.2}$$

where $k = T$ for the test product, $k = R$ for the reference product, μ_T and μ_R are fixed product effects, ε_{jk}'s are independent random measurement errors distributed as $N(0, \sigma_k^2)$, $k = T, R$. Under model (5.6.2), the parameter θ in (5.6.1) is equal to

$$\theta = \frac{(\mu_T - \mu_R)^2 + \sigma_T^2 - \sigma_R^2}{\max\{\sigma_0^2, \sigma_R^2\}} \tag{5.6.3}$$

and $\theta < \theta_{BE}$ if and only if $\zeta < 0$, where

$$\zeta = (\mu_T - \mu_R)^2 + \sigma_T^2 - \sigma_R^2 - \theta_{BE} \max\{\sigma_0^2, \sigma_R^2\}. \tag{5.6.4}$$

Under model (5.6.2), the best unbiased estimator of $\delta = \mu_T - \mu_R$ is

$$\hat{\delta} = \bar{y}_T - \bar{y}_R \sim N\left(\delta, \frac{\sigma_T^2}{m_T} + \frac{\sigma_R^2}{m_R}\right),$$

where $\bar{y}_k$ is the average of y_{jk} over j for a fixed k. The best unbiased estimator of σ_k^2 is

$$s_k^2 = \frac{1}{m_k - 1} \sum_{j=1}^{m_k} (y_{jk} - \bar{y}_k)^2 \sim \frac{\sigma_k^2 \chi_{m_k-1}^2}{m_k - 1}, \quad k = T, R.$$

Using the method for IBE testing (§5.3.2), an approximate 95% upper confidence bound for ζ in (5.6.4) is

$$\tilde{\zeta}_U = \hat{\delta}^2 + s_T^2 - s_R^2 - \theta_{BE} \max\{\sigma_0^2, s_R^2\} + \sqrt{U_0},$$

where U_0 is the sum of the following three quantities:

$$\left[\left(|\hat{\delta}| + z_{0.95}\sqrt{\frac{s_T^2}{m_T} + \frac{s_R^2}{m_R}}\right)^2 - \hat{\delta}^2\right]^2,$$

$$s_T^4 \left(\frac{m_T - 1}{\chi_{0.05;m_T-1}^2} - 1\right)^2,$$

and

$$(1 + c\theta_{BE})^2 s_R^4 \left(\frac{m_R - 1}{\chi_{0.95;m_R-1}^2} - 1\right)^2,$$

$c = 1$ if $s_R^2 \geq \sigma_0^2$ and $c = 0$ if $s_R^2 < \sigma_0^2$, z_a is the ath quantile of the standard normal distribution, and $\chi_{t;a}^2$ is the ath quantile of the central chi-square distribution with t degrees of freedom. Note that the estimation method in §5.3.2 for determining the use of the reference-scaled criterion or the constant-scaled criterion is applied here. *In vitro* bioequivalence can be claimed if $\tilde{\zeta}_U < 0$. This procedure is recommended by the FDA guidance.

To ensure that the previously described test has a significant level close to the nominal level 5% with a desired power, the FDA requires that at least 30 canisters of each of the test and reference products be tested. However, $m_k = 30$ may not be enough to achieve a desired power of the bioequivalence test in some situations (see Chow, Shao, and Wang, 2001c). Increasing m_k can certainly increase the power, but in some situations, obtaining replicates from each canister may be more practical, and/or cost-effective. With replicates from each canister, however, the previously described test procedure is necessarily modified in order to address the between- and within-canister variabilities.

Suppose that there are n_k replicates from each canister for product k. Let y_{ijk} be the ith replicate in the jth canister under product k, b_{jk} be the between-canister variation, and e_{ijk} be the within-canister measurement error. Then

$$y_{ijk} = \mu_k + b_{jk} + e_{ijk}, \quad i = 1, ..., n_k, \ j = 1, ..., m_k, \qquad (5.6.5)$$

where $b_{jk} \sim N(0, \sigma_{Bk}^2)$, $e_{ijk} \sim N(0, \sigma_{Wk}^2)$, and b_{jk}'s and e_{ijk}'s are independent. Under model (5.6.5), the total variances σ_T^2 and σ_R^2 in (5.6.3) and (5.6.4) are equal to $\sigma_{BT}^2 + \sigma_{WT}^2$ and $\sigma_{BR}^2 + \sigma_{WR}^2$, respectively, i.e., the sums of between-canister and within-canister variances. The parameter θ in (5.6.1) is still given by (5.6.3) and $\theta < \theta_{BE}$ if and only if $\zeta < 0$, where ζ is given in (5.6.4).

Under model (5.6.5), the best unbiased estimator of $\delta = \mu_T - \mu_R$ is

$$\hat{\delta} = \bar{y}_T - \bar{y}_R \sim N\left(\delta, \ \frac{\sigma_{BT}^2}{m_T} + \frac{\sigma_{BR}^2}{m_R} + \frac{\sigma_{WT}^2}{m_T n_T} + \frac{\sigma_{WR}^2}{m_R n_R}\right),$$

where $\bar{y}_k$ is the average of y_{ijk} over i and j for a fixed k.

To construct a confidence bound for ζ in (5.6.4) using the approach in IBE testing, we need to find independent, unbiased, and chi-square distributed estimators of σ_T^2 and σ_R^2. These estimators, however, are not available when $n_k > 1$. Note that

$$\sigma_k^2 = \sigma_{Bk}^2 + n_k^{-1}\sigma_{Wk}^2 + (1 - n_k^{-1})\sigma_{Wk}^2, \quad k = T, R;$$

$\sigma_{Bk}^2 + n_k^{-1}\sigma_{Wk}^2$ can be estimated by

$$s_{Bk}^2 = \frac{1}{m_k - 1} \sum_{j=1}^{m_k} (\bar{y}_{jk} - \bar{y}_k)^2 \sim \frac{(\sigma_{Bk}^2 + n_k^{-1}\sigma_{Wk}^2)\chi_{m_k-1}^2}{m_k - 1},$$

where $\bar{y}_{jk}$ is the average of y_{ijk} over i; σ^2_{Wk} can be estimated by

$$s^2_{Wk} = \frac{1}{m_k(n_k-1)} \sum_{j=1}^{m_k} \sum_{i=1}^{n_k} (y_{ijk} - \bar{y}_{jk})^2 \sim \frac{\sigma^2_{Wk} \chi^2_{m_k(n_k-1)}}{m_k(n_k-1)};$$

and $\hat{\delta}$, s^2_{Bk}, s^2_{Wk}, $k = T, R$, are independent. Thus, an approximate 95% upper confidence bound for ζ in (5.6.4) is:

$$\hat{\zeta}_U = \hat{\delta}^2 + s^2_{BT} + (1 - n_T^{-1})s^2_{WT} - s^2_{BR} - (1 - n_R^{-1})s^2_{WR}$$
$$- \theta_{BE} \max\{\sigma_0^2, s^2_{BR} + (1 - n_R^{-1})s^2_{WR}\} + \sqrt{U},$$

where U is the sum of the following five quantities,

$$\left[\left(|\hat{\delta}| + z_{0.95} \sqrt{\frac{s^2_{BT}}{m_T} + \frac{s^2_{BR}}{m_R}} \right)^2 - \hat{\delta}^2 \right]^2,$$

$$s^4_{BT} \left(\frac{m_T - 1}{\chi^2_{0.05;m_T-1}} - 1 \right)^2,$$

$$(1 - n_T^{-1})^2 s^4_{WT} \left(\frac{m_T(n_T-1)}{\chi^2_{0.05;m_T(n_T-1)}} - 1 \right)^2,$$

$$(1 + \theta_{BE})^2 s^4_{BR} \left(\frac{m_R - 1}{\chi^2_{0.95;m_R-1}} - 1 \right)^2,$$

and

$$(1 + c\theta_{BE})^2 (1 - n_R^{-1})^2 s^4_{WR} \left(\frac{m_R(n_R-1)}{\chi^2_{0.95;m_R(n_R-1)}} - 1 \right)^2,$$

and $c = 1$ if $s^2_{BR} + (1 - n_R^{-1})s^2_{WR} \geq \sigma_0^2$ and $c = 0$ if $s^2_{BR} + (1 - n_R^{-1})s^2_{WR} < \sigma_0^2$. In vitro bioequivalence can be claimed if $\hat{\zeta}_U < 0$ provided that the observed ratio of geometric means is within the limits of 90% and 110%.

If the difference between model (5.6.2) and model (5.6.5) is ignored and the confidence bound $\tilde{\zeta}_U$ with m_k replaced by $m_k n_k$ (instead of $\hat{\zeta}_U$) is used, then the asymptotic size of the test procedure is not 5%.

5.6.3 Profile Analysis

The profile analysis applies to cascade impactor (CI) or multistage liquid impriger (MSLI) for particle size distribution. As indicated in the 1999

FDA draft guidance, bioequivalence may be assessed by comparing the profile variation between test product and reference product bottles with the profile variation between reference product bottles. The profile variation between test and reference product bottles can be assessed by the chi-square difference

$$d_{TR} = \sum_{s=1}^{S} \frac{(\bar{y}_{Ts} - \bar{y}_{Rs})^2}{(\bar{y}_{Ts} + \bar{y}_{Rs})/2},$$

where $\bar{y}_{ks}$ represent the sample mean profiles over a batch at stage s, $s = 1, ..., S$ and $k = T, R$. Similarly, the profile variation between any two bottles of the reference product is given by

$$d_{RR'} = \sum_{s=1}^{S} \frac{(\bar{y}_{Rs} - \bar{y}_{R's})^2}{(\bar{y}_{Rs} + \bar{y}_{R's})/2}.$$

The test and reference products are considered to be *in vitro* bioequivalent if $r < r_{BE}$, where

$$r = \frac{E(d_{TR})}{E(d_{RR'})}$$

and r_{BE} is a bioequivalence limit specified by the FDA. If $\hat{r}_U$ is an approximate 95% upper confidence bound for r, then bioequivalence can be claimed if $\hat{r}_U < r_{BE}$. An approximate 95% upper confidence bound can be obtained using a resampling procedure (e.g., bootstrapping without replacement) as specified in the FDA draft guidance (FDA, 1999b).

5.7   Sample Size Determination

In this section we consider sample size calculation for assessment of IBE, PBE, and *in vitro* bioequivalence based on the test procedures introduced in §5.3-5.6. Sample size calculation for assessment of ABE under a standard 2×2 crossover design or under a higher-order crossover design can be found in Liu and Chow (1992b) and Chen, Chow, and Li (1997). More details regarding sample size calculation based on either raw data or log-transformed data under either a crossover design or a parallel design can be found in Chow and Wang (2001).

5.7.1   Sample Size for IBE Testing

Typically, we would choose $n_1 = n_2 = n$ so that the power of the IBE test reaches a given level β when the unknown parameters are set at some initial guessing values $\tilde{\delta}$, $\tilde{\sigma}_D^2$, $\tilde{\sigma}_{WT}^2$, and $\tilde{\sigma}_{WR}^2$.

For the IBE test based on the confidence bound $\hat{\gamma}_U$, its power is given by

$$P_n = P(\hat{\gamma}_U < 0)$$

when $\gamma < 0$. Consider first the case where $\tilde{\sigma}_{WR}^2 > \sigma_0^2$. Let U be given in the definition of the reference-scaled bound $\hat{\gamma}_U$ and U_β be the same as U but with 5% and 95% replaced by $1 - \beta$ and β, respectively. Since

$$P(\hat{\gamma}_U < \gamma + \sqrt{U} + \sqrt{U_\beta}) \approx \beta,$$

the power P_n is approximately larger than β if

$$\gamma + \sqrt{U} + \sqrt{U_\beta} \leq 0.$$

Let $\tilde{\gamma}$, $\tilde{U}$ and $\tilde{U}_\beta$ be γ, U and U_β, respectively, with parameter values and their estimators replaced by $\tilde{\delta}$, $\tilde{\sigma}_D^2$, $\tilde{\sigma}_{WT}^2$, and $\tilde{\sigma}_{WR}^2$. Then, the required sample size n to have approximately power β is the smallest integer satisfying

$$\tilde{\gamma} + \sqrt{\tilde{U}} + \sqrt{\tilde{U}_\beta} \leq 0, \tag{5.7.1}$$

assuming that $n_1 = n_2 = n$ and $\tilde{\delta}$, $\tilde{\sigma}_D^2$, $\tilde{\sigma}_{WT}^2$, and $\tilde{\sigma}_{WR}^2$ are true parameter values. When $\tilde{\sigma}_{WR}^2 < \sigma_0^2$, the previous procedure can be modified by replacing U by U_0 in the definition of constant-scaled bound $\hat{\gamma}_U$. If $\tilde{\sigma}_{WR}^2$ is equal or close to σ_0^2, then we recommend the use of U instead of U_0 to produce a more conservative sample size and the use of the test approach in the IBE test (see the discussion in §5.3.2).

This procedure can be applied to any of the 2×3 and 2×4 designs described in §5.2-5.4.

Since the IBE tests are based on the asymptotic theory, n should be reasonably large to ensure the asymptotic convergence. Hence, we suggest that the solution greater than 10 from (5.7.1) be used. In other words, a sample size of more than $n=10$ per sequence that satisfies (5.7.1) is recommended.

To study the performance of formula (5.7.1) for sample size determination, Chow, Shao, and Wang (2002) computed the sample size n according to (5.7.1) with some given parameter values and $\beta = 80\%$ and then computed (with 10,000 simulations) the actual power P_n of the IBE test using n as the sample size for both sequences. The results for the 2×3 extra-reference design and 2×4 crossover design are given in Table 5.7.1. For each selected n that is smaller than 10, the power of the IBE test using $n^* = \max(n, 10)$ as the sample size, which is denoted by P_{n^*}, is also included.

It can be seen from Table 5.7.1 that the actual power P_n is larger than the target value of 80% in most cases and only in a few cases where n determined from (5.7.1) is very small, the power P_n is lower than 75%. n

Table 5.7.1. Sample Size n Selected Using (5.7.1) with $\beta = 80\%$ and the Power P_n of the IBE Test Based on 10,000 Simulations

σ_D	σ_{WT}	σ_{WR}	δ	n	P_n	n^*	P_{n^*}	n	P_n	n^*	P_{n^*}
				\multicolumn{4}{c}{2 × 3 extra-reference}		\multicolumn{4}{c}{2 × 4 crossover}	
0	.15	.15	0	5	.7226	10	.9898	4	.7007	10	.9998
			.1	6	.7365	10	.9572	5	.7837	10	.9948
			.2	13	.7718	13		9	.7607	10	.8104
0	.2	.15	0	9	.7480	10	.8085	7	.7995	10	.9570
			.1	12	.7697	12		8	.7468	10	.8677
			.2	35	.7750	35		23	.7835	23	
0	.15	.2	0	9	.8225	10	.8723	8	.8446	10	.9314
			.1	12	.8523	12		10	.8424	10	
			.2	26	.8389	26		23	.8506	23	
0	.2	.2	0	15	.8206	15		13	.8591	13	
			.1	20	.8373	20		17	.8532	17	
			.2	52	.8366	52		44	.8458	44	
0	.3	.2	0	91	.8232	91		71	.8454	71	
.2	.15	.15	0	20	.7469	20		17	.7683	17	
			.1	31	.7577	31		25	.7609	25	
.2	.15	.2	0	31	.8238	31		28	.8358	28	
			.1	43	.8246	43		39	.8296	39	
.2	.2	.2	0	59	.8225	59		51	.8322	51	
			.2	91	.8253	91		79	.8322	79	
0	.15	.3	0	7	.8546	10	.9607	6	.8288	10	.9781
			.1	7	.8155	10	.9401	7	.8596	10	.9566
			.2	10	.8397	10		9	.8352	10	.8697
			.3	16	.7973	16		15	.8076	15	
			.4	45	.8043	45		43	.8076	43	
0	.3	.3	0	15	.7931	15		13	.8162	13	
			.1	17	.7942	17		14	.8057	14	
			.2	25	.8016	25		21	.8079	21	
			.3	52	.7992	52		44	.8009	44	
0	.2	.5	0	6	.8285	10	.9744	6	.8497	10	.9810
			.1	6	.8128	10	.9708	6	.8413	10	.9759
			.2	7	.8410	10	.9505	7	.8600	10	.9628
			.3	8	.8282	10	.9017	8	.8548	10	.9239
			.4	10	.8147	10		10	.8338	10	
			.5	14	.8095	14		14	.8248	14	
			.6	24	.8162	24		23	.8149	23	
			.7	51	.8171	51		49	.8170	49	
0	.5	.5	0	15	.7890	15		13	.8132	13	
			.1	16	.8000	16		13	.7956	13	
			.2	18	.7980	18		15	.8033	15	
			.3	23	.8002	23		19	.8063	19	
			.5	52	.7944	52		44	.8045	44	
.2	.2	.3	0	13	.7870	13		12	.7970	12	
			.1	15	.8007	15		14	.8144	14	
			.2	21	.7862	21		20	.8115	20	
			.3	43	.8037	43		40	.8034	40	
.2	.3	.3	0	26	.7806	26		22	.7877	22	
			.1	30	.7895	30		26	.8039	26	
.2	.3	.5	0	9	.8038	10	.8502	8	.8050	10	.8947
			.1	9	.7958	10	.8392	9	.8460	10	.8799
			.2	10	.7966	10		9	.7954	10	.8393
			.3	12	.7929	12		11	.8045	11	
			.4	16	.7987	16		15	.8094	15	

$n^* = \max(n, 10)$

Using $n^* = \max(n, 10)$ as the sample size produces better results when selected by (5.7.1) is very small, but in most cases it results in a power much larger than 80%.

5.7.2 Sample Size for PBE Testing

For PBE testing, we only consider the 2×2 crossover design. Based on an asymptotic analysis, Chow, Shao and Wang (2001b) proposed the following formula for sample size determination assuming that $n_1 = n_2 = n$:

$$n \geq \frac{\zeta(z_{0.95} + z_\beta)^2}{\lambda^2},\qquad(5.7.2)$$

where

$$\zeta = 2\delta^2\sigma_{1,1}^2 + \sigma_{TT}^4 + (1+a)^2\sigma_{TR}^4 - 2(1+a)\rho^2\sigma_{BT}^2\sigma_{BR}^2,$$

δ, $\sigma_{1,1}^2$, σ_{TT}^2, σ_{TR}^2, σ_{BT}^2, σ_{BR}^2 and ρ are given initial values, z_t is the tth quantile of the standard normal distribution, β is the desired power, $a = \theta_{PBE}$ if $\sigma_{TR} \geq \sigma_0$ and $a = 0$ if $\sigma_{TR} < \sigma_0$.

A simulation study similar to that in §5.7.1 was conducted to study the performance of formula (5.7.2). The results are shown in Table 5.7.2. It can be seen from Table 5.7.2 that the actual power P_n corresponding to each selected n is larger than the target value of 80%, although the sample size obtained by formula (5.7.2) is conservative since P_n is much larger than 80% in some cases.

When the value of $\delta > 0.233$ and the value of $\lambda < 0$, the two formulations are PBE but not ABE. In such a case the required sample size n may be very large, although PBE can still be claimed with a power larger than 80%.

When the variation of the test formulation is larger than that of the reference formulation, it is difficult to claim PBE even when the two formulations are both PBE and ABE. When $\delta = 0$ and $(\sigma_{BT}, \sigma_{BR}, \sigma_{WT}, \sigma_{WR}) = (0.4, 0.4, 0.6, 0.4)$ or $(0.6, 0.4, 0.4, 0.4)$, for example, the required sample size n for demonstration of PBE ranges from 35 to 46.

5.7.3 Sample Size for In Vitro Bioequivalence Testing

In the nonprofile analysis for *in vitro* bioequivalence, the FDA requires that $m_k \geq 30$ canisters be sampled (see §5.6). Since $m_k = 30$ and $n_k = 1$ observation from each canister may not produce a test with sufficient power, Chow, Shao, and Wang (2001c) proposed a procedure for determining sample sizes $m = m_T = m_R$ and $n = n_T = n_R$, using the same technique in

Table 5.7.2. Sample Size n Selected Using (5.7.2) with $\beta = 80\%$ and the Power P_n of the PBE Test Based on 10,000 Simulations

	Parameter					$\rho = .75$		$\rho = 1$	
σ_{BT}	σ_{BR}	σ_{WT}	σ_{WR}	δ	λ	n	P_n	n	P_n
.1	.1	.1	.4	.4726	-.2233	37	.8447	36	.8337
				.4227	-.2679	24	.8448	24	.8567
				.2989	-.3573	12	.8959	12	.9035
				.0000	-.4466	7	.9863	7	.9868
.1	.4	.1	.1	.4726	-.2233	34	.8492	32	.8560
				.3660	-.3127	16	.8985	15	.8970
				.2113	-.4020	9	.9560	8	.9494
.1	.1	.4	.4	.2983	-.2076	44	.8123	43	.8069
				.1722	-.2670	23	.8381	23	.8337
				.0000	-.2966	17	.8502	17	.8531
.1	.4	.4	.4	.5323	-.4250	36	.8305	35	.8290
				.4610	-.4958	25	.8462	24	.8418
				.2661	-.6375	13	.8826	13	.8872
				.0000	-.7083	10	.9318	10	.9413
.1	.4	.6	.4	.3189	-.4066	39	.8253	38	.8131
				.2255	-.4575	29	.8358	28	.8273
				.0000	-.5083	22	.8484	22	.8562
.1	.4	.6	.6	.6503	-.6344	44	.8186	44	.8212
				.4598	-.8459	22	.8424	22	.8500
				.3252	-.9515	16	.8615	16	.8689
				.0000	-1.057	12	.8965	12	.9000
.4	.4	.1	.1	.3445	-.1779	37	.8447	22	.8983
				.2436	-.2373	20	.8801	12	.9461
				.1722	-.2670	15	.8951	9	.9609
				.0000	-.2966	12	.9252	7	.9853
.4	.4	.1	.4	.5915	-.3542	44	.8354	38	.8481
				.4610	-.4958	21	.8740	18	.8851
				.2661	-.6375	12	.9329	11	.9306
				.0000	-.7083	9	.9622	9	.9698
.4	.4	.6	.4	.0000	-.3583	46	.8171	43	.8213
.4	.4	.6	.6	.5217	-.6351	41	.8246	39	.8252
				.3012	-.8166	22	.8437	21	.8509
				.0000	-.9073	17	.8711	16	.8755
.4	.6	.4	.4	.6655	-.6644	33	.8374	30	.8570
				.5764	-.7751	23	.8499	21	.8709
				.3328	-.9965	13	.9062	12	.9258
				.0000	-1.107	10	.9393	9	.9488
.4	.6	.4	.6	.9100	-.8282	45	.8403	42	.8447
				.7049	-1.159	21	.8684	20	.8874
				.4070	-1.491	11	.9081	11	.9295
				.0000	-1.656	9	.9608	8	.9577
.6	.4	.1	.4	.3905	-.3558	41	.8334	32	.8494
				.3189	-.4066	30	.8413	24	.8649
				.2255	-.4575	23	.8584	18	.8822
				.0000	-.3583	17	.8661	14	.9009
.6	.4	.4	.4	.0000	-.3583	42	.8297	35	.8403
.6	.6	.1	.4	.7271	-.5286	47	.8335	36	.8584
				.5632	-.7401	23	.8785	18	.9046
				.3252	-.9515	13	.9221	10	.9474
				.0000	-1.057	10	.9476	8	.9780
.6	.6	.4	.4	.6024	-.5444	47	.8246	38	.8455
				.3012	-.8166	19	.8804	15	.8879
				.0000	-.9073	14	.8903	12	.9147

§5.7.1. Let $\psi = (\delta, \sigma^2_{BT}, \sigma^2_{BR}, \sigma^2_{WT}, \sigma^2_{WR})$ be the vector of unknown parameters under model (5.6.5). Let U be given in the definition of $\hat{\zeta}_U$ and U_β be the same as U but with 5% and 95% replaced by $1 - \beta$ and β, respectively, where β is a given power. Let $\tilde{U}$ and $\tilde{U}_\beta$ be U and U_β, respectively, with $(\hat{\delta}, s^2_{BT}, s^2_{BR}, s^2_{WT}, s^2_{WR})$ replaced by $\tilde{\psi}$, an initial guessing value for which the value of ζ (denoted by $\tilde{\zeta}$) is negative. From the results in Chow, Shao, and Wang (2001c), it is advangeous to have a large m and a small n when mn, the total number of observations for one treatment, is fixed. Thus, the sample sizes m and n can be determined as follows.

Step 1. Set $m = 30$ and $n = 1$. If

$$\tilde{\zeta} + \sqrt{\tilde{U}} + \sqrt{\tilde{U}_\beta} \leq 0 \qquad (5.7.3)$$

holds, stop and the required sample sizes are $m = 30$ and $n = 1$; otherwise, go to step 2.

Step 2. Let $n = 1$ and find a smallest integer m_* such that (5.7.3) holds. If $m_* \leq m_+$ (the largest possible number of canisters in a given problem), stop and the required sample sizes are $m = m_*$ and $n = 1$; otherwise, go to step 3.

Step 3. Let $m = m_+$ and find a smallest integer n_* such that (5.7.3) holds. The required sample sizes are $m = m_+$ and $n = n_*$.

If in practice it is much easier and inexpensive to obtain more replicates than to sample more canisters, then Steps 2-3 in the previous procedure can be replaced by

Step 2'. Let $m = 30$ and find a smallest integer n_* such that (5.7.3) holds. The required sample sizes are $m = 30$ and $n = n_*$.

Table 5.7.3 contains selected m_* and n_* according to Steps 1-3 or Steps 1 and 2' with $\beta = 80\%$ and the simulated power p of the *in vitro* bioequivalence test using these sample sizes.

Table 5.7.3. Selected Sample Sizes m_* and n_* and
the Actual Power p (10,000 Simulations)

σ_{BT}	σ_{BR}	σ_{WT}	σ_{WR}	δ	Step 1 p	Step 2 m_*,n_*	Step 2 p	Step 2' m_*,n_*	Step 2' p
0	0	.25	.25	.0530	.4893	55,1	.7658	30,2	.7886
				0	.5389	47,1	.7546	30,2	.8358
		.25	.50	.4108	.6391	45,1	.7973	30,2	.8872
				.2739	.9138	–	–	–	–
		.50	.50	.1061	.4957	55,1	.7643	30,2	.7875
				0	.5362	47,1	.7526	30,2	.8312
.25	.25	.25	.25	.0750	.4909	55,1	.7774	30,3	.7657
				0	.5348	47,1	.7533	30,2	.7323
		.25	.50	.4405	.5434	57,1	.7895	30,3	.8489
				.2937	.8370	–	–	–	–
		.50	.50	.1186	.4893	55,1	.7683	30,2	.7515
				0	.5332	47,1	.7535	30,2	.8091
.50	.25	.25	.50	.1186	.4903	55,1	.7660	30,4	.7586
				0	.5337	47,1	.7482	30,3	.7778
.25	.50	.25	.25	.2937	.8357	–	–	–	–
		.50	.25	.1186	.5016	55,1	.7717	30,4	.7764
				0	.5334	47,1	.7484	30,3	.7942
		.25	.50	.5809	.6416	45,1	.7882	30,2	.7884
				.3873	.9184	–	–	–	–
		.50	.50	.3464	.6766	38,1	.7741	30,2	.8661
				.1732	.8470	–	–	–	–
.50	.50	.25	.50	.3464	.6829	38,1	.7842	30,2	.8045
				.1732	.8450	–	–	–	–
		.50	.50	.1500	.4969	55,1	.7612	30,3	.7629
				0	.5406	47,1	.7534	30,2	.7270

In step 1, $m_* = 30$, $n_* = 1$.

Chapter 6

Randomization and Blinding

In drug development, the efficacy and safety of a study drug can only be established through the conduct of adequate and well-controlled clinical trials (see §1.2.5). For demonstration of the efficacy and safety of a study drug product, a typical approach is to show, based on results from clinical trials, that there is a significant difference between the study drug product and a control (e.g., a placebo or a standard therapy) with some statistical assurance, and that a clinically meaningful difference between the study drug and the placebo can be detected. *Randomization* plays an important role in the conduct of clinical trials. Randomization not only generates comparable groups of patients who constitute representative samples from the intended patient population, but also enable valid statistical tests for clinical evaluation of the study drug. Several randomization models are introduced in §6.1. Randomization methods for treatment assignment are discussed in §6.2. In §6.3, statistical justification for a rule of thumb for selection of the number of centers is provided. The effect of mixing up treatment assignment, a problem that is commonly encountered in practice, is studied in §6.4.

Clinical results may be directly or indirectly distorted when either the investigators or the patients know which treatment the patients receive, although randomization is applied to assign treatments. *Blinding* is commonly used to eliminate such a problem by blocking the identity of treatments. The concept of blinding is introduced in §6.5. Testing for the integrity of blinding is discussed in §6.6. The related issue of making statistical inference when the integrity of blinding is questionable is considered in §6.7.

147

6.1   Randomization Models

Randomization in clinical trials involves random recruitment of the patients from the targeted patient population and random assignment of patients to the treatments. For a valid statistical assessment of the efficacy and safety of a study drug, it is important that a representative sample of qualified patients be randomly selected from the targeted patient population. A qualified patient is referred to as a patient who meets the inclusion and exclusion criteria and has signed the informed consent form. Randomization avoids subjective selection bias for the integrity and scientific and/or statistical validity of the intended clinical trials. Patients participated in the clinical trials are randomly assigned to one of the treatments under study, which avoids subjective assignment of treatments. When there are heterogeneity in demographics and/or patient characteristics, randomization with blocking and/or stratification is helpful in removing the potential bias that might occur due to the differences in demographics and/or patient characteristics. Under randomization, statistical inference can be drawn under some probability distribution assumption of the intended patient population. The probability distribution assumption depends on the method of randomization under a randomization (population) model. A study without randomization will result in the violation of the probability distribution assumption and consequently no accurate and reliable statistical inference on the evaluation of the safety and efficacy of the study drug can be drawn.

In practice, the selection of patients may be performed under different principles of randomization. Lachin (1988a) provided a comprehensive summarization of randomization basis for statistical tests under various models, which are summarized in this section.

6.1.1   The Population Model

The concept for selecting a representative sample from a patient population by some random procedures for obtaining statistical inference by which clinicians can draw conclusions regarding the patient population is called the *population* model (Lehmann, 1975; Lachin, 1988a). Under the assumption of a homogeneous population, the clinical responses of all patients in the trial are independent and have the same distribution. Lachin (1988a) pointed out that the significance level and power will not be affected by random assignment of patients to the treatments as long as the patients in the trial represents a random sample from the homogeneous population. If we split a random sample into two subsamples, statistical inferential procedures are still valid even the first half patients are assigned to the study drug and the other half are assigned to a placebo.

6.1.2   The Invoked Population Model

When planning a clinical trial, we usually subjectively select investigators
first and then recruit/enroll qualified patients at each selected investigator's
site sequentially. As a result, neither the selection of investigators (or study
centers) nor the recruitment of patients is random. However, patients who
enter the trial are assigned to treatment groups at random. In practice,
the collected clinical data are usually analyzed as if they were obtained
under the assumption that the sample is randomly selected from a homogeneous patient population. Lachin (1988a) referred to this process as the
invoked population model because the population model is invoked as the
basis for statistical analysis as if a formal sampling procedure were actually
performed. In current practice, the invoked population model is commonly
employed in data analysis for most clinical trials. It should be noted, however, that the invoked population model is based on the assumption that is
inherently intestable.

6.1.3   The Randomization Model

For current practice, although the process for study site selection and patient recruitment is not random, the assignment of treatments to patients
is performed based on some random mechanism. Thus, treatment comparisons can be made based on the so-called randomization or permutation
tests. We will refer this process as the *randomization model.* Since the
statistical procedures based on the concept of permutation require the enumeration of all possible permutations, it is feasible only for small samples.
When the sample size increases, the probability distribution derived under
permutation will approach to a normal distribution according to the Central
Limit Theorem. Lachin (1988b) indicated that the probability distributions
for the family of linear rank statistics for large samples are equivalent to
those of the tests obtained under the assumption of the population model.
As a result, if patients are randomly assigned to the treatments, statistical
tests for evaluation of treatments should be based on permutation tests because the exact p-value can be easily calculated for small samples. For large
samples, the data can be analyzed by the methods derived under the population model as if the patients were randomly selected from a homogeneous
population.

6.2   Randomization Methods

In general, randomization methods for treatment assignment can be classified into three types according to the restriction of the randomization and

the change in probability for randomization with respect to the previous treatment assignments. These randomization methods include complete randomization, permuted-block randomization, and adaptive randomization. In what follows, we will describe these randomization methods and compare their relative merits and limitations whenever possible.

6.2.1   Complete Randomization

Simple randomization or complete randomization is the procedure in which no restrictions are enforced on the nature of the randomization sequence except for the number of patients required for achieving the desired statistical power and the ratio of patient allocation between treatments. For a clinical trial comparing a study drug with a placebo, the method of simple randomization is referred to as a completely binomial design (Blackwell and Hodges, 1957) or a simply complete randomization (Lachin, 1988b) if it has the properties of (i) the chance that a patient receives either the test drug or the placebo is 50% and (ii) randomization of assignments are performed independently for each patient. The randomization codes based on the method of complete randomization can be generated either by random numbers (Pocock, 1983) or by some statistical computing software such as SAS. However, it should be realized that a computer can not generate *true* random numbers but *pseudo* random numbers because only a fixed number of different long series of almost unpredictable permuted numbers are generated. Therefore, Lehmann (1975) recommended that a run test be performed to verify the randomness of the generated randomization codes.

6.2.2   Permuted-Block Randomization

One of the major disadvantages of simple randomization is that treatment imbalance may occur periodically. One resolution to this major disadvantage of simple randomization is to force balance of the number of patients assignment to each treatment periodically. In other words, we first divide the whole series of patients, who are to enroll into the trial, into blocks with appropriate (typically equal) blocking sizes. We then randomize the patients within each block to ensure that an equal number of patients will be assigned to each of the two treatment groups. For example, a blocking size of two guarantees that each treatment group will be assigned one patient for the first two patients enrolled into the study. A blocking size of four indicates that two patients of the first four patients who enter the study will be randomly assigned to each of the two treatment groups. This method of randomization is known as *permuted-block randomization*. Permuted-block randomization is probably the most frequently employed method for the assignment of patients to treatments in clinical trials.

Permuted-block randomization is in fact a stratified randomization. Therefore, a stratified analysis should be performed with blocks as strata to properly control the overall type I error rate and hence to provide the optimal power for detection of a possible treatment effect. In practice, the block effect is usually ignored when performing data analysis. Matts and Lachin (1988) showed that the test statistic ignoring the block is equal to 1 minus the intrablock correlation coefficient times the test statistic that takes the block into account. Since the patients within the same block are usually more homogeneous than those between blocks, the intrablock correlation coefficient is often positive. As a result, the tests which ignore block will produce more conservative results. However, since most clinical trials are multicenter studies with a moderate block size, it is not clear from their discussion whether a saturated model with factors treatment, center, and block and their corresponding two-factor and three-factor interactions should be included in the analysis of variance. It is also not clear whether the Mantel-Haenszel test and linear rank statistics based on permutation model are adequate for a complete combination of all levels of all strata with a very small number of patients in each stratum. In addition, when block size is large, there is a high possibility that a moderate number of patients fall in the last block at which the randomization codes are not entirely used up. If the trial is also stratified according to some covariates, the number of patients in such incomplete block will become quite sizable. Therefore, a stratified analysis will be quite complicated because of these incomplete blocks from all strata and possible presence of intrablock correlation coefficient.

A practical issue related to permuted-block randomization is the choice of block size. A small blocking size such as two may prevent treatment imbalance, but it may result in a high intra-block correlation coefficient and thus a large loss of power. Note that a smaller block size leads to a higher probability of guessing the treatment code right, which may decrease the reliability of blinding and consequently the integrity of the study (see §6.5-6.6).

6.2.3   Adaptive Randomization

In addition to permuted-block randomization, it is also of interest to adjust the probability of assignment of patients to treatments during the study. This type of randomization is called *adaptive randomization* because the probability for the assignment of current patients is adjusted based on the assignment of previous patients. Unlike other randomization methods described above, the randomization codes based on the method of adaptive randomization cannot be prepared before the conduct of the study. This is because that the randomization process is actually performed at the time when a patient is enrolled into the study and because adaptive randomization requires information about previous randomized patients. In clinical trials, the method of adaptive randomization is often applied with respect to treatment, covariate, or clinical response. Therefore, adaptive randomization is also known as the treatment adaptive randomization, the covariate adaptive randomization, or the response adaptive randomization. Treatment adaptive randomization has been discussed in literature by many researchers. See, for example, Efron (1971), Wei (1977, 1978), and Wei and Lachin (1988). The response adaptive randomization has also received much attention since introduced by Zelen (1969) (see, for example, Wei et al., 1990; Rosenburger and Lachin, 1993). More details regarding the covariate adaptive randomization can be found in Taves (1974), Pocock (1983), and Spilker (1991).

6.2.4   Discussion

In some situations, deliberate unequal allocation of patients between treatment groups may be desirable. For example, it may be of interest to allocate patients to the treatment and a control in a ratio of 2 to 1. Such situations include that (i) the patient population is small, (ii) previous experience with the study drug is limited, (iii) the response profile of the competitor is well known, and (iv) there are missing values and their rates depend on the treatment groups.

Randomization is a key element in the success of clinical trials intended to address scientific and/or medical questions. It, however, should be noted that in many situations, randomization may not be feasible in clinical research. For example, nonrandomized observational or case-controlled studies are often conducted to study the relationship between smoking and cancer. However, if the randomization is not used for some medical considerations, the FDA requires that statistical justification should be provided with respect to how systematic selection bias can be avoided.

6.3   The Number of Centers

An important practical issue in planning a multicenter trial is the determination of the number of centers used in the study and the number of patients in each selected center, when the total number of patients is fixed. For example, if the intended clinical trial calls for 100 patients, the sponsor may choose to have 5 centers with 20 patients in each, 10 centers with 10 patients in each, or 20 centers with 5 patients in each. This question, however, does not have a definite answer. It is desirable to utilize as many centers as possible to expedite patients' enrollment in order to complete the trials within a relatively short period of time. However, too many centers may decrease the power of statistical tests for treatment effects and may increase the chance of observing treatment imbalance and treatment-by-center interaction.

In the following we argue (in the viewpoint of randomization and statistical efficiency) that it is generally a good idea to keep the number of centers as small as possible.

Let the total number of patients be n. Consider for simplicity the case where all study centers have the same number of patients. Suppose that there are $a \geq 2$ treatments to be compared. Thus, $n = acm$, where c is the number of centers and m is the number of patients in each treatment group at each center. Let x_{ijk} be the response from the kth patient in the jth study center under treatment i, $\bar{x}_{ij.}$ be the sample mean of patients in center j under treatment i, $\bar{x}_{i..}$ be the sample mean of patients under treatment i, $\bar{x}_{.j.}$ be the sample mean of patients in center j, and $\bar{x}$ is the sample mean of all patients. Define

$$SS(T) = cm \sum_{i=1}^{a} (\bar{x}_{i..} - \bar{x})^2,$$

$$SS(C) = am \sum_{j=1}^{c} (\bar{x}_{.j.} - \bar{x})^2,$$

$$SS(TC) = m \sum_{i=1}^{a} \sum_{j=1}^{c} (\bar{x}_{ij.} - \bar{x}_{i..} - \bar{x}_{.j.} + \bar{x})^2,$$

and

$$SSE = \sum_{i=1}^{a} \sum_{j=1}^{c} \sum_{k=1}^{m} (x_{ijk} - \bar{x}_{ij.})^2.$$

A typical two-way balanced ANOVA table, which can be used to test effects from treatment, center, and treatment-by-center interaction, is given in Table 6.3.1.

If randomization is properly used so that the population model holds (see §6.1.1), then testing treatment effect can be done by using the fact that the F-ratio MS(T)/MSE in the ANOVA table has an F-distribution. As indicated earlier, however, in multicenter clinical trials the centers usually are not randomly selected, but based on convenience and availability. If selected patients are randomly assigned to treatment groups at each center, then the randomization model (see §6.1.2) holds and the distribution of the F-ratio MS(T)/MSE under the null hypothesis of no treatment difference can be obtained by enumeration of all possible permutations. This enumeration, however, is computationally difficult when the sample sizes are

Table 6.3.1. ANOVA Table for Treatment and Center Effects

Source	Sum of squares	Degrees of freedom	Mean squares	F-ratio
Treatment	SS(T)	$a-1$	$MS(T) = \frac{SS(C)}{a-1}$	$\frac{MS(T)}{MSE}$
Center	SS(C)	$c-1$	$MS(C) = \frac{SS(C)}{c-1}$	$\frac{MS(C)}{MSE}$
Interaction	SS(TC)	$(a-1)(c-1)$	$MS(TC) = \frac{SS(TC)}{(a-1)(c-1)}$	$\frac{MS(TC)}{MSE}$
Error	SSE	$n-ac$	$MSE = \frac{SSE}{n-ac}$	
Total	SS(TO)	$n-1$		

moderate and the center effect and/or treatment-by-center interaction are present. In practice, methods based on F-distributions (i.e., the population models) are still employed for convenience. This can be justified when the number of patients in each center is large (see §6.1.3). Thus, the violation of randomization in selecting study centers may have a substantial effect on statistical analysis based on F-distributions if there are many study centers and a relatively small number of patients at each center. Selecting a small number of centers may minimize the effect of the violation of randomization. A rule-of-thumb is that the number of patients in each center should not be less than the number of centers (Shao and Chow, 1993; Chow and Liu, 1998, p. 219). Furthermore, a smaller sample size at a study center leads to a higher chance for the investigator at the center to correctly guess the treatment code, which may result in a higher chance of distorting statistical analysis (see §6.5).

Suppose that the population model is approximately valid. For testing the treatment effect, the F-ratio MS(T)/MSE in the ANOVA table has the F-distribution with $a-1$ and $n-ac$ degrees of freedom. With a and n fixed, it follows that if testing treatment effect is the main concern, then the most efficient analysis can be achieved if c is at its smallest possible value (i.e., the F-distribution has the largest degrees of freedom).

A similar discussion can be made when the number of patients in each treatment group at each center varies, which results in a two-way unbalanced ANOVA.

6.4   Effect of Mixed-Up Treatment Codes

A problem commonly encountered during the conduct of a clinical trial is that a proportion of treatment codes are mixed-up in randomization schedules. Mixing up treatment codes can distort the statistical analysis based on the population or randomization model. In this section we make an attempt to quantatively study the effect of mixed-up treatment codes on the analysis based on the intention-to-treat (ITT) population.

Consider a two-group parallel design for comparing a test drug and a control (placebo), where n_1 patients are randomly assigned to the treatment group and n_2 patients are randomly assigned to the control group. When randomization is properly applied, the population model holds and responses from patients are normally distributed. Consider the simple case where two patient populations (treatment and control) have the same variance σ^2. Let μ_1 and μ_2 be the population means for the treatment and the control, respectively. The null hypothesis that $\mu_1 = \mu_2$ (i.e., there is no treatment effect) is rejected at the 5% level of significance if

$$T = \frac{|\bar{x}_1 - \bar{x}_2|}{\hat{\sigma}\sqrt{\frac{1}{n_1} + \frac{1}{n_2}}} > t_{0.975;n_1+n_2-2}, \tag{6.4.1}$$

where

$$\hat{\sigma}^2 = \frac{(n_1-1)s_1^2 + (n_2-1)s_2^2}{n_1+n_2-2},$$

$\bar{x}_1$ and s_1^2 are respectively the sample mean and variance of responses from patients in the treatment group, $\bar{x}_2$ and s_2^2 are respectively the sample mean and variance of responses from patients in the control group, and $t_{0.975;n_1+n_2-2}$ is the 97.5th percentile of the t-distribution with $n_1 + n_2 - 2$ degrees of freedom. The power of the test defined by (6.4.1), i.e., the probability of correctly detecting a treatment difference when $\mu_1 \neq \mu_2$, is

$$
\begin{aligned}
p(\theta) &= P\left(T > t_{0.975;n_1+n_2-2}\right) \\
&= 1 - \mathcal{T}_{n_1+n_2-2}(t_{0.975;n_1+n_2-2}|\theta) + \mathcal{T}_{n_1+n_2-2}(-t_{0.975;n_1+n_2-2}|\theta),
\end{aligned}
$$

where

$$\theta = \frac{\mu_1 - \mu_2}{\sigma\sqrt{\frac{1}{n_1} + \frac{1}{n_2}}}$$

and $\mathcal{T}_{n_1+n_2-2}(\cdot|\theta)$ is the noncentral t-distribution function with $n_1 + n_2 - 2$ degrees of freedom and the noncentrality parameter θ. This follows from the fact that under the population model, $\bar{x}_1 - \bar{x}_2$ has the normal distribution with mean $\mu_1 - \mu_2$ and variance $\sigma^2\left(\frac{1}{n_1} + \frac{1}{n_2}\right)$; $(n_1 + n_2 - 2)\hat{\sigma}^2$ has the chi-square distribution with $n_1 + n_2 - 2$ degrees of freedom, and $\bar{x}_1 - \bar{x}_2$ and $\hat{\sigma}^2$ are independent. When $n_1 + n_2$ is large,

$$p(\theta) \approx \Phi(\theta - 1.96) + \Phi(-\theta - 1.96),$$

where Φ is the standard normal distribution function.

Suppose that in each treatment group, patients independently have probability p to mix up their treatment codes. A straightforward calculation shows that the mean of $\bar{x}_1 - \bar{x}_2$ is

$$E(\bar{x}_1 - \bar{x}_2) = (1 - 2p)(\mu_1 - \mu_2)$$

and the variance of $\bar{x}_1 - \bar{x}_2$ is

$$\text{Var}(\bar{x}_1 - \bar{x}_2) = [\sigma^2 + p(1 - p)(\mu_1 - \mu_2)^2] \left(\frac{1}{n_1} + \frac{1}{n_2} \right).$$

Under the null hypothesis that $\mu_1 = \mu_2$, the distributions of $\bar{x}_1 - \bar{x}_2$ and $\hat{\sigma}^2$ are the same as those in the case of no mixed-up treatment codes and, hence, mixing up codes does not have any effect on the significance level of the test defined by (6.4.1). When $\mu_1 \neq \mu_2$ and $p > 0$, $\bar{x}_1 - \bar{x}_2$ is no longer normally distributed but is approximately normal when both n_1 and n_2 are large. Also, $\hat{\sigma}^2$ is a consistent estimator of $\sigma^2 + p(1 - p)(\mu_1 - \mu_2)^2$ when $n_i \to \infty$, $i = 1, 2$. Thus, the power of the test defined by (6.4.1) is approximately

$$p(\theta_m) = \Phi(\theta_m - 1.96) + \Phi(-\theta_m - 1.96), \qquad (6.4.2)$$

where

$$\theta_m = \frac{(1 - 2p)(\mu_1 - \mu_2)}{\sqrt{[\sigma^2 + p(1 - p)(\mu_1 - \mu_2)^2] \left(\frac{1}{n_1} + \frac{1}{n_2} \right)}}$$

$$= \frac{(1 - 2p)\theta}{\sqrt{1 + \frac{p(1-p)(\mu_1 - \mu_2)^2}{\sigma^2}}}$$

$$= \frac{(1 - 2p)\theta}{\sqrt{1 + p(1 - p)\theta^2 \left(\frac{1}{n_1} + \frac{1}{n_2} \right)}}$$

(assuming that $0 < p < 0.5$). Note that $\theta_m = \theta$ if $p = 0$, i.e., there is no mixed-up treatment codes.

The effect of mixed-up treatment codes can be measured by comparing $p(\theta)$ with $p(\theta_m)$. Suppose that $n_1 = n_2 = 100$ and, when there is no mixed-up treatment codes, $p(\theta) = 80\%$, which gives that $|\mu_1 - \mu_2|/\sigma = 0.397$ and $|\theta| = 2.81$. When 5% of treatment codes are mixed up, i.e., $p = 5\%$, $p(\theta_m) = 71.23\%$. When $p = 10\%$, $p(\theta_m) = 60.68\%$. Hence, a small proportion of mixed-up treatment codes may seriously affect the probability of detecting treatment effect when such an effect exists. The effect of mixed-up treatment codes is higher when n_1 and n_2 are not large. Table 6.4.1 lists simulation approximations to the values of power of the test defined by (6.4.1) when $n_1 = n_2 = n_0$ is 10, 15, 20, or 30 and $p = 1\%$, 3%, 5%, or 10%. It can be seen that when $n_0 \leq 30$, the actual power is substantially lower than that given by formula (6.4.2) with $n_0 = 100$.

When $n_1 = n_2 = n_0$ is large, we may plan ahead to ensure a desired power when the maximum proportion of mixed-up treatment codes is known. Assume that the maximum proportion of mixed-up treatment codes is p and the desired power is 80%, i.e., $|\theta| = 2.81$. Let n_w be the sample size for which the power is equal to 80% when there are 5% of mixed-up treatment codes. Then

$$\frac{(1 - 2p)\left|\frac{\mu_1 - \mu_2}{\sigma}\right|\sqrt{\frac{n_w}{2}}}{\sqrt{1 + p(1 - p)\left|\frac{\mu_1 - \mu_2}{\sigma}\right|^2}} = \left|\frac{\mu_1 - \mu_2}{\sigma}\right|\sqrt{\frac{n_0}{2}},$$

which is the same as

$$(1 - 2p)^2 n_w = n_0\left[1 + p(1 - p)\left|\frac{\mu_1 - \mu_2}{\sigma}\right|^2\right]$$

$$= n_0 + 2p(1 - p)\theta^2.$$

Therefore,

$$n_w = \frac{n_0}{(1 - 2p)^2} + \frac{2p(1 - p)\theta^2}{(1 - 2p)^2}$$

will maintain the desired power when the proportion of mixed-up treatment codes is no larger than p. For example, if $p = 5\%$ and 80% power is desired, then $\theta^2 = 2.81^2$ and $n_w = 1.235 n_0 + 1.026$. Hence, $n_w = 1.24 n_0$, i.e., a 24% increase of the sample size will offset a 5% mix-up in randomization schedules.

Table 6.4.1. Power of the Two-Sample t-Test
Approximated by Monte Carlo of Size 10,000

n_0	$\frac{\mu_1 - \mu_2}{\sigma}$	θ	p in %				
			0	1	3	5	10
10	1.26	2.81	0.7584	0.7372	0.6844	0.6359	0.5156
	1.45	3.24	0.8671	0.8490	0.8015	0.7410	0.6120
15	1.03	2.81	0.7727	0.7518	0.7052	0.6650	0.5449
	1.19	3.24	0.8751	0.8647	0.8261	0.7818	0.6602
20	0.89	2.81	0.7828	0.7649	0.7170	0.6796	0.5619
	1.03	3.24	0.8903	0.8549	0.8378	0.7918	0.6762
30	0.73	2.81	0.7892	0.7747	0.7429	0.7032	0.5834
	0.84	3.24	0.8945	0.8791	0.8423	0.8101	0.6963

When n_1 and n_2 are small, it is difficult to estimate a new sample size to ensure a desired power even when the maximum proportion of mixed-up treatment codes is known. A simulation study may be helpful. For example, suppose that $n_1 = n_2 = n_0 = 10$ and $(\mu_1 - \mu_2)/\sigma = 1.26$, which results in a power of 75.84% when $p = 0$ (Table 6.4.1). If $p = 5\%$, then the power is 63.59%. According to the results in Table 6.4.1, the power is 74.1% when $p = 5\%$ and $\theta = 3.24$. Hence, we need to increase the sample size so that $\theta = 3.24$ in order to ensure a power comparable to the original power 75.84%, i.e., the new sample size should be $n_w = 2(3.24/1.26)^2 = 13.22$. Thus, a recommended new sample size is $n_1 = n_2 = 14$.

6.5   Blinding

Although randomization is used to prevent bias from a statistical assessment of the study drug, it does not guarantee that there will be no bias caused by subjective judgment in reporting, evaluation, data processing, and statistical analysis due to the knowledge of the identity of the treatments. Since this subjective and judgmental bias is directly or indirectly related to treatment, it can seriously distort statistical inference on the treatment effect. In practice, it is extremely difficult to quantitatively assess such bias and its impact on the assessment of the treatment effect. In clinical trials, it is therefore important to consider an approach to eliminate such bias by blocking the identity of treatments. Such an approach is referred to as blinding.

Basically, blinding in clinical trials can be classified into four types: open-label, single-blind, double-blind, and triple-blind (Chow and Liu, 1998). An open-label study is a clinical trial in which no blinding is employed; that is, both the investigators and the patients know which treatment the patients receive. Since patients may psychologically react in favor of the treatments they receive if they are aware of which treatment they receive, serious bias may occur. Therefore, open-label trials are generally not recommended for comparative clinical trials. In current practice, open-label trials are not accepted as adequate well-controlled clinical trials for providing substantial evidence for approval by most regulatory agencies including the FDA. However, under certain circumstances, open-label trials are necessarily conducted. Spilker (1991) provided a list of situations and circumstances in which open-label trials may be conducted. Ethical consideration is always an important factor, or perhaps the only factor that is used to determine whether a trial should be conducted in an open-label fashion. For example, phase I dose-escalating studies for determination of the maximum tolerable dose of drugs in treating terminally ill cancer patients are usually open-labelled. Clinical trials for evaluation of the effectiveness and safety of a new surgical procedure are usually conducted in an open-label fashion because it is clearly unethical to conduct a double-blind trial with a concurrent control group in which patients are incised under a general anesthesia to simulate a surgical procedure. Note that premarketing and postmarketing surveillance studies are usually open-labelled. The purpose of premarketing surveillance studies is to collect the data of efficacy and safety with respect to the duration of exposure of a broader patient population to the test drug, while the objective of postmarketing surveillance studies is to monitor the safety and tolerability of the drug product.

In practice, a single-blind trial is referred to as a trail in which only the patient is unaware of his or her treatment assignment. As compared with open-label trials, single-blind studies offer a certain degree of control and the assurance of the validity of clinical trials. However, the investigator may bias his or her clinical evaluation by knowing which treatment the patients receive.

A double-blind trial is a trial in which neither the patients nor the investigators (study centers) are aware of patients' treatment assignments. Note that the *investigator* could mean all of the health care personnel involved, including the study center, contract laboratories, and other consulting experts for evaluation of effectiveness and safety of patients in a broader sense. In addition to the patients and the investigators, if all members of clinical project team associated with the study are also blinded, then the clinical trial is said to be triple-blinded. These members include the project clinicians, clinical research associates (CRA), statisticians, programmers, and data coordinators. In addition to patients' treatment assignments, the blindness also applies to concealment of the overall results of the trial. In practice, although the project clinicians, CRA, statisticians, programmers, and data coordinators usually have access to an individual patient's data, they are generally not aware of the treatment assignment for each patient. In addition, the overall treatment results, if any (such as interim analyses), will not be made available to the patients, the investigators, the project clinicians, CRA, statisticians, programmers, and data coordinators until a decision is made at an appropriate time. A triple-blind study with respect to blindness can provide the highest degree of validity for a controlled clinical trial. Hence, it provides the most conclusive unbiased evidence for the evaluation of the effectiveness and safety of the therapeutic intervention under investigation.

Note that a triple-blinding is generally reserved for large cooperative, multicenter studies monitored by a committee; however, it has been applied to company monitors to ensure that they remain unaware of treatment allocation. For current practice, double-blinding has become the gold standard for clinical research since it provides the greatest probability for reducing bias.

6.6   The Integrity of Blinding

In practice, even with the best intention for preserving blindness throughout a clinical trial, blindness can sometimes be breached for various reasons.
One method to determine whether the blindness is seriously violated is to
ask patients to guess their treatment codes during the study or at the conclusion of the trial prior to unblinding. In some cases, investigators are also
asked to guess patients' treatment codes. Once the guesses are recorded on
the case report forms and entered into the database, the integrity of blinding can be tested. When the integrity of blinding is doubtful, adjustments
to statistical analysis should be made (see §6.7).

Data on guessing treatment codes are typically of the form given in
Tables 6.6.1 and 6.6.2 in the following two examples.

The first example is a one-year double-blind placebo-controlled study
conducted by the National Institutes of Health (NIH) to evaluate the difference between the prophylactic and the therapeutic effects of ascorbic acid
for the common cold (Karlowski et al., 1975). A two-group parallel design
was used. At the completion of the study, a questionnaire was distributed
to everyone enrolled in the study so that they could guess which treatment
they had been taking. Results from the 190 subjects who completed the
study are given in Table 6.6.1.

The second example is a double-blind placebo-controlled trial with a
two-group parallel design for evaluation of the effectiveness of an appetite
suppressant in weight loss in obese women (Brownell and Stunkard, 1982).
Table 6.6.2 lists the data on patients' guesses of the treatment codes.

To test the integrity of blinding we need to define a null hypothesis
H_0. Consider a single-site parallel design comparing $a \geq 2$ treatments.
Let A_i be the event that a patient guesses that he/she is in the ith group,
$i = 1, ..., a$, A_{a+1} be the event that a patient does not guess (or answers
"do not know"), and B_j be the event that a patient is assigned to the jth
group, $j = 1, ..., a$. If the hypothesis

$$H_0 : A_i \text{ and } B_j \text{ are independent for any } i \text{ and } j$$

holds, then the blindness is considered to be preserved. The hypothesis
H_0 can be tested using the well-known Pearson's chi-square test under the
contingency tables constructed based on observed counts such as those given
by Tables 6.6.1 and 6.6.2. Analysis on investigators' guesses of patients'
treatment codes can be performed similarly.

A straightforward calculation using data in Tables 6.6.1 and 6.6.2 results
in observed Pearson's chi-square statistics 31.3 and 22.5, respectively. Thus,
the null hypothesis of independence of A_i and B_j is rejected at a very high

Table 6.6.1. Observed Number of Patients on
Treatment for the Prophylactic Use

	Actual assignment	
Patient's guess	Ascorbic acid	Placebo
Ascorbic acid	40	11
Placebo	12	39
Do not know	49	39
Total	101	89

Source: Karlowski et al. (1975)

Table 6.6.2. Observed Number of Patients on
Treatment for Weight Loss

	Actual assignment	
Patient's guess	Active drug	Placebo
Active drug	19	3
Placebo	3	16
Do not know	2	6
Total	24	25

Source: Brownell and Stunkard (1982)

significance level (the p-values are smaller than 0.001). That is, in both examples the blindness is not preserved.

6.7 Analysis Under Breached Blindness

When the test of the integrity of blinding in §6.6 resulted in a significant result (i.e., the integrity of blinding is doubtful), analyzing data by ignoring this result may lead to a biased result. In this section we introduce a method of testing treatment effects by incorporating the data of patients' guesses of their treatment codes (Chow and Shao, 2001b). The idea is to include the patient's guess as a factor in the analysis of variance (ANOVA) for the treatment effects.

Suppose that the study design is a single-site parallel design comparing $a \geq 2$ treatments. If the blindness is preserved, then treatment effects can be tested using the one-way ANOVA. Let γ be the factor of guessing treatment codes, which has b levels. Including factor γ in the analysis with patients' guessing data and assuming that patients' guessing is independent of their response value, we can test treatment effects by using a two-way ANOVA. If the study is a multicenter trial, then including factor γ leads to a three-way ANOVA.

There are different ways to construct the variable γ. One way is to use guessing treatment i, $i = 1, ..., a$, as the first a levels of γ and not guessing (do not know) as the last level. Hence, $b = a + 1$. Another way is to use guessing correctly, guessing incorrectly, and not guessing as three levels for γ and, thus, $b = 3$.

Even if the original design is balanced, i.e., each treatment (and center) has the same number of patients, the two-way ANOVA or three-way ANOVA after including factor γ is not balanced. Hence, methods for unbalanced ANOVA are necessarily considered. In the following we illustrate the idea using a single study site (i.e., two-way ANOVA).

Let x_{ijk} be the response from the kth patient under the ith treatment with the jth guessing status, where $i = 1, ..., a$, $j = 1, ..., b$, $k = 1, ..., n_{ij}$, and n_{ij} is the number of patients in the (i,j)th cell. Let $\bar{x}_{ij.}$ be the sample mean of the patients in the (i,j)th cell, $\bar{x}_{i..}$ be the sample mean of the patients under treatment i, $\bar{x}_{.j.}$ be the sample mean of patients with guessing status j, $\bar{x}$ be the sample mean of all patients, $n_{i.}$ be the number of patients under treatment i, $n_{.j}$ be the number of patients with guessing status j, and n be the total number of patients. Define

$$R(\mu) = n\bar{x}^2,$$

$$R(\mu, \tau) = \sum_{i=1}^{a} n_{i.} \bar{x}_{i..}^2$$

(where τ denotes treatment effect and μ denotes the overall mean),

$$R(\mu, \gamma) = \sum_{j=1}^{b} n_{.j} \bar{x}_{.j.}^2,$$

$$R(\mu, \tau, \gamma, \tau \times \gamma) = \sum_{i=1}^{a} \sum_{j=1}^{b} n_{ij} \bar{x}_{ij.}^2$$

(where $\tau \times \gamma$ denotes the interaction between τ and γ), and

$$R(\mu, \tau, \gamma) = \sum_{i=1}^{a} n_{i.} \bar{x}_{i..}^2 + Z'C^{-1}Z,$$

where Z is a $(b-1)$-vector whose jth component is

$$n_{.j}\bar{x}_{.j.} - \sum_{i=1}^{a} n_{ij}\bar{x}_{i..}, \quad j = 1, ..., b-1$$

and C is a $(b-1) \times (b-1)$ matrix whose jth diagonal element is

$$n_{.j} - \sum_{i=1}^{a} n_{ij}^2/n_{i.}$$

and (j,l)th off-diagonal element is

$$-\sum_{i=1}^{a} n_{ij} n_{il}/n_{i..}$$

Let

$$R(\tau \times \gamma | \mu, \tau, \gamma) = R(\mu, \tau, \gamma, \tau \times \gamma) - R(\mu, \tau, \gamma),$$

$$R(\tau | \mu) = R(\mu, \tau) - R(\mu),$$

$$R(\gamma | \mu) = R(\mu, \gamma) - R(\mu),$$

$$R(\tau | \mu, \gamma) = R(\mu, \tau, \gamma) - R(\mu, \gamma),$$

$$R(\gamma | \mu, \tau) = R(\mu, \tau, \gamma) - R(\mu, \tau),$$

$$\text{SSE} = \sum_{i=1}^{a} \sum_{j=1}^{3} \sum_{k=1}^{n_{ij}} x_{ijk}^2 - R(\mu, \tau, \gamma, \tau \times \gamma),$$

and s be the number of nonzero n_{ij}'s. An ANOVA table according to Searle (1971, Chapter 7) can be constructed (Table 6.7.1).

Table 6.7.1. ANOVA for Treatment Effects Under Breached Blindness

Source	Sum of squares	Degrees of freedom	F-ratio
τ after μ	$R(\tau\|\mu)$	$a-1$	$F(\tau\|\mu) = \frac{R(\tau\|\mu)/(a-1)}{\text{SSE}/(n-s)}$
γ after μ and τ	$R(\gamma\|\mu,\tau)$	$b-1$	$F(\gamma\|\mu,\tau) = \frac{R(\gamma\|\mu,\tau)/(b-1)}{\text{SSE}/(n-s)}$
γ after μ	$R(\gamma\|\mu)$	$b-1$	$F(\gamma\|\mu) = \frac{R(\gamma\|\mu)/(b-1)}{\text{SSE}/(n-s)}$
τ after μ and γ	$R(\tau\|\mu,\gamma)$	$a-1$	$F(\tau\|\mu,\gamma) = \frac{R(\tau\|\mu,\gamma)/(a-1)}{\text{SSE}/(n-s)}$
Interaction	$R(\tau\times\gamma\|\mu,\tau,\gamma)$	$s-a-b+1$	$F(\tau\times\gamma\|\mu,\tau,\gamma)$
			$= \frac{R(\tau\times\gamma\|\mu,\tau,\gamma)/(s-a-b+1)}{\text{SSE}/(n-s)}$
Error	SSE	$n-s$	
Total	SS(TO)	$n-1$	

An F-ratio (in the last column of Table 6.7.1) is said to be significant at level α if it is larger than the $(1 - \alpha)$th quantile of the F-distribution with denominator degrees of freedom $n - s$ and the numerator degrees of freedom given by the number in the third column of the same row. Note that $F(\tau|\mu)$ is the F-ratio for testing τ-effect (treatment effect) adjusted for μ and ignoring γ, whereas $F(\tau|\mu,\gamma)$ is the F-ratio for testing τ-effect adjusted for both μ and γ. These two F-ratios are the same in a balanced model but are different in an unbalanced model. Similar discussion can be made for $F(\gamma|\mu)$ and $F(\gamma|\mu,\tau)$.

Because of its imbalance, the interpretation of the results given by F-ratios in the ANOVA table is not straightforward. Consider first the case where the interaction $F(\tau \times \gamma|\mu,\tau,\gamma)$ is not significant. Table 6.7.2 lists a total of 14 possible cases according to the significance of F-ratios $F(\tau|\mu)$, $F(\tau|\mu,\gamma)$, $F(\gamma|\mu)$, and $F(\gamma|\mu,\tau)$. The suggestion from Searle (1971, Chapter 7) regarding which effects should be included in the model is given in the second last column of Table 6.7.2. However, our purpose is slightly different, i.e., we are interested in whether the treatment effect τ is significant regardless of the presence of the effect γ. Our recommendations in these 14 cases are given in the last column of Table 6.7.2, which is

Table 6.7.2. Conclusions on the Significance of the Treatment Effect
When $F(\tau \times \gamma|\mu,\tau,\gamma)$ is Insignificant

Significance of F-ratio				Effects to be included in the model (Searle, 1971)	Conclusion: significance of the treatment effect
Fitting τ and then γ after τ		Fitting γ and then τ after γ			
$F(\tau|\mu)$	$F(\gamma|\mu,\tau)$	$F(\gamma|\mu)$	$F(\tau|\mu,\gamma)$		
Yes	Yes	Yes	Yes	τ, γ	Yes
Yes	Yes	No	Yes	τ, γ	Yes
Yes	No	Yes	Yes	τ	Yes
Yes	No	No	Yes	τ	Yes
No	Yes	Yes	Yes	τ, γ	Yes
No	Yes	No	Yes	τ, γ	Yes
No	No	No	Yes	τ, γ	Yes
No	Yes	Yes	No	γ	No
No	No	Yes	No	γ	No
Yes	Yes	Yes	No	γ	No
Yes	No	Yes	No	τ, γ	No
Yes	No	No	No	τ	Yes
No	Yes	No	No	τ, γ	No
No	No	No	No	None	No

interpreted as follows. When both $F(\tau|\mu)$ and $F(\tau|\mu,\gamma)$ are significant (the first 4 rows of Table 6.7.2), regardless of whether γ-effect is significant or not, the conclusion is easy to make, i.e., the treatment effect is significant. In the next three cases (rows 5-7 of Table 6.7.2), $F(\tau|\mu)$ is not significant but $F(\tau|\mu,\gamma)$ is significant, indicating that the treatment effect cannot be clearly detected by ignoring γ but once γ is included in the model as a blocking variable, the treatment effect is significant. In these three cases we conclude that the treatment effect is significant. When $F(\tau|\mu,\gamma)$ is not significant but $F(\gamma|\mu)$ is significant, it indicates that once γ is fitted into the model, the treatment effect is not significant, i.e., the treatment effect is distorted by the γ-effect. In such cases (rows 8-11 in Table 6.7.2), we can not conclude that the treatment effect is significant. In the last three cases (rows 12-14 of Table 6.7.2), both $F(\gamma|\mu)$ and $F(\tau|\mu,\gamma)$ are not significant. If $F(\tau|\mu)$ is significant but $F(\gamma|\mu,\tau)$ is not (row 12 of Table 6.7.2), it indicates that γ has no effect and the treatment effect is significant. On the other hand, if $F(\gamma|\mu,\tau)$ is significant but $F(\tau|\mu)$ is not (row 13 of Table 6.7.2; a case "should happen somewhat infrequently" according to Searle, 1971), we can not conclude that the treatment effect is significant. Finally, when neither $F(\tau|\mu)$ nor $F(\gamma|\mu,\tau)$ is significant, then neither treatment effect nor γ-effect is significant (row 14 of Table 6.7.2).

The analysis is difficult when the interaction $F(\tau \times \gamma|\mu,\tau,\gamma)$ is significant. In general, we can not conclude that the treatment effect is significant when $F(\tau \times \gamma|\mu,\tau,\gamma)$ is significant. Analysis conditional on the value of γ may be carried out to draw some partial conclusions. An illustration is given in Example 6.7.1.

Example 6.7.1. Observed mean weight loss (kg) in the problem of the effectiveness of an appetite suppressant in weight loss in obese women (Brownell and Stunkard, 1982) is shown in Table 6.7.3. Recall that the analysis in §6.6 shows that in this example, the blindness is not preserved with a high significance.

Table 6.7.3. Mean Weight Loss (kg) in Example 6.7.1

	Actual assignment	
Patient's guess	Active drug	Placebo
Active drug	9.6	2.6
Placebo	3.9	6.1
Do not know	12.2	5.8
Total	9.1	5.6

Source: Brownell and Stunkard (1982)

First, consider the analysis with γ = guessing correctly, guessing incorrectly, and not guessing. Then,

$$
\begin{array}{llll}
\bar{x}_{11.} = 9.6, & n_{11} = 19, & \bar{x}_{21.} = 6.1, & n_{21} = 16, \\
\bar{x}_{12.} = 3.9, & n_{12} = 3, & \bar{x}_{22.} = 2.6, & n_{22} = 3, \\
\bar{x}_{13.} = 12.2, & n_{13} = 2, & \bar{x}_{23.} = 5.8, & n_{23} = 6, \\
\bar{x}_{1..} = 9.1, & n_{1.} = 24, & \bar{x}_{.1.} = 8.0, & n_{.1} = 35, \\
\bar{x}_{2..} = 5.6, & n_{2.} = 25, & \bar{x}_{.2.} = 3.3, & n_{.2} = 6, \\
\bar{x} = 7.3, & n = 49, & \bar{x}_{.3.} = 7.4, & n_{.3} = 8.
\end{array}
$$

The resulting ANOVA table (see Table 6.7.1) is given by

Source	R	df	R/df	F-ratio	p-value
τ after μ	$R(\tau\|\mu)$	1	160.2	6.43	0.015
γ after μ and τ	$R(\gamma\|\mu,\tau)$	2	72.1	2.90	0.066
γ after μ	$R(\gamma\|\mu)$	2	32.6	1.31	0.280
τ after μ and γ	$R(\tau\|\mu,\gamma)$	1	115.2	4.63	0.037
Interaction	$R(\tau\times\gamma\|\mu,\tau,\gamma)$	2	12.6	0.51	0.604
Error	SSE	43	24.9		

It seems that the interaction $F(\tau \times \gamma|\mu,\tau,\gamma)$ is not significant and both treatment effect F-ratios $F(\tau|\mu)$ and $F(\tau|\mu,\gamma)$ are significant. Thus, according to the previous discussion (see Table 6.7.2), we can conclude that the treatment effect is significant, regardless of whether the effect of γ is significant or not.

However, the conclusion may be different if we consider the levels of γ to be guessing active drug, guessing placebo, and not guessing. With this choice of levels of γ, the sample means are given by

$$
\begin{array}{llll}
\bar{x}_{11.} = 9.6, & n_{11} = 19, & \bar{x}_{21.} = 2.6, & n_{21} = 3, \\
\bar{x}_{12.} = 3.9, & n_{12} = 3, & \bar{x}_{22.} = 6.1, & n_{22} = 16, \\
\bar{x}_{13.} = 12.2, & n_{13} = 2, & \bar{x}_{23.} = 5.8, & n_{23} = 6, \\
\bar{x}_{1..} = 9.1, & n_{1.} = 24, & \bar{x}_{.1.} = 8.7, & n_{.1} = 22, \\
\bar{x}_{2..} = 5.6, & n_{2.} = 25, & \bar{x}_{.2.} = 5.7, & n_{.2} = 19, \\
\bar{x} = 7.3, & n = 49, & \bar{x}_{.3.} = 7.4, & n_{.3} = 8.
\end{array}
$$

Note that $\bar{x}_{1i.}$ are unchanged but $\bar{x}_{2j.}$ are changed with this new choice of levels of γ. The corresponding ANOVA table is given by

Source	R	df	R/df	F-ratio	p-value
τ after μ	$R(\tau\|\mu)$	1	160.2	6.43	0.015
γ after μ and τ	$R(\gamma\|\mu,\tau)$	2	47.2	1.90	0.162
γ after μ	$R(\gamma\|\mu)$	2	41.9	1.68	0.198
τ after μ and γ	$R(\tau\|\mu,\gamma)$	1	17.9	0.72	0.401
Interaction	$R(\tau{\times}\gamma\|\mu,\tau,\gamma)$	2	61.3	2.46	0.097
Error	SSE	43	24.9		

Although $F(\tau|\mu)$ remains the same, the value of $F(\tau \times \gamma|\mu,\tau,\gamma)$ is much larger than that in the previous case. The p-value corresponding to $F(\tau \times \gamma|\mu,\tau,\gamma)$ is 0.097, which indicates that the interaction between the treatment and γ is marginally significant. If this interaction is ignored, then we may conclude that the treatment effect is significant, since the only significant F-ratio is $F(\tau|\mu)$. But no conclusion can be made if the interaction effect can not be ignored. In the presence of interaction, a subgroup analysis (according to the levels of γ) may be useful.

Subgroup sample mean comparisons can be made as indicated by Figure 6.7.1. Figure 6.7.1 displays six subgroup sample means $\bar{x}_{ij}.$, $i = 1, 2$, $j = 1, 2, 3$. Part (A) of Figure 6.7.1 considers the situation where $\gamma =$ guessing correctly, guessing incorrectly, and not guessing, while part (B) of Figure 6.7.1 considers the situation where $\gamma =$ guessing active drug, guessing placebo, and not guessing. The two sample means (dots) corresponding to the same γ level are connected by a straight line segment. In part (A) of the figure, although the three line segments have different slopes, the slopes have the same sign; furthermore, every pair of two line segments either does not cross or crosses slightly. This indicates that in the situation considered by part (A) of the figure, there is no significant interaction (see also the discussion in §10.1.4) and the treatment effect is evident. On the other hand, the slopes of the line segments in part (B) of Figure 6.7.1 have different signs and two line segments cross considerably, which indicates that interaction is significant and we cannot draw an overall conclusion on the treatment effect in the situation considered by part (B) of the figure.

(A)

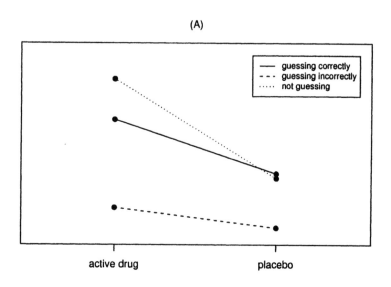

(B)

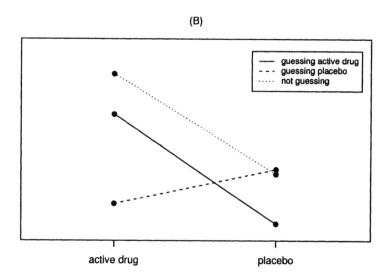

Figure 6.7.1. Subgroup Sample Mean Comparison

Chapter 7

Substantial Evidence in Clinical Development

For marketing approval of a new drug product, the FDA requires that at least two adequate and well-controlled clinical trials be conducted to provide substantial evidence regarding the effectiveness of the drug product under investigation (FDA, 1988). However, under certain circumstances, the FDA Modernization Act (FDAMA) of 1997 includes a provision (Section 115 of FDAMA) to allow data from one adequate and well-controlled clinical trial investigation and confirmatory evidence to establish effectiveness for risk/benefit assessment of drug and biological candidates for approval. The purpose of requiring at least two clinical studies is not only to assure the *reproducibility* but also to provide valuable information regarding *generalizability*. Reproducibility is referred to as whether the clinical results are reproducible from location (e.g., study site) to location within the same region or from region to region, while generalizability is referred to as whether the clinical results can be generalized to other similar patient populations within the same region or from region to region. When the sponsor of a newly developed or approved drug product is interested in getting the drug product into the marketplace from one region (e.g., where the drug product is developed and approved) to another region, it is a concern that differences in ethnic factors could alter the efficacy and safety of the drug product in the new region. As a result, it is recommended that a bridging study be conducted to generate a limited amount of clinical data in the new region in order to extrapolate the clinical data between the two regions (ICH, 1998a).

In practice, it is often of interest to determine whether a clinical trial that produced positive clinical results provides substantial evidence to assure reproducibility and generalizability of the clinical results. In this chapter, the reproducibility of a positive clinical result is studied by evaluating the probability of observing a positive result in a future clinical study with the same study protocol, given that a positive clinical result has been observed. The generalizability of clinical results observed from a clinical trial will be evaluated by means of a sensitivity analysis with respect to changes in mean and standard deviation of the primary clinical endpoints of the study.

In §7.1, the concept of reproducibility probability of a positive clinical result is introduced. Three different approaches of evaluating the reproducibility probability, the estimated power approach, the confidence bound approach, and the Bayesian approach, are discussed in §7.2-7.4, respectively. Applications and extensions of the derived results are discussed in §7.5. For example, if the reproducibility probability is high (e.g., 95%) with some statistical assurance based on the results from the first clinical trial, then it may not be necessary to require the sponsor to conduct the second clinical trial. The problem of sample size determination for the second trial is also discussed. Finally, the concept of generalizability probability of a positive clinical result is introduced in §7.6.

7.1 Reproducibility Probability

Throughout this chapter we consider adequate and well-controlled clinical trials (see §1.2.5). Let H_0 be the null hypothesis that the mean response of the drug product is the same as the mean response of a control (e.g., placebo). When H_0 is concluded, the drug product is considered to be not effective. Let T be the test statistic based on the responses from a clinical trial. The clinical trial produces a positive clinical result if the observed value of T leads to the rejection of the null hypothesis H_0.

Let H_1 be the alternative hypothesis that H_0 is not true. Suppose that the null hypothesis H_0 is rejected if and only if $|T| > c$, where c is a positive known constant. This is usually related to a two-sided alternative hypothesis. The discussion for one-sided alternative hypotheses is similar. In statistical theory, the probability of observing a positive clinical result when H_1 is indeed true, which is commonly denoted by

$$P(|T| > c|H_1), \qquad (7.1.1)$$

is referred to as the power of the test procedure. Typically the power is a function of unknown parameters.

Consider two independent clinical trials of the same study protocol and sample size. The power for each trial is given by (7.1.1), whereas the probability that *both* trials yield positive results when H_1 is true is

$$[P(|T| > c|H_1)]^2,$$

since the two trials are independent. For example, if the power for a single study is 80%, then the probability of observing two positive clinical results when H_1 is true is $(80\%)^2 = 64\%$.

Suppose now that one clinical trial was conducted and the result is positive. What is the probability that the second trial will produce a positive result, i.e., the positive result from the first trial is reproducible? Mathematically, since the two trials are independent, the probability of observing a positive result in the second trial when H_1 is true is still given by (7.1.1), regardless of whether the result from the first trial is positive or not. However, information from the first clinical trial should be useful in the evaluation of the probability of observing a positive result in the second trial. This leads to the concept of reproducibility probability, which is different from the power defined by (7.1.1).

In general, the reproducibility probability is a person's subjective probability of observing a positive clinical result from the second trial, when he/she observes a positive result from the first trial. For example, the reproducibility probability can be defined as the probability in (7.1.1) with all unknown parameters replaced by their estimates from the first trial (Goodman, 1992). In other words, the reproducibility probability is defined to be an estimated power of the second trial using the data from the first trial. More discussions of this approach will be given in §7.2-7.3.

Perhaps a more sensible definition of reproducibility probability can be obtained by using the Bayesian approach (Shao and Chow, 2002). Under the Bayesian approach, the unknown parameter under H_1, denoted by θ, is a random vector with a prior distribution $\pi(\theta)$ assumed to be known. Thus,

$$P(|T| > c|H_1) = P(|T| > c|\theta)$$

and the reproducibility probability can be defined as the conditional probability of $|T| > c$ in the second trial, given the dataset x observed from the first trial, i.e.,

$$P(|T| > c|x) = \int P(|T| > c|\theta)\pi(\theta|x)d\theta, \qquad (7.1.2)$$

where $T = T(y)$ is based on the dataset y from the second trial and $\pi(\theta|x)$ is the posterior density of θ, given x. More discussions of this Bayesian approach will be given in §7.4.

7.2   The Estimated Power Approach

To study the reproducibility probability, we need to specify the test procedure, i.e., the form of the test statistic T. We first consider the simplest design of two parallel groups with equal variances. The case of unequal variances is considered next. The parallel-group design is discussed at the end of this section.

7.2.1   Two Samples with Equal Variances

Suppose that a total of $n = n_1 + n_2$ patients are randomly assigned to two groups, a treatment group and a control group. In the treatment group, n_1 patients receive the treatment (or a test drug) and produce responses $x_{11}, ..., x_{1n_1}$. In the control group, n_2 patients receive the placebo (or a reference drug) and produce responses $x_{21}, ..., x_{2n_2}$. This design is a typical two-group parallel design in clinical trials. We assume that x_{ij}'s are independent and normally distributed with means μ_i, $i = 1, 2$, and a common variance σ^2. Suppose that the hypotheses of interest are

$$H_0 : \mu_1 - \mu_2 = 0 \quad \text{versus} \quad H_1 : \mu_1 - \mu_2 \neq 0. \qquad (7.2.1)$$

The discussion for a one sided H_1 is similar.

When σ^2 is known, we reject H_0 at the 5% level of significance if and only if

$$|T| > z_{0.975}, \qquad (7.2.2)$$

where $z_{0.975}$ is the 97.5th percentile of the standard normal distribution,

$$T = \frac{\bar{x}_1 - \bar{x}_2}{\sigma\sqrt{\frac{1}{n_1} + \frac{1}{n_2}}}, \qquad (7.2.3)$$

and $\bar{x}_i$ is the sample mean based on the data in the ith group.

Consider two independent clinical trials of the same design. Let x denote the data observed from the first trial and y be the data to be observed from the second trial. The test statistics for two trials are denoted by $T(x)$ and $T(y)$, respectively. For T given by (7.2.3), the power of T for the second trial is

$$P(|T(y)| > z_{0.975}) = \Phi(\theta - z_{0.975}) + \Phi(-\theta - z_{0.975}), \qquad (7.2.4)$$

where Φ is the standard normal distribution function and

$$\theta = \frac{\mu_1 - \mu_2}{\sigma\sqrt{\frac{1}{n_1} + \frac{1}{n_2}}}. \qquad (7.2.5)$$

If we replace θ in (7.2.4) by its estimate based on the data from the first trial, $T(x)$, then an estimated power, which can be defined as the reproducibility probability, is given by

$$\hat{P} = \Phi(T(x) - z_{0.975}) + \Phi(-T(x) - z_{0.975}). \qquad (7.2.6)$$

Note that $\hat{P}$ is a function of $|T(x)|$. When $|T(x)| > z_{0.975}$ (i.e., the first trial yields a positive clinical result),

$$\hat{P} \approx \Phi(|T(x)| - z_{0.975}),$$

which is the formula for reproducibility probability given by Goodman (1992). Values of $\hat{P}$ in (7.2.6) for several different values of $|T(x)|$ (and the related p-values) are listed in the third column of Table 7.2.1. As it can be seen from Table 7.2.1, if the p-value observed from the first trial is less than 0.001, there is more than 90% chance that the clinical result will be reproducible in the second trial under the same protocol and clinical trial environments.

In practice, σ^2 is usually unknown and, thus, the test given by (7.2.2)-(7.2.3) needs to be replaced by the commonly used two sample t-test which rejects H_0 if and only if

$$|T| > t_{0.975;n-2},$$

where $t_{0.975;n-2}$ is the 97.5th percentile of the t-distribution with $n - 2$ degrees of freedom,

$$T = \frac{\bar{x}_1 - \bar{x}_2}{\sqrt{\frac{(n_1-1)s_1^2+(n_2-1)s_2^2}{n-2}}\sqrt{\frac{1}{n_1} + \frac{1}{n_2}}}, \qquad (7.2.7)$$

and s_i^2 is the sample variance based on the data from the ith group. Then the power of T for the second trial is

$$\begin{aligned}
p(\theta) &= P(|T(y)| > t_{0.975;n-2}) \\
&= 1 - \mathcal{T}_{n-2}(t_{0.975;n-2}|\theta) + \mathcal{T}_{n-2}(-t_{0.975;n-2}|\theta), \qquad (7.2.8)
\end{aligned}$$

where θ is given by (7.2.5) and $\mathcal{T}_{n-2}(\cdot|\theta)$ denotes the distribution function of the noncentral t-distribution with $n - 2$ degrees of freedom and the noncentrality parameter θ. Note that $p(\theta) = p(|\theta|)$. Values of $p(\theta)$ as a function of $|\theta|$ is provided in Table 7.2.2. Using the same idea of replacing θ by its estimate $T(x)$, where T is now defined by (7.2.7), we obtain the following reproducibility probability:

$$\hat{P} = 1 - \mathcal{T}_{n-2}(t_{0.975;n-2}|T(x)) + \mathcal{T}_{n-2}(-t_{0.975;n-2}|T(x)), \qquad (7.2.9)$$

Table 7.2.1. Reproducibility Probability $\hat{P}$

$|T(x)|$	Known σ^2		Unknown σ^2 $(n=30)$	
	p-value	$\hat{P}$	p-value	$\hat{P}$
1.96	0.050	0.500	0.060	0.473
2.05	0.040	0.536	0.050	0.508
2.17	0.030	0.583	0.039	0.554
2.33	0.020	0.644	0.027	0.614
2.58	0.010	0.732	0.015	0.702
2.81	0.005	0.802	0.009	0.774
3.30	0.001	0.910	0.003	0.890

which is a function of $|T(x)|$. Again, when $|T(x)| > t_{0.975;n-2}$,

$$\hat{P} \approx \begin{cases} 1 - \mathcal{T}_{n-2}(t_{0.975;n-2}|T(x)) & \text{if } T(x) > 0 \\ \mathcal{T}_{n-2}(-t_{0.975;n-2}|T(x)) & \text{if } T(x) < 0. \end{cases}$$

For comparison, values of $\hat{P}$ in (7.2.9) for $n = 30$ corresponding to $\hat{P}$ in (7.2.6) are listed in the fifth column of Table 7.2.1. It can be seen that with the same value of $T(x)$, the reproducibility probability for the case of unknown σ^2 is lower than that for the case of known σ^2.

Table 7.2.2 can be used to find the reproducibility probability $\hat{P}$ in (7.2.9) with a fixed sample size n. For example, if $T(x) = 2.9$ was observed in a clinical trial with $n = n_1 + n_2 = 40$, then the reproducibility probability is 0.807. If $|T(x)| = 2.9$ was observed in a clinical trial with $n = 36$, then an extrapolation of the results in Table 7.2.2 (for $n = 30$ and 40) leads to a reproducibility probability of 0.803.

7.2.2 Two Samples with Unequal Variances

Consider the problem of testing hypotheses (7.2.1) under the two-group parallel design without the assumption of equal variances. That is, x_{ij}'s are independently distributed as $N(\mu_i, \sigma_i^2)$, $i = 1, 2$.

When $\sigma_1^2 \neq \sigma_2^2$, there exists no exact testing procedure for the hypotheses in (7.2.1). When both n_1 and n_2 are large, an approximate 5% level test rejects H_0 when $|T| > z_{0.975}$, where

$$T = \frac{\bar{x}_1 - \bar{x}_2}{\sqrt{\frac{s_1^2}{n_1} + \frac{s_2^2}{n_2}}}. \tag{7.2.10}$$

Table 7.2.2. Values of the Power Function $p(\theta)$ in (7.2.8)

$|\theta|$	10	20	30	40	50	60	100	∞
1.96	0.407	0.458	0.473	0.480	0.484	0.487	0.492	0.500
1.98	0.414	0.466	0.481	0.488	0.492	0.495	0.500	0.508
2.00	0.421	0.473	0.489	0.496	0.500	0.503	0.508	0.516
2.02	0.429	0.481	0.496	0.504	0.508	0.511	0.516	0.524
2.04	0.435	0.488	0.504	0.511	0.516	0.518	0.524	0.532
2.06	0.442	0.496	0.512	0.519	0.523	0.526	0.532	0.540
2.08	0.448	0.503	0.519	0.527	0.531	0.534	0.540	0.548
2.10	0.455	0.511	0.527	0.535	0.539	0.542	0.548	0.556
2.12	0.462	0.519	0.535	0.542	0.547	0.550	0.555	0.563
2.14	0.469	0.526	0.542	0.550	0.555	0.557	0.563	0.571
2.16	0.476	0.534	0.550	0.558	0.562	0.565	0.571	0.579
2.18	0.483	0.541	0.558	0.565	0.570	0.573	0.579	0.587
2.20	0.490	0.549	0.565	0.573	0.578	0.581	0.586	0.594
2.22	0.497	0.556	0.573	0.581	0.585	0.588	0.594	0.602
2.24	0.504	0.563	0.580	0.588	0.593	0.596	0.602	0.610
2.26	0.511	0.571	0.588	0.596	0.601	0.604	0.609	0.618
2.28	0.518	0.578	0.595	0.603	0.608	0.611	0.617	0.625
2.30	0.525	0.586	0.603	0.611	0.616	0.619	0.625	0.633
2.32	0.532	0.593	0.610	0.618	0.623	0.626	0.632	0.640
2.34	0.538	0.600	0.618	0.626	0.630	0.634	0.639	0.648
2.36	0.545	0.608	0.625	0.633	0.638	0.641	0.647	0.655
2.38	0.552	0.615	0.632	0.640	0.645	0.648	0.654	0.662
2.40	0.559	0.622	0.640	0.648	0.652	0.655	0.661	0.670
2.42	0.566	0.629	0.647	0.655	0.660	0.663	0.669	0.677
2.44	0.573	0.636	0.654	0.662	0.667	0.670	0.676	0.684
2.46	0.580	0.643	0.661	0.669	0.674	0.677	0.683	0.691
2.48	0.586	0.650	0.668	0.676	0.681	0.684	0.690	0.698
2.50	0.593	0.657	0.675	0.683	0.688	0.691	0.697	0.705
2.52	0.600	0.664	0.682	0.690	0.695	0.698	0.704	0.712
2.54	0.606	0.671	0.689	0.697	0.702	0.705	0.711	0.719
2.56	0.613	0.678	0.695	0.704	0.708	0.711	0.717	0.725
2.58	0.620	0.685	0.702	0.710	0.715	0.718	0.724	0.732
2.60	0.626	0.691	0.709	0.717	0.722	0.725	0.731	0.739
2.62	0.632	0.698	0.715	0.724	0.728	0.731	0.737	0.745
2.64	0.639	0.704	0.722	0.730	0.735	0.738	0.743	0.751
2.66	0.646	0.711	0.728	0.736	0.741	0.744	0.750	0.758

Table 7.2.2. Continued

				n				
$\lvert\theta\rvert$	10	20	30	40	50	60	100	∞
2.68	0.652	0.717	0.735	0.743	0.747	0.750	0.756	0.764
2.70	0.659	0.724	0.741	0.749	0.754	0.757	0.762	0.770
2.72	0.665	0.730	0.747	0.755	0.760	0.763	0.768	0.776
2.74	0.671	0.736	0.753	0.761	0.766	0.769	0.774	0.782
2.76	0.678	0.742	0.759	0.767	0.772	0.775	0.780	0.788
2.78	0.684	0.748	0.765	0.773	0.778	0.780	0.786	0.794
2.80	0.690	0.754	0.771	0.779	0.783	0.786	0.792	0.799
2.82	0.696	0.760	0.777	0.785	0.789	0.792	0.797	0.804
2.84	0.702	0.766	0.783	0.790	0.795	0.798	0.803	0.810
2.86	0.708	0.772	0.788	0.796	0.800	0.803	0.808	0.815
2.88	0.714	0.777	0.794	0.801	0.806	0.808	0.814	0.820
2.90	0.720	0.783	0.799	0.807	0.811	0.814	0.819	0.825
2.92	0.725	0.789	0.805	0.812	0.816	0.819	0.824	0.830
2.94	0.731	0.794	0.810	0.817	0.821	0.824	0.829	0.833
2.96	0.737	0.799	0.815	0.822	0.826	0.829	0.834	0.840
2.98	0.742	0.805	0.820	0.827	0.831	0.834	0.839	0.845
3.00	0.748	0.810	0.825	0.832	0.836	0.839	0.844	0.850
3.02	0.753	0.815	0.830	0.837	0.841	0.844	0.849	0.854
3.04	0.759	0.820	0.835	0.842	0.846	0.848	0.853	0.860
3.06	0.764	0.825	0.840	0.847	0.850	0.853	0.858	0.864
3.08	0.770	0.830	0.844	0.851	0.855	0.857	0.862	0.867
3.10	0.775	0.834	0.849	0.856	0.859	0.862	0.866	0.872
3.12	0.780	0.839	0.853	0.860	0.864	0.866	0.871	0.876
3.14	0.785	0.843	0.858	0.864	0.868	0.870	0.875	0.880
3.16	0.790	0.848	0.862	0.868	0.872	0.874	0.879	0.884
3.18	0.795	0.852	0.866	0.873	0.876	0.878	0.883	0.888
3.20	0.800	0.857	0.870	0.877	0.880	0.882	0.887	0.891
3.22	0.805	0.861	0.874	0.881	0.884	0.886	0.890	0.895
3.24	0.809	0.865	0.878	0.884	0.888	0.890	0.894	0.899
3.26	0.814	0.869	0.882	0.888	0.891	0.894	0.898	0.902
3.28	0.819	0.873	0.886	0.892	0.895	0.897	0.901	0.906
3.30	0.823	0.877	0.890	0.895	0.899	0.901	0.904	0.910
3.32	0.827	0.881	0.893	0.899	0.902	0.904	0.908	0.913
3.34	0.832	0.884	0.897	0.902	0.905	0.907	0.911	0.916
3.36	0.836	0.888	0.900	0.906	0.909	0.911	0.914	0.919
3.38	0.840	0.892	0.904	0.909	0.912	0.914	0.917	0.923

Table 7.2.2. Continued

$|\theta|$	10	20	30	40	50	60	100	∞
				n				
3.40	0.844	0.895	0.907	0.912	0.915	0.917	0.920	0.925
3.42	0.849	0.898	0.910	0.915	0.918	0.920	0.923	0.928
3.44	0.853	0.902	0.913	0.918	0.921	0.923	0.926	0.930
3.46	0.856	0.905	0.916	0.921	0.924	0.925	0.929	0.932
3.48	0.860	0.908	0.919	0.924	0.926	0.928	0.931	0.935
3.50	0.864	0.911	0.922	0.927	0.929	0.931	0.934	0.937
3.52	0.868	0.914	0.925	0.929	0.932	0.933	0.936	0.940
3.54	0.871	0.917	0.927	0.932	0.934	0.936	0.939	0.942
3.56	0.875	0.920	0.930	0.934	0.937	0.938	0.941	0.944
3.58	0.879	0.923	0.933	0.937	0.939	0.941	0.943	0.947
3.60	0.882	0.925	0.935	0.939	0.941	0.943	0.946	0.949
3.62	0.885	0.928	0.937	0.941	0.944	0.945	0.948	0.951
3.64	0.889	0.931	0.940	0.944	0.946	0.947	0.950	0.953
3.66	0.892	0.933	0.942	0.946	0.948	0.949	0.952	0.955
3.68	0.895	0.935	0.944	0.948	0.950	0.951	0.954	0.957
3.70	0.898	0.938	0.946	0.950	0.952	0.953	0.956	0.959
3.72	0.901	0.940	0.948	0.952	0.954	0.955	0.958	0.961
3.74	0.904	0.942	0.950	0.954	0.956	0.957	0.959	0.963
3.76	0.907	0.944	0.952	0.956	0.958	0.959	0.961	0.965
3.78	0.910	0.946	0.954	0.958	0.959	0.961	0.963	0.966
3.80	0.913	0.949	0.956	0.959	0.961	0.962	0.964	0.968
3.82	0.915	0.950	0.958	0.961	0.963	0.964	0.966	0.969
3.84	0.918	0.952	0.960	0.963	0.964	0.965	0.967	0.971
3.86	0.920	0.954	0.961	0.964	0.966	0.967	0.969	0.972
3.88	0.923	0.956	0.963	0.966	0.967	0.968	0.970	0.973
3.90	0.925	0.958	0.964	0.967	0.969	0.970	0.971	0.975
3.92	0.928	0.959	0.966	0.968	0.970	0.971	0.973	0.976
3.94	0.930	0.961	0.967	0.970	0.971	0.972	0.974	0.977
3.96	0.932	0.963	0.969	0.971	0.973	0.973	0.975	0.978
3.98	0.935	0.964	0.970	0.972	0.974	0.975	0.976	0.979
4.00	0.937	0.966	0.971	0.974	0.975	0.976	0.977	0.980
4.02	0.939	0.967	0.972	0.975	0.976	0.977	0.978	0.981
4.04	0.941	0.968	0.974	0.976	0.977	0.978	0.979	0.982
4.06	0.943	0.970	0.975	0.977	0.978	0.979	0.980	0.983
4.08	0.945	0.971	0.976	0.978	0.979	0.980	0.981	0.984

Since T is approximately distributed as $N(\theta, 1)$ with

$$\theta = \frac{\mu_1 - \mu_2}{\sqrt{\frac{\sigma_1^2}{n_1} + \frac{\sigma_2^2}{n_2}}}, \tag{7.2.11}$$

the reproducibility probability obtained by using the estimated power approach is given by (7.2.6) with T defined by (7.2.10).

    When the variances under different treatments are different and the sample sizes are not large, a different study design, such as a matched-pair parallel design or a 2×2 crossover design is recommended. A matched-pair parallel design involves m pairs of matched patients. One patient in each pair is assigned to the treatment group and the other is assigned to the control group. Let x_{ij} be the observation from the jth pair and the ith group. It is assumed that the differences $x_{1j} - x_{2j}$, $j = 1, ..., m$, are independent and identically distributed as $N(\mu_1 - \mu_2, \sigma_D^2)$. Then, the null hypothesis H_0 is rejected at the 5% level of significance if $|T| > t_{0.975;m-1}$, where

$$T = \frac{\sqrt{m}(\bar{x}_1 - \bar{x}_2)}{\hat{\sigma}_D} \tag{7.2.12}$$

and $\hat{\sigma}_D^2$ is the sample variance based on the differences $x_{1j} - x_{2j}$, $j = 1, ..., m$. Note that T has the noncentral t-distribution with $n - 1$ degrees of freedom and the noncentrality parameter

$$\theta = \frac{\sqrt{m}(\mu_1 - \mu_2)}{\sigma_D}. \tag{7.2.13}$$

Consequently, the reproducibility probability obtained by using the estimated power approach is given by (7.2.9) with T defined by (7.2.14) and $n - 2$ replaced by $m - 1$.

    Suppose that the study design is a 2×2 crossover design in which n_1 patients receive the treatment at the first period and the placebo at the second period and n_2 patients receive the placebo at the first period and the treatment at the second period. Let x_{lij} be the normally distributed observation from the jth patient at the ith period and lth sequence. Then the treatment effect μ_D can be unbiasedly estimated by

$$\hat{\mu}_D = \frac{\bar{x}_{11} - \bar{x}_{12} - \bar{x}_{21} + \bar{x}_{22}}{2} \sim N\left(\mu_D, \frac{\sigma_{1,1}^2}{4}\left(\frac{1}{n_1} + \frac{1}{n_2}\right)\right),$$

where $\bar{x}_{li}$ is the sample mean based on x_{lij}, $j = 1, ..., n_l$, and $\sigma_{1,1}^2$ is a function of variance components (see formula (5.3.3)). An unbiased estimator of $\sigma_{1,1}^2$ is

$$\hat{\sigma}_{1,1}^2 = \frac{1}{n_1 + n_2 - 2} \sum_{l=1}^{2} \sum_{j=1}^{n_l} (x_{l1j} - x_{l2j} - \bar{x}_{l1} + \bar{x}_{l2})^2,$$

which is independent of $\hat{\mu}_D$ and distributed as $\sigma_{1,1}^2/(n_1 + n_2 - 2)$ times the chi-square distribution with $n_1 + n_2 - 2$ degrees of freedom. Thus, the null hypothesis $H_0 : \mu_D = 0$ is rejected at the 5% level of significance if $|T| > t_{0.975;n-2}$, where $n = n_1 + n_2$ and

$$T = \frac{\hat{\mu}_D}{\frac{\hat{\sigma}_{1,1}}{2}\sqrt{\frac{1}{n_1} + \frac{1}{n_2}}}. \tag{7.2.14}$$

Note that T has the noncentral t-distribution with $n - 2$ degrees of freedom and the noncentrality parameter

$$\theta = \frac{\mu_D}{\frac{\sigma_{1,1}}{2}\sqrt{\frac{1}{n_1} + \frac{1}{n_2}}}. \tag{7.2.15}$$

Consequently, the reproducibility probability obtained by using the estimated power approach is given by (7.2.9) with T defined by (7.2.14).

7.2.3 Parallel-Group Designs

Parallel-group designs are often employed in clinical trials to compare more than one treatments with a placebo control or to compare one treatment, one placebo control, and one active control. Let $a \geq 3$ be the number of groups and x_{ij} be the observation from the jth patient in the ith group, $j = 1, ..., n_i$, $i = 1, ..., a$. Assume that x_{ij}'s are independently distributed as $N(\mu_i, \sigma^2)$. The null hypothesis H_0 is then

$$H_0 : \mu_1 = \mu_2 = \cdots = \mu_a,$$

which is rejected at the 5% level of significance if $T > F_{0.95;a-1,n-a}$, where $F_{0.95;a-1,n-a}$ is the 95th percentile of the F-distribution with $a - 1$ and $n - a$ degrees of freedom, $n = n_1 + \cdots + n_a$,

$$T = \frac{\text{SST}/(a-1)}{\text{SSE}/(n-a)}, \tag{7.2.16}$$

$$\text{SST} = \sum_{i=1}^{a} n_i(\bar{x}_i - \bar{x})^2, \qquad \text{SSE} = \sum_{i=1}^{a}\sum_{j=1}^{n_i}(x_{ij} - \bar{x}_i)^2,$$

$\bar{x}_i$ is the sample mean based on the data in the ith group, and $\bar{x}$ is the overall sample mean.

Note that T has the noncentral F-distribution with $a - 1$ and $n - a$ degrees of freedom and the noncentrality parameter

$$\theta = \sum_{i=1}^{a} \frac{n_i(\mu_i - \bar{\mu})^2}{\sigma^2}, \tag{7.2.17}$$

where $\bar{\mu} = \sum_{i=1}^{a} n_i \mu_i / n$. Let $\mathcal{F}_{a-1,n-a}(\cdot|\theta)$ be the distribution function of T. Then, the power of the second clinical trial is

$$P(T(y) > F_{0.95;a-1,n-a}) = 1 - \mathcal{F}_{a-1,n-a}(F_{0.95;a-1,n-a}|\theta).$$

Thus, the reproducibility probability obtained by using the estimated power approach is

$$\hat{P} = 1 - \mathcal{F}_{a-1,n-a}(F_{0.95;a-1,n-a}|T(x)),$$

where $T(x)$ is the observed T based on the data x from the first clinical trial.

7.3   The Confidence Bound Approach

Since $\hat{P}$ in (7.2.6) or (7.2.9) is an estimated power, it provides a rather optimistic result. Alternatively, we may consider a more conservative approach, which considers a 95% lower confidence bound of the power as the reproducibility probability (Shao and Chow, 2002).

Consider first the case of the two-group parallel design with a known common variance σ^2 (§7.2.1). Note that a 95% lower confidence bound for $|\theta|$, where θ is given by (7.2.5), is

$$|T(x)| - z_{0.975},$$

where T is given by (7.2.3). Since

$$P(|T(y)| > z_{0.975}) \geq \Phi(|\theta| - z_{0.975})$$

and Φ is a strictly increasing function, a 95% lower confidence bound for the power is

$$\hat{P}_- = \Phi(|T(x)| - 2z_{0.975}). \tag{7.3.1}$$

Note that the lower confidence bound in (7.3.1) is not useful unless $|T(x)| \geq 2z_{0.975}$, i.e., the positive clinical result from the first trial is highly significant.

When σ^2 is unknown, it is more difficult to obtain a confidence bound for θ in (7.2.5). Note that $T(x)$ defined by (7.2.7) has the noncentral t-distribution with $n - 2$ degrees of freedom and the noncentrality parameter θ. Let $\mathcal{T}_{n-2}(\cdot|\theta)$ be the distribution function of $T(x)$ for any given θ. It can be shown that $\mathcal{T}_{n-2}(t|\theta)$ is a strictly decreasing function of θ for any fixed t. Consequently, a 95% confidence interval for θ is $(\hat{\theta}_-, \hat{\theta}_+)$, where $\hat{\theta}_-$ is the unique solution of

$$\mathcal{T}_{n-2}(T(x)|\theta) = 0.975$$

and $\hat{\theta}_+$ is the unique solution of

$$T_{n-2}(T(x)|\theta) = 0.025$$

(see, e.g., Theorem 7.1 in Shao, 1999). Then, a 95% lower confidence bound for $|\theta|$ is

$$\widehat{|\theta|}_- = \begin{cases} \hat{\theta}_- & \text{if } \hat{\theta}_- > 0 \\ -\hat{\theta}_+ & \text{if } \hat{\theta}_+ < 0 \\ 0 & \text{if } \hat{\theta}_- \leq 0 \leq \hat{\theta}_+, \end{cases} \qquad (7.3.2)$$

and a 95% lower confidence bound for the power $p(\theta)$ in (7.2.8) is

$$\hat{P}_- = 1 - T_{n-2}(t_{0.975;n-2}|\widehat{|\theta|}_-) + T_{n-2}(-t_{0.975;n-2}|\widehat{|\theta|}_-) \qquad (7.3.3)$$

if $\widehat{|\theta|}_- > 0$ and $\hat{P}_- = 0$ if $\widehat{|\theta|}_- = 0$. Again, the lower confidence bound in (7.3.3) is useful when the clinical result from the first trial is highly significant.

Table 7.3.1 contains values of the lower confidence bound $\widehat{|\theta|}_-$ corresponding to $|T(x)|$ values ranging from 4.0 to 6.5. If $4 \leq |T(x)| \leq 6.5$ and the value of $\widehat{|\theta|}_-$ is found from Table 7.3.1, the reproducibility probability $\hat{P}_-$ in (7.3.3) can be obtained from Table 7.2.2. For example, suppose that $|T(x)| = 5$ was observed from a clinical trial with $n = 30$. From Table 7.3.1, $\widehat{|\theta|}_- = 2.6$. Then, by Table 7.2.2, $\hat{P}_- = 0.709$.

While $\hat{P}$ in (7.2.9) is rather optimistic, $\hat{P}_-$ in (7.3.3) may be too conservative. A compromise is to reduce the significance level of the lower confidence bound $\widehat{|\theta|}_-$ to 90%. Table 7.3.2 contains values of the 90% lower confidence bound for $|\theta|$. For $n = 30$ and $|T(x)| = 5$, $\widehat{|\theta|}_-$ is 2.98, which leads to $\hat{P}_- = 0.82$.

Consider next the two-group parallel design with unequal variances σ_1^2 and σ_2^2. When both n_1 and n_2 are large, T given by (7.2.10) is approximately distributed as $N(\theta, 1)$ with θ given by (7.2.11). Hence, the reproducibility probability obtained by using the lower confidence bound approach is given by (7.3.1) with T defined by (7.2.10).

For the matched-pair parallel design described in §7.2.2, T given by (7.2.12) has the noncentral t-distribution with $m-1$ degrees of freedom and the noncentrality parameter θ given by (7.2.13). Hence, the reproducibility probability obtained by using the lower confidence bound approach is given by (7.3.3) with T defined by (7.2.12) and $n - 2$ replaced by $m - 1$.

Suppose now that the study design is the 2×2 crossover design described in §7.2.2. Since T defined by (7.2.14) has the noncentral t-distribution with $n - 2$ degrees of freedom and the noncentrality parameter θ given by (7.2.15), the reproducibility probability obtained by using the lower confidence bound approach is given by (7.3.3) with T defined by (7.2.14).

Finally, consider the parallel-group design described in §7.2.3. Since T in (7.2.16) has the noncentral F-distribution with $a - 1$ and $n - a$ degrees of freedom and the noncentrality parameter θ given by (7.2.17) and $\mathcal{F}_{a-1,n-a}(t|\theta)$ is a strictly decreasing function of θ, the reproducibility probability obtained by using the lower confidence bound approach is

$$\hat{P}_- = 1 - \mathcal{F}_{a-1,n-a}(F_{0.95;a-1,n-a}|\hat{\theta}_-),$$

where $\hat{\theta}_-$ is the solution of

$$\mathcal{F}_{a-1,n-a}(T(x)|\theta) = 0.95.$$

Table 7.3.1. 95% Lower Confidence Bound $\widehat{|\theta|}_-$

$|T(x)|$	n							
	10	20	30	40	50	60	100	∞
4.5	1.51	2.01	2.18	2.26	2.32	2.35	2.42	2.54
4.6	1.57	2.09	2.26	2.35	2.41	2.44	2.52	2.64
4.7	1.64	2.17	2.35	2.44	2.50	2.54	2.61	2.74
4.8	1.70	2.25	2.43	2.53	2.59	2.63	2.71	2.84
4.9	1.76	2.33	2.52	2.62	2.68	2.72	2.80	2.94
5.0	1.83	2.41	2.60	2.71	2.77	2.81	2.90	3.04
5.1	1.89	2.48	2.69	2.80	2.86	2.91	2.99	3.14
5.2	1.95	2.56	2.77	2.88	2.95	3.00	3.09	3.24
5.3	2.02	2.64	2.86	2.97	3.04	3.09	3.18	3.34
5.4	2.08	2.72	2.95	3.06	3.13	3.18	3.28	3.44
5.5	2.14	2.80	3.03	3.15	3.22	3.27	3.37	3.54
5.6	2.20	2.88	3.11	3.24	3.31	3.36	3.47	3.64
5.7	2.26	2.95	3.20	3.32	3.40	3.45	3.56	3.74
5.8	2.32	3.03	3.28	3.41	3.49	3.55	3.66	3.84
5.9	2.39	3.11	3.37	3.50	3.58	3.64	3.75	3.94
6.0	2.45	3.19	3.45	3.59	3.67	3.73	3.85	4.04
6.1	2.51	3.26	3.53	3.67	3.76	3.82	3.94	4.14
6.2	2.57	3.34	3.62	3.76	3.85	3.91	4.03	4.24
6.3	2.63	3.42	3.70	3.85	3.94	4.00	4.13	4.34
6.4	2.69	3.49	3.78	3.93	4.03	4.09	4.22	4.44
6.5	2.75	3.57	3.86	4.02	4.12	4.18	4.32	4.54

Table 7.3.2. 90% Lower Confidence Bound $\widehat{|\theta|}_-$

$\|T(x)\|$	n							
	10	20	30	40	50	60	100	∞
4.5	1.95	2.40	2.54	2.62	2.67	2.70	2.76	2.86
4.6	2.02	2.48	2.63	2.71	2.76	2.79	2.85	2.96
4.7	2.09	2.56	2.72	2.80	2.85	2.88	2.95	3.06
4.8	2.16	2.64	2.81	2.89	2.94	2.98	3.05	3.16
4.9	2.22	2.73	2.90	2.98	3.03	3.07	3.14	3.26
5.0	2.29	2.81	2.98	3.07	3.13	3.16	3.24	3.36
5.1	2.36	2.89	3.07	3.16	3.22	3.26	3.33	3.46
5.2	2.43	2.97	3.16	3.25	3.31	3.35	3.43	3.56
5.3	2.49	3.05	3.24	3.34	3.40	3.44	3.52	3.66
5.4	2.56	3.13	3.33	3.43	3.49	3.54	3.62	3.76
5.5	2.63	3.21	3.42	3.52	3.59	3.63	3.72	3.86
5.6	2.69	3.30	3.50	3.61	3.68	3.72	3.81	3.96
5.7	2.76	3.38	3.59	3.70	3.77	3.81	3.91	4.06
5.8	2.83	3.46	3.68	3.79	3.86	3.91	4.00	4.16
5.9	2.89	3.54	3.76	3.88	3.95	3.00	4.10	4.26
6.0	2.96	3.62	3.85	3.97	4.04	4.09	4.19	4.36
6.1	3.02	3.70	3.93	4.06	4.13	4.18	4.29	4.46
6.2	3.09	3.78	4.02	4.15	4.22	4.28	4.38	4.56
6.3	3.15	3.86	4.11	4.23	4.31	4.37	4.48	4.66
6.4	3.22	3.94	4.19	4.32	4.40	4.46	4.57	4.76
6.5	3.28	4.02	4.28	4.41	4.49	4.55	4.67	4.86

7.4   The Bayesian Approach

As discussed in §7.1, the reproducibility probability can be viewed as the posterior mean of the power function $p(\theta) = P(|T| > c|\theta)$ for the second trial. Thus, under the Bayesian approach, it is essential to construct the posterior density $\pi(\theta|x)$ in formula (7.1.2), given the dataset x observed from the first trial (Shao and Chow, 2002).

7.4.1   Two Samples with Equal Variances

Consider the two-group parallel design described in §7.2.1 with equal variances, i.e., x_{ij}'s are independent and normally distributed with means μ_1 and μ_2 and a common variance σ^2.

If σ^2 is known, then the power for testing hypotheses in (7.2.1) is given by (7.2.4) with θ defined by (7.2.5). A commonly used prior for (μ_1, μ_2) is the noninformative prior $\pi(\mu_1, \mu_2) \equiv 1$. Consequently, the posterior density for θ is $N(T(x), 1)$, where T is given by (7.2.3), and the posterior mean given by (7.1.2) is

$$\int [\Phi(\theta - z_{0.975}) + \Phi(-\theta - z_{0.975})]\pi(\theta|x)d\theta$$

$$= \Phi\left(\frac{T(x) - z_{0.975}}{\sqrt{2}}\right) + \Phi\left(\frac{-T(x) - z_{0.975}}{\sqrt{2}}\right).$$

When $|T(x)| > z_{0.975}$, this probability is nearly the same as

$$\Phi\left(\frac{|T(x)| - z_{0.975}}{\sqrt{2}}\right), \tag{7.4.1}$$

which is exactly the same as that in formula (1) in Goodman (1992).

For the more realistic situation where σ^2 is unknown, we need a prior for σ^2. A commonly used noninformative prior for σ^2 is the Lebesgue (improper) density $\pi(\sigma^2) = \sigma^{-2}$. Assume that the priors for μ_1, μ_2, and σ^2 are independent. The posterior density for (δ, u^2) is

$$\pi(\delta|u^2, x)\pi(u^2|x),$$

where

$$\delta = \frac{\mu_1 - \mu_2}{\sqrt{\frac{(n_1-1)s_1^2 + (n_2-1)s_2^2}{n-2}}\sqrt{\frac{1}{n_1} + \frac{1}{n_2}}},$$

$$u^2 = \frac{(n-2)\sigma^2}{(n_1-1)s_1^2 + (n_2-1)s_2^2},$$

$$\pi(\delta|u^2, x) = \frac{1}{u}\phi\left(\frac{\delta - T(x)}{u}\right),$$

ϕ is the density function of the standard normal distribution, T is given by (7.2.7), and $\pi(u^2|x) = f(u)$ with

$$f(u) = \left[\Gamma\left(\frac{n-2}{2}\right)\right]^{-1}\left(\frac{n-2}{2}\right)^{(n-2)/2}u^{-n}e^{-(n-2)/(2u^2)}.$$

Since θ in (7.2.5) is equal to δ/u, the posterior mean of $p(\theta)$ in (7.2.8) is

$$\hat{P} = \int_0^\infty \left[\int_{-\infty}^\infty p\left(\frac{\delta}{u}\right)\phi\left(\frac{\delta - T(x)}{u}\right)d\delta\right]2f(u)du, \tag{7.4.2}$$

which is the reproducibility probability under the Bayesian approach. It is clear that $\hat{P}$ depends on the data x through the function $T(x)$.

The probability $\hat{P}$ in (7.4.2) can be evaluated numerically. A Monte Carlo method can be applied as follows. First, generate a random variate γ_j from the gamma distribution with the shape parameter $(n-2)/2$ and the scale parameter $2/(n-2)$, and generate a random variate δ_j from $N(T(x), u_j^2)$, where $u_j^2 = \gamma_j^{-1}$. Repeat this process independently N times to obtain (δ_j, u_j^2), $j = 1, ..., N$. Then $\hat{P}$ in (7.4.2) can be approximated by

$$\hat{P}_N = 1 - \frac{1}{N} \sum_{j=1}^{N} \left[T_{n-2} \left(t_{0.975;n-2} \Big| \frac{\delta_j}{u_j} \right) - T_{n-2} \left(-t_{0.975;n-2} \Big| \frac{\delta_j}{u_j} \right) \right].$$

(7.4.3)

Values of $\hat{P}_N$ for $N = 10,000$ and some selected values of $T(x)$ and n are given by Table 7.4.1. It can be seen that in assessing reproducibility, the Bayesian approach is more conservative than the estimated power approach, but less conservative than the confidence bound approach.

7.4.2   Two Samples with Unequal Variances

Consider first the two-group parallel design with unequal variance and large n_i's. The approximate power for the second trial is

$$p(\theta) = \Phi(\theta - z_{0.975}) + \Phi(-\theta - z_{0.975}), \qquad \theta = \frac{\mu_1 - \mu_2}{\sqrt{\frac{\sigma_1^2}{n_1} + \frac{\sigma_2^2}{n_2}}}.$$

Suppose that we use the following noninformative prior density for $(\mu_1, \mu_2, \sigma_1^2, \sigma_2^2)$:

$$\pi(\mu_1, \mu_2, \sigma_1^2, \sigma_2^2) = \sigma_1^{-2} \sigma_2^{-2}, \qquad \sigma_1^2 > 0, \sigma_2^2 > 0.$$

Let $\tau_i^2 = \sigma_i^{-2}$, $i = 1, 2$, and $\zeta^2 = \frac{1}{n_1 \tau_1^2} + \frac{1}{n_2 \tau_2^2}$. Then, the posterior density $\pi(\mu_1 - \mu_2 | \tau_1^2, \tau_2^2, x)$ is the normal density with mean $\bar{x}_1 - \bar{x}_2$ and variance ζ^2 and the posterior density

$$\pi(\tau_1^2, \tau_2^2 | x) = \pi(\tau_1^2 | x) \pi(\tau_2^2 | x),$$

where $\pi(\tau_i^2 | x)$ is the gamma density with the shape parameter $(n_i - 1)/2$ and the scale parameter $2/[(n_i - 1)s_i^2]$, $i = 1, 2$. Consequently, the posterior mean of $p(\theta)$ is

$$\iiint \Phi(\theta - z_{0.975}) \pi(\mu_1 - \mu_2 | \tau_1^2, \tau_2^2, x) d(\mu_1 - \mu_2) \pi(\tau_1^2, \tau_2^2 | x) d\tau_1^2 d\tau_2^2$$

$$+ \iiint \Phi(-\theta - z_{0.975}) \pi(\mu_1 - \mu_2 | \tau_1^2, \tau_2^2, x) d(\mu_1 - \mu_2) \pi(\tau_1^2, \tau_2^2 | x) d\tau_1^2 d\tau_2^2.$$

Table 7.4.1. Reproducibility Probability $\hat{P}_N$ given by (7.4.3)

$|T(x)|$	10	20	30	40	50	60	100	∞
2.02	0.435	0.482	0.495	0.501	0.504	0.508	0.517	0.519
2.08	0.447	0.496	0.512	0.515	0.519	0.523	0.532	0.536
2.14	0.466	0.509	0.528	0.530	0.535	0.543	0.549	0.553
2.20	0.478	0.529	0.540	0.547	0.553	0.556	0.565	0.569
2.26	0.487	0.547	0.560	0.564	0.567	0.571	0.577	0.585
2.32	0.505	0.558	0.577	0.580	0.581	0.587	0.590	0.602
2.38	0.519	0.576	0.590	0.597	0.603	0.604	0.610	0.618
2.44	0.530	0.585	0.610	0.611	0.613	0.617	0.627	0.634
2.50	0.546	0.609	0.624	0.631	0.634	0.636	0.640	0.650
2.56	0.556	0.618	0.638	0.647	0.648	0.650	0.658	0.665
2.62	0.575	0.632	0.654	0.655	0.657	0.664	0.675	0.680
2.68	0.591	0.647	0.665	0.674	0.675	0.677	0.687	0.695
2.74	0.600	0.660	0.679	0.685	0.686	0.694	0.703	0.710
2.80	0.608	0.675	0.690	0.702	0.705	0.712	0.714	0.724
2.86	0.629	0.691	0.706	0.716	0.722	0.723	0.729	0.738
2.92	0.636	0.702	0.718	0.730	0.733	0.738	0.742	0.752
2.98	0.649	0.716	0.735	0.742	0.744	0.748	0.756	0.765
3.04	0.663	0.726	0.745	0.753	0.756	0.759	0.765	0.778
3.10	0.679	0.738	0.754	0.766	0.771	0.776	0.779	0.790
3.16	0.690	0.754	0.767	0.776	0.781	0.786	0.792	0.802
3.22	0.701	0.762	0.777	0.790	0.792	0.794	0.804	0.814
3.28	0.708	0.773	0.793	0.804	0.806	0.809	0.820	0.825
3.34	0.715	0.784	0.803	0.809	0.812	0.818	0.828	0.836
3.40	0.729	0.793	0.815	0.819	0.829	0.830	0.838	0.846
3.46	0.736	0.806	0.826	0.832	0.837	0.839	0.847	0.856
3.52	0.745	0.816	0.834	0.843	0.845	0.846	0.855	0.865
3.58	0.755	0.828	0.841	0.849	0.857	0.859	0.867	0.874
3.64	0.771	0.833	0.854	0.859	0.863	0.865	0.872	0.883
3.70	0.778	0.839	0.861	0.867	0.870	0.874	0.884	0.891
3.76	0.785	0.847	0.867	0.874	0.882	0.883	0.890	0.898
3.82	0.795	0.857	0.878	0.883	0.889	0.891	0.898	0.906
3.88	0.800	0.869	0.881	0.891	0.896	0.899	0.904	0.913
3.94	0.806	0.873	0.890	0.897	0.904	0.907	0.910	0.919
4.00	0.812	0.883	0.896	0.905	0.908	0.911	0.916	0.925
4.06	0.822	0.888	0.902	0.910	0.915	0.917	0.924	0.931

Note that

$$\int \Phi(\theta - z_{0.975})\pi(\mu_1 - \mu_2|\tau_1^2, \tau_2^2, x)d(\mu_1 - \mu_2) = \Phi\left(\frac{\bar{x}_1 - \bar{x}_2}{\sqrt{2\zeta}} - \frac{z_{0.975}}{\sqrt{2}}\right)$$

and

$$\int \Phi(-\theta - z_{0.975})\pi(\mu_1 - \mu_2|\tau_1^2, \tau_2^2, x)d(\mu_1 - \mu_2) = \Phi\left(-\frac{\bar{x}_1 - \bar{x}_2}{\sqrt{2\zeta}} - \frac{z_{0.975}}{\sqrt{2}}\right).$$

Hence, the reproducibility probability based on the Bayesian approach is

$$\hat{P} = \int \left[\Phi\left(\frac{\bar{x}_1 - \bar{x}_2}{\sqrt{2\zeta}} - \frac{z_{0.975}}{\sqrt{2}}\right) + \Phi\left(-\frac{\bar{x}_1 - \bar{x}_2}{\sqrt{2\zeta}} - \frac{z_{0.975}}{\sqrt{2}}\right)\right]\pi(\zeta|x)d\zeta,$$

where $\pi(\zeta|x)$ is the posterior density of ζ constructed using $\pi(\tau_i^2|x)$, $i = 1, 2$.

The following Monte Carlo method can be applied to evaluate $\hat{P}$. Generate independent random variates τ_{1j}^2 and τ_{2j}^2 respectively from the gamma densities $\pi(\tau_1^2|x)$ and $\pi(\tau_2^2|x)$ as previously specified. Repeat this process independently N times to obtain $(\tau_{1j}^2, \tau_{2j}^2)$, $j = 1, ..., N$. Then $\hat{P}$ can be approximated by

$$\hat{P}_N = \frac{1}{N}\sum_{j=1}^{N}\left[\Phi\left(\frac{\bar{x}_1 - \bar{x}_2}{\sqrt{2\zeta_j}} - \frac{z_{0.975}}{\sqrt{2}}\right) + \Phi\left(-\frac{\bar{x}_1 - \bar{x}_2}{\sqrt{2\zeta_j}} - \frac{z_{0.975}}{\sqrt{2}}\right)\right],$$

where

$$\zeta_j = \frac{1}{n_1\tau_{1j}^2} + \frac{1}{n_2\tau_{2j}^2}, \qquad j = 1, ..., N.$$

For the matched-pairs parallel design described in §7.2.2, the power function is

$$p(\theta) = 1 - \mathcal{T}_{m-1}(t_{0.975;m-1}|\theta) + \mathcal{T}_{m-1}(-t_{0.975;m-1}|\theta)$$

with θ given by (7.2.13). Under the noninformative prior $\pi(\mu, \sigma_D^2) = \sigma_D^{-1}$, the reproducibility probability, the posterior mean of $p(\theta)$, is given by (7.4.2) with T given by (7.2.12), $n - 2$ replaced by $m - 1$, and δ and u^2 defined by

$$\delta = \frac{\sqrt{n}(\mu_1 - \mu_2)}{\sigma_D} \qquad \text{and} \qquad u^2 = \frac{\sigma_D^2}{\hat{\sigma}_D^2},$$

respectively.

For the 2×2 crossover design described in §7.2.2, the power function is

$$p(\theta) = 1 - \mathcal{T}_{n-2}(t_{0.975;n-2}|\theta) + \mathcal{T}_{n-2}(-t_{0.975;n-2}|\theta)$$

with θ given by (7.2.15). If we use the noninformative prior $\pi(\mu_D, \sigma_{1,1}^2) = \sigma_{1,1}^{-2}$, then the reproducibility probability is still given by (7.4.2) with T given by (7.2.14), δ and u^2 defined by

$$\delta = \frac{\mu_D}{\frac{\hat{\sigma}_{1,1}^2}{2}\sqrt{\frac{1}{n_1} + \frac{1}{n_2}}} \qquad \text{and} \qquad u^2 = \frac{\sigma_{1,1}^2}{\hat{\sigma}_{1,1}^2},$$

respectively.

7.4.3 Parallel-Group Designs

Consider the a-group parallel design in §7.2.3, where the power is given by

$$p(\theta) = 1 - \mathcal{F}_{a-1,n-a}(F_{0.95;a-1,n-a}|\theta)$$

with θ given by (7.2.17). Under the noninformative prior

$$\pi(\mu_1, ..., \mu_a, \sigma^2) = \sigma^{-2}, \qquad \sigma^2 > 0,$$

the posterior density $\pi(\theta|\tau^2, x)$, where $\tau^2 = \text{SSE}/[(n-a)\sigma^2]$, is the density of the noncentral chi-square distribution with $a - 1$ degrees of freedom and the noncentrality parameter $\tau^2(a-1)T(x)$. The posterior density $\pi(\tau^2|x)$ is the gamma distribution with the shape parameter $(n-a)/2$ and the scale parameter $2/(n-a)$. Consequently, the reproducibility probability under the Bayesian approach is

$$\hat{P} = \int_0^\infty \left[\int_0^\infty p(\theta)\pi(\theta|\tau^2, x)d\theta \right] \pi(\tau^2|x)d\tau^2.$$

A Monte Carlo method similar to that in §7.4.1 can be applied to compute $\hat{P}$.

7.5 Applications and Extensions

In this section we discuss some applications and extensions of the results obtained in §7.2-7.4.

7.5.1 Substantial Evidence with a Single Trial

An important application of the results derived in the previous sections is to address the following question: is it necessary to conduct a second clinical trial when the first trial produces a relatively strong positive clinical result (e.g., a relatively small p-value is observed)? As indicated earlier, the FDA *Modernization Act* of 1997 includes a provision stating that under certain circumstances, data from one adequate and well-controlled clinical investigation and confirmatory evidence may be sufficient to establish effectiveness for risk/benefit assessment of drug and biological candidates for approval. This provision essentially codified an FDA policy that had existed for several years but whose application had been limited to some biological products approved by the Center for Biologic Evaluation and Research (CBER) of the FDA and a few pharmaceuticals, especially orphan drugs such as zidovudine and lamotrigine. As it can be seen from Table 7.2.1, a relatively strong significant result observed from a single clinical trial (say, p-value is less than 0.001) would have about 90% chance of reproducing the result in future clinical trials. Consequently, a single clinical trial is sufficient to provide substantial evidence for demonstration of efficacy and safety of the medication under study. In 1998, FDA published a guidance which shed the light on this approach despite that the FDA has recognized that advances in sciences and practice of drug development may permit an expanded role for the single controlled trial in contemporary clinical development (FDA, 1988).

Suppose that it is agreed that the second trial is not needed if the probability for reproducing a positive clinical result in the second trial is equal to or higher than 90%. If a positive clinical result is observed in the first trial and the confidence bound $\hat{P}_-$ derived in §7.3 is equal to or higher than 90%, then we have 95% statistical assurance that, with a probability of at least 90%, the positive result will be reproduced in the second trial. For example, under the two-group parallel design with a common unknown variance and $n = 40$, the 95% lower confidence bound $\hat{P}_-$ given by (7.3.1) is equal to or higher than 90% if and only if $|T(x)| \geq 5.7$, i.e., the clinical result in the first trial is highly significant. Alternatively, if the Bayesian approach is applied to the same situation, the reproducibility probability in (7.4.1) is equal to or higher than 90% if and only if $|T(x)| \geq 3.96$.

On the other hand, if the reproducibility probability is very low (e.g., $\hat{P}$ in (7.2.9) is less than 50%), it may also indicate that a clinically meaningful difference between the placebo and the drug product under study can not be detected through the intended trials and, thus, there is no need to run the second trial.

7.5.2 Sample Size Adjustments

When the reproducibility probability based on the result from the first trial is high but not high enough, the second trial must be conducted. The results on the reproducibility probability derived in §7.2-7.4 can be used to adjust the sample size for the second trial. If the sample size for the first trial was determined based on a power analysis with some initial guessing values of the unknown parameters, then it is reasonable to make a sample size adjustment for the second trial based on the results from the first trial. If the reproducibility probability is too low, then the sample size should be increased. On the other hand, if the reproducibility probability is high, then the sample size may be decreased to reduce costs. In the following we illustrate the idea using the two-group parallel design with a common unknown variance.

Suppose that $\hat{P}$ in (7.2.9) is used as the reproducibility probability when $T(x)$ given by (7.2.7) is observed from the first trial. For simplicity, consider the case where the sample size $n^*/2$ is used for two treatment groups in the second trial, where n^* is the total sample size in the second trial. With fixed $\bar{x}_i$ and $\hat{\sigma}^2 = [(n_1 - 1)s_1^2 + (n_2 - 1)s_2^2]/(n - 2)$ but a new sample size n^*, the T-statistic becomes

$$T^* = \frac{\sqrt{n^*}(\bar{x}_1 - \bar{x}_2)}{2\hat{\sigma}}$$

and the reproducibility probability is $\hat{P}$ with T replaced by T^*. By letting T^* be the value to achieve a desired power, the new sample size n^* should be

$$n^* = \left(\frac{T^*}{T}\right)^2 \bigg/ \left(\frac{1}{4n_1} + \frac{1}{4n_2}\right). \tag{7.5.1}$$

For example, suppose that the desired reproducibility probability is 80%. If $T = 2.58$ is observed in the first trial with $n_1 = n_2 = 15$, which yields $\hat{P} = 0.702$ (see Table 7.2.2), then T^* needs to be 2.91, which yields $n^* \approx 1.27n \approx 38$, i.e., the sample size should be increased by about 27%. On the other hand, if $T = 3.30$ is observed in the first trial with $n_1 = n_2 = 15$, then $n^* \approx 0.78n \approx 24$, i.e., the sample size can be reduced by about 22%.

7.5.3   Trials with Different Designs

The results in §7.2-7.4 can be easily extended to situations where two trials have different designs. For example, suppose that the first trial uses a two-group parallel design (§7.2.1) and the second trial uses a 2 × 2 crossover design (§7.2.2). We can still use formula (7.2.9) or (7.3.3) with T given by (7.2.7) for the reproducibility probability. On the other hand, if the first trial uses a 2 × 2 crossover design and the second trial uses a two-group parallel design, then formula (7.2.9) or (7.3.3) should be used with T given by (7.2.14).

Furthermore, the results in §7.2-7.4 are still valid when the observations in the first and the second trials are dependent. For example, (7.2.9) or (7.3.3) with T given by (7.2.7) can be applied to the case where the first trial uses a two-group parallel design and the design for the second trial is obtained by adding a period to the first design, i.e., the design for the second trial is a 2×2 crossover design with the first period being the first trial. Another example is the two-stage design for cancer trials in which the sample from the first trial is a part of the sample for the second trial.

7.5.4 Reproducibility Probabilities for k Trials

Consider the situation where a number of clinical trials are conducted in a sequential manner. Our interest is the reproducibility probability for the kth trial, given that all previous $k-1$ trials produce positive clinical results.

The extension of the results in §7.4 under the Bayesian approach is straightforward. Let $\pi_0(\theta|x_0) = \pi(\theta)$ be the prior for θ (which is usually a noninformative prior) and $\pi_k(\theta|x_k)$ be the posterior after observing the data from the kth trial, $k = 1, 2, ...$ Then $\pi_k(\theta|x_k)$ can be used as the prior for the $(k+1)$th trial. The reproducibility probability for the $(k+1)$th trial is

$$P(|T| > c|x_k) = \int P(|T| > c|\theta)\pi_k(\theta|x_k)d\theta, \qquad k = 0, 1, ...,$$

where x_k is the dataset containing all data up to the kth trial.

For the non-Bayesian approach, the simplest way of constructing a reproducibility probability for the $(k+1)$th trial is to apply the procedures in §7.2-7.3 with $x = x_k$, assuming that all trials have the same design.

7.5.5 Binary Data

In some clinical trials data are binary and μ_i's are proportions. Consider a two-group parallel design. For binary data, sample sizes n_1 and n_2 are usually large so that the Central Limit Theorem can be applied to sample proportions $\bar{x}_1$ and $\bar{x}_2$, i.e., $\bar{x}_i$ is approximately $N(\mu_i, \mu_i(1-\mu_i)/n_i)$. Thus, the results in §7.2-7.4 for the case of unequal variances with large n_i's can be applied.

7.6 Generalizability

Consider the situation where the target patient population of the second clinical trial is similar but slightly different (e.g., due to difference in ethnic factors) from the population of the first clinical trial. The difference in population may be reflected by the difference in mean, variance, or both mean and variance of the primary study endpoints. For example, the population means may be different when the patient populations in two trials are of different race. When a pediatric population is used for the first trial and adult patients or elderly patients are considered in the second trial, the population variance is likely to be different.

The reproducibility probability considered in the previous sections with the population of the second trial slightly deviated from the population of the first trial is referred to as the generalizability probability. In this section we illustrate how to obtain generalizability probabilities in the case where the study design is a two-group parallel design with a common variance. Other cases can be similarly treated.

7.6.1 The Frequentist Approach

Consider the two-group parallel design described in §7.2.1. Let $\mu_1 - \mu_2$ be the population mean difference and σ^2 be the common population variance of the first trial. Suppose that in the second trial, the population mean difference is changed to $\mu_1 - \mu_2 + \varepsilon$ and the population variance is changed to $C^2\sigma^2$, where $C > 0$. If $|\mu_1 - \mu_2|/\sigma$ is the signal-to-noise ratio for the population difference in the first trial, then the signal-to-noise ratio for the population difference in the second trial is

$$\frac{|\mu_1 - \mu_2 + \varepsilon|}{C\sigma} = \frac{|\Delta(\mu_1 - \mu_2)|}{\sigma},$$

where

$$\Delta = \frac{1 + \varepsilon/(\mu_1 - \mu_2)}{C} \tag{7.6.1}$$

is a measure of change in the signal-to-noise ratio for the population difference. For most practical problems, $|\varepsilon| < |\mu_1 - \mu_2|$ and, thus, $\Delta > 0$. Then, the power for the second trial is

$$1 - \mathcal{T}_{n-2}(t_{0.975;n-2}|\Delta\theta) + \mathcal{T}_{n-2}(-t_{0.975;n-2}|\Delta\theta),$$

where

$$\theta = \frac{\mu_1 - \mu_2}{\sigma\sqrt{\frac{1}{n_1} + \frac{1}{n_2}}}.$$

Note that the power for the second trial is the same as the power for the first trial if and only if Δ in (7.6.1) equals 1. Define

$$T = \frac{\bar{x}_1 - \bar{x}_2}{\sqrt{\frac{(n_1-1)s_1^2 + (n_2-1)s_2^2}{n-2}}\sqrt{\frac{1}{n_1} + \frac{1}{n_2}}},$$

where $\bar{x}_i$'s and s_i^2's are the sample means and variances based on the data from the first trial. Then, the generalizability probability on the estimated power approach can be obtained in the same way that the reproducibility probability is obtained in §7.2, with T replaced by ΔT, assuming that Δ is known, i.e.,

$$\hat{P}_\Delta = 1 - \mathcal{T}_{n-2}(t_{0.975;n-2}|\Delta T) + \mathcal{T}_{n-2}(-t_{0.975;n-2}|\Delta T),$$

where $\mathcal{T}_{n-2}(\cdot|\theta)$ is the noncentral t-distribution with $n-2$ degrees of freedom and the noncentrality parameter θ. The generalizability probability based on the confidence bound approach is

$$\hat{P}_{\Delta-} = 1 - \mathcal{T}_{n-2}(t_{0.975;n-2}|\Delta\widehat{|\theta|}_-) + \mathcal{T}_{n-2}(-t_{0.975;n-2}|\Delta\widehat{|\theta|}_-)$$

if $\widehat{|\theta|}_- > 0$ and $\hat{P}_{\Delta-} = 0$ if $\widehat{|\theta|}_- = 0$, where $\widehat{|\theta|}_-$ is the same as that given in (7.3.2).

Values of $\hat{P}_\Delta$ and $\hat{P}_{\Delta-}$ can be obtained using Tables 7.2.2 and 7.3.1 once n, Δ, and $T(x)$ are known. In practice, the value of Δ may be unknown. We may either consider a maximum possible value of $|\Delta|$ or a set of Δ-values to carry out a sensitivity analysis.

7.6.2   The Bayesian Approach

For the Bayesian approach with a known Δ given by (7.6.1), the generalizability probability is

$$\hat{P}_\Delta = \int_0^\infty \left[\int_{-\infty}^\infty p\left(\frac{\Delta\delta}{u}\right) \phi\left(\frac{\delta - T(x)}{u}\right) d\delta \right] 2f(u)du,$$

where $p(\delta/u)$, u, and $f(u)$ are the same as those in (7.4.2).

Table 7.4.1 can be used to obtain values of $\hat{P}_\Delta$ once n, Δ, and $T(x)$ are known. When Δ is unknown, the method considered in §7.6.1 can be applied. Alternatively, we may consider the average of $\hat{P}_\Delta$ over a noninformative prior density $\pi(\Delta)$, i.e.,

$$\hat{P} = \int \hat{P}_\Delta \pi(\Delta)d\Delta.$$

7.6.3   Applications

In clinical development, after the investigational drug product has been shown to be effective and safe with respect to a target patient population (e.g., adults), it is often of interest to study how likely the clinical result is reproducible in a similar but slightly different patient population (e.g., elderly patient population with the same disease under study or a patient population with different ethnic factors). This information is useful in regulatory submission or supplement new drug application (e.g., when generalizing the clinical results from adults to elderly patient population) and regulatory evaluation for bridging studies (e.g., when generalizing clinical results from Caucasian to Asian patient population). Detailed information regarding bridging studies can be found in ICH (1998a).

Example 7.6.1. A double-blind randomized trial was conducted in patients with schizophrenia for comparing the efficacy of a test drug with a standard therapy. A total of 104 chronic schizophrenic patients participated in this study. Patients were randomly assigned to receive the treatment of the test drug or the standard therapy for at least one year, where the test drug group has 56 patients and the standard therapy group has 48 patients. The primary clinical endpoint of this trial was the total score of Positive and Negative Symptom Scales (PANSS). No significant differences in demographics and baseline characteristics were observed for baseline comparability.

Mean changes from baseline in total PANSS for the test drug and the standard therapy are $\bar{x}_1 = -3.51$ and $\bar{x}_2 = 1.41$, respectively, with $s_1^2 = 76.1$ and $s_2^2 = 74.86$. The difference $\mu_1 - \mu_2$ is estimated by $\bar{x}_1 - \bar{x}_2 = -4.92$ and is considered to be statistically significant with $T = -2.88$, a p-value of 0.004, and a reproducibility probability of 0.814 under the estimated power approach or 0.742 under the Bayesian approach.

The sponsor of this trial would like to evaluate the probability for reproducing the clinical result in a different population where Δ, the change in the signal-to-noise ratio, ranges from 0.75 to 1.2. The generalizability probabilities are given in Table 7.6.1 (since $|T| < 4$, the confidence bound

Table 7.6.1. Generalizability Probabilities and Sample Sizes
for Clinical Trials in a New Population (Example 7.6.1)

Δ	The Estimated Power Approach			The Bayesian Approach		
	$\hat{P}_\Delta$	New Sample Size n^*		$\hat{P}_\Delta$	New Sample Size n^*	
		70% Power	80% Power		70% Power	80% Power
1.20	0.929	52	66	0.821	64	90
1.10	0.879	62	80	0.792	74	102
1.00	0.814	74	96	0.742	86	118
0.95	0.774	84	106	0.711	98	128
0.90	0.728	92	118	0.680	104	140
0.85	0.680	104	132	0.645	114	154
0.80	0.625	116	150	0.610	128	170
0.75	0.571	132	170	0.562	144	190

approach is not considered). In this example, $|T|$ is not very large and, thus, a clinical trial is necessary to evaluate in the new population. The generalizability probability can be used to determine the sample size n^* for such a clinical trial. The results are given in Table 7.6.1. For example, if $\Delta = 0.9$ and the desired power (reproducibility probability) is 80%, then $n^* = 118$ under the estimated power approach and 140 under the Bayesian approach; if the desired power (reproducibility probability) is 70%, then $n^* = 92$ under the estimated power approach and 104 under the Bayesian approach. A sample size smaller than that of the original trial is allowed if $\Delta \geq 1$, i.e., the new population is less variable.

The sample sizes n^* in Table 7.6.1 are obtained as follows. Under the estimated power approach,

$$n^* = \left(\frac{T^*}{\Delta T}\right)^2 \Big/ \left(\frac{1}{4n_1} + \frac{1}{4n_2}\right),$$

where T^* is the value obtained from Table 7.2.2 for which the reproducibility probability has the desired level (e.g., 70% or 80%). Under the Bayesian approach, for each given Δ we first compute the value T^*_Δ at which the reproducibility probability has the desired level and then use

$$n^* = \left(\frac{T^*_\Delta}{T}\right)^2 \Big/ \left(\frac{1}{4n_1} + \frac{1}{4n_2}\right).$$

Chapter 8

Therapeutic Equivalence and Noninferiority

In drug research and development, *equivalence* and *noninferiority* trials have become increasingly popular. The definition of equivalence is not unique. It often includes the concepts of bioequivalence as described in Chapter 5 and therapeutic equivalence/noninferiority. For example, the sponsors may want to show that a capsule is equivalent to a tablet (bioequivalence) or a 10-day of therapy is as effective as a 14-day therapy (therapeutic equivalence/noninferiority). Equivalence/noninferiority trials usually involve the comparison with a control. Section 314.126 in Part 21 of CFR indicates that there are four kinds of controls including placebo control, no treatment control, positive control, and historical control. The assessment of equivalence/noninferiority depends upon the definition of a clinically meaningful difference, which may vary from indication to indication and therapy to therapy. Little information or discussion regarding the clinically meaningful difference is provided in regulatory guidelines such as the FDA and ICH guidelines. Clinical judgment based on previous experience or historical data is often used. In practice, active control trials are often conducted for establishment of therapeutic equivalence and noninferiority using the two one-sided tests procedure or the confidence interval approach.

In §8.1, some basic concepts and important issues for equivalence/noninferiority trials are introduced. The corresponding statistical methods are discussed in §8.2. The primary objectives for establishment of therapeutic equivalence and noninferiority through the conduct of active control trials in clinical development are introduced in §8.3. Some statistical methods for assessment of drug efficacy under active control trials are discussed in

§8.4. In §8.5, active control equivalence trials are introduced and statistical methods for assessment of drug efficacy are discussed, including the establishment of therapeutic equivalence and noninferiority among a test drug, an active control agent, and a placebo. A Bayesian approach for analyzing data from an active control trial is introduced in §8.6. The last section contains some discussions.

8.1   Equivalence/Noninferiority Trials

In clinical trials, it is often of interest to show that the study drug is as effective as, superior to, or equivalent to a standard therapy or an active control agent that has been demonstrated to be effective and safe for the intended indication. Two drug products are considered equivalent if they are therapeutically equivalent, i.e., they have equal therapeutic effect. Noninferiority of the study drug is referred to as that the study drug is not inferior to or as effective as the standard therapy or the active control agent. This study objective in clinical trials is not uncommon especially when the study drug is considered less toxic, easier to administer, inducing better compliance, or less expensive than the established standard therapy or active control agent. In what follows, some basic considerations regarding the selection of controls, hypotheses for testing equivalence/noninferiority, the choice of noninferiority margin, design strategy, and sample size calculation in equivalence/noninferiority trials are provided.

8.1.1   Selection of Controls

As indicated in the ICH Draft Guideline on Choice of Control Group in Clinical Trials (ICH, 1999), control groups in clinical trials can be classified on the basis of two clinical attributes: (i) the type of treatment received and (ii) the method of determining who will be in the control group. Based on the type of treatment received, the control groups include placebo, no treatment, different dose or regimen of the study treatment, or different active treatment. The principal methods of determining who will be in the control group are either by randomization or by selection of a control population separate from the population treated in the trial. The ICH guideline refers to the latter control group as external or historical control. As a result, control groups can be classified into five types. The first four control groups, namely, placebo concurrent control, no-treatment control, dose-response concurrent control, and active concurrent control, are concurrent controlled because the control groups and test groups are chosen from the same population and treated concurrently. The fifth type of control group is the external or historical control group, which compares a group of subjects receiving the test treatment with a group of subjects external to the study.

Placebo control trials are almost always double-blind studies. Subjects are randomly assigned to a test treatment or to an identical-appearing inactive treatment (placebo). Placebo control trials seek to show a difference in efficacy between treatments or to show lack of difference (of specified size) in safety between treatments. In a no-treatment control study, subjects and investigators are not blinded to treatment assignment. No-treatment control trials are needed and suitable when it is difficult or impossible to double-blind and there is reasonable confidence that the study endpoints are objective and that the results of the study are unlikely to be influenced. Dose-response concurrent controls are usually considered in randomized, fixed-dose, dose response studies. Subjects are randomized to one of several fixed-dose groups. Although subjects may either be placed on their fixed dose initially or be raised to that dose gradually, the intended comparison is between the groups on their final dose. Dose-response control studies, which may include a placebo (zero dose) and/or active control, are usually double-blind. For active (or positive) control trials, subjects are randomly assigned to the teat treatment or to an active control drug. In practice, it is preferred to have double-blinded active control trials. However, it is not always possible. For example, many oncology studies are considered not possible to blind because of different regimens, different routes of administration, and different recognizable toxicities. External controls could be a group of patients treated at an earlier time, which is referred to as historical control, or during the same time period but in another setting.

In practice, it is often possible and advantageous to use more than one kind of controls in a single study, e.g., use of both active control and placebo control. Similarly, clinical trials may use several doses of the test drug and several doses of active control with or without placebo. We refer to these studies as multiple control trials. Multiple control trials may be useful for active drug comparisons where the relative potency of the test drug and the active control is not well established.

8.1.2   Hypotheses of Equivalence/Noninferiority

Let μ_T and μ_S denote respectively the mean responses of a primary study endpoint for the test drug and the standard therapy. Also, let $\delta > 0$ be the magnitude of difference of clinical importance. That is, if the absolute value of the difference between μ_T and μ_S is less than δ, then the test drug is considered to be equivalent to the standard therapy. Thus, the following interval hypotheses should be considered for evaluation of equivalence between the test drug and the standard therapy:

$$H_0 : |\mu_T - \mu_S| \geq \delta \quad \text{versus} \quad H_1 : |\mu_T - \mu_S| < \delta. \qquad (8.1.1)$$

We conclude that the difference between the test drug and the standard therapy is of no clinical importance and, hence, they are therapeutically equivalent if the null hypothesis H_0 is rejected at a given level of significance.

On the other hand, one may wish to show that the test drug is not inferior to or at least as effective as the standard therapy. In this case, Blackwelder (1982) suggested testing the following hypotheses for noninferiority:

$$H_0 : \mu_T \leq \mu_S - \delta \quad \text{versus} \quad H_1 : \mu_T > \mu_S - \delta.$$

The concept is to reject the null hypothesis of inferiority and conclude that the difference between the test drug and the standard therapy is less than a clinically meaningful difference and, hence, the test drug is at least as effective as or noninferior to the standard therapy. Note that most active control equivalence trials are really noninferiority trials, which are intended to establish the efficacy of a test drug.

Similarly, if one wishes to show that the test drug is superior to the standard therapy, the following hypotheses should be considered:

$$H_0 : \mu_T \leq \mu_S + \delta \quad \text{versus} \quad H_1 : \mu_T > \mu_S + \delta.$$

The rejection of the null hypothesis H_0 suggests that the difference between the test drug and the standard therapy is greater than a clinically meaningful difference and, hence, the test drug is superior to the standard therapy. In practice, it is suggested that the superiority be established after the noninferiority is concluded.

The hypotheses for testing noninferiority and superiority are also known as hypotheses for testing one-sided equivalence. The relationship among therapeutical equivalence, noninferiority, and superiority is summarized in Figure 8.1.1. Note that when $\delta = 0$, the previously discussed therapeutical (or clinical) equivalence, noninferiority, and superiority reduce to strict (or statistical) equivalence, noninferiority, and superiority, respectively.

8.1.3 Equivalence Limits and Noninferiority Margins

As it can be seen from the previous section, the choice of δ, a clinically meaningful difference, is critical in equivalence/noninferiority or superiority trials. In equivalence trials, δ is known as the equivalence limit, while δ is referred to as the noninferiority margin in noninferiority trials. The noninferiority margin reflects the degree of inferiority of the test drug compared to the standard therapy that the trials attempts to exclude.

A different choice of δ may affect the sample size calculation and may alter the conclusion of clinical results. Thus, the choice of δ is critical

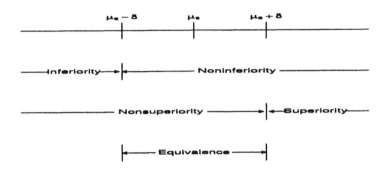

Figure 8.1.1. Regions of Therapeutical Equivalence,
Noninferiority, and Superiority

in clinical trials. In practice, there is no gold rule for determination of
δ in equivalence/noninferiority trials. As indicated in the ICH E10 Draft
Guideline, the noninferiority margin cannot be chosen to be greater than
the smallest effect size that the active drug would be reliably expected to
have compared with placebo in the setting of the planned trial, but may
be smaller based on clinical judgment. The ICH E10 Guideline suggests
that the noninferiority margin be identified based on past experience in
placebo control trials of adequate design under conditions similar to those
planned for the new trial. In addition, the ICH E10 Guideline emphasizes
that the determination of δ should be based on both statistical reasoning
and clinical judgment, which should not only reflect uncertainties in the
evidence on which the choice is based, but also be suitably conservative.

In some cases, regulatory agencies do provide clear guidelines for selection of an appropriate δ for equivalence/noninferiority trials. For example,
as indicated by Huque and Dubey (1990), the FDA proposed some noninferiority margins for some clinical endpoints (binary responses) such as
cure rate for drug products (e.g., topical antifungals or vaginal antifungals). These limits are given in Table 8.1.1. For example, if the cure rate
is between 80% and 90%, it is suggested that the noninferiority margin be
chosen as $\delta = 15\%$. For bioequivalence trials, the margin of $\delta = \log(1.25)$
for mean difference on log-transformed data such as area under the blood or
plasma concentration-time curve (AUC) or maximum concentration C_{max}
is considered (FDA, 2001).

Table 8.1.1. Noninferiority Margins for Binary Responses

δ (%)	Response Rate for the Active Control (%)
20	50-80
15	80-90
10	90-95
5	> 95

Source: FDA Anti-Infectives Drug Guideline

In clinical trials, the choice of δ may depend upon absolute change, percent change, or effect size of the primary study endpoint. In practice, a standard effect size (i.e., effect size adjusted for standard deviation) between 0.25 and 0.5 is usually chosen as δ if no prior knowledge regarding clinical performance of the test drug is available. This recommendation is made based on the fact that the standard effect size of clinical importance observed from most clinical trials are within the range of 0.25 and 5.0.

8.1.4 Design Strategy

In clinical development, different designs may be employed depending upon the study objectives of the intended clinical trial. Fleming (1990) discussed the following design strategies that are commonly used in equivalence/noninferiority and superiority trials.

Design	Description
Classical	STD + TEST versus STD
Active Control	TEST versus STD
Dual Purpose	TEST versus STD versus STD + TEST

The classical design is to compare the combination of a test drug (TEST) and a standard therapy (STD) (i.e., STD + TEST) against STD to determine whether STD+TEST yields superior efficacy. When the intent is to determine whether a test drug could be used as an alternative to a standard therapy, one may consider an active control design involving direct randomization to either TEST or STD. This occurs frequently when STD is quite toxic and the intent is to develop alternative therapy that are less toxic, yet equally efficacious. To achieve both objectives, a dual purpose design strategy is useful.

As indicated in the ICH E10 Draft Guideline, two purposes of clinical trials should be distinguished: (1) assessment of the efficacy and/or safety of a treatment and (2) assessment of the relative (comparative) efficacy, safety, benefit/risk relationship or utility of two treatments. As a result, it is suggested that the following study objectives related to efficacy and safety be clarified before choosing an appropriate design strategy for the intended trial.

		Safety		
		Equivalence	Noninferiority	Superiority
	Equivalence	E/E	E/N	E/S
Efficacy	Noninferiority	N/E	N/N	N/S
	Superiority	S/E	S/N	S/S

For example, if the intent is to develop an alternative therapy to the standard therapy that is quite toxic, then we may consider the strategy of E/S, which is to show that the test drug has equal efficacy but less toxicity (superior safety).

8.2 Assessing Therapeutic Equivalence

From the discussion in §8.1, the assessment of therapeutic noninferiority or superiority involves a one-sided null hypothesis and, thus, standard statistical tests for one-sided null hypotheses can be applied. In this section we focus on the assessment of therapeutic equivalence, which involves some two-sided or interval null and alternative hypotheses.

8.2.1 Two Commonly Used Approaches

For assessment of therapeutic equivalence, there are two commonly employed statistical methods. One is the procedure of two one-sided tests (TOST) and the other is the approach of confidence interval. The TOST approach is based on the fact that the null hypothesis H_0 in (8.1.1) is the union of the following two one-sided hypotheses:

$$H_{01} : \mu_T - \mu_S \geq \delta \quad \text{and} \quad H_{02} : \mu_T - \mu_S \leq -\delta.$$

Hence, we may reject the null hypothesis H_0 at a given level α when both H_{01} and H_{02} are rejected at level α. For example, when observed responses are normally distributed with a constant variance, the TOST procedure rejects H_0 in (8.1.1) if

$$\frac{\bar{y}_T - \bar{y}_S + \delta}{\text{se}} > t_\alpha \quad \text{and} \quad \frac{\bar{y}_T - \bar{y}_S - \delta}{\text{se}} < -t_\alpha, \qquad (8.2.1)$$

where $\bar{y}_T$ and $\bar{y}_S$ are the sample means of the test product and the standard therapy, respectively, se is an estimated standard deviation of $\bar{y}_T - \bar{y}_S$, and

t_α is the upper αth percentile of a central t-distribution with appropriate degrees of freedom.

Note that the TOST approach is adopted in average bioequivalence testing (§5.3.1) and is in fact a special case of the method of intersection-union tests (Berger and Hsu, 1996).

The approach of confidence interval (or, more generally, confidence set) can actually be used to construct a statistical test for any problem in which the null and alternative hypotheses can be expressed as $H_0 : \theta \in \Theta_0$ and $H_1 : \theta \in \Theta_1$, where θ is an unknown parameter, Θ_0 and Θ_1 are two disjoint subsets of Θ, the set of all possible values of θ, and $\Theta_0 \cup \Theta_1 = \Theta$. If C is a level $1 - \alpha$ confidence set (not necessary an interval) for θ based on the observed data, then a level α test for H_0 versus H_1 rejects H_0 if and only if $C \cap \Theta_0 = \emptyset$ (see Berger and Hsu, 1996, Theorem 4).

Consequently, in the problem of testing hypotheses in (8.1.1) (assessing therapeutic equivalence), if C is a level $1 - \alpha$ confidence interval for $\mu_T - \mu_S$, then a level α test rejects H_0 if and only if C falls within the interval $(-\delta, \delta)$.

The following confidence intervals are commonly considered in the confidence interval approach:

Type	Confidence Level	Confidence Interval
CI_W	$1 - \alpha$	$[\bar{y}_T - \bar{y}_S - t_{\alpha_1}\mathrm{se},\ \bar{y}_T - \bar{y}_S + t_{\alpha_2}\mathrm{se}]$
CI_L	$1 - \alpha$	$[-|\bar{y}_T - \bar{y}_S| - t_\alpha\mathrm{se},\ |\bar{y}_T - \bar{y}_S| + t_\alpha\mathrm{se}]$
CI_E	$1 - \alpha$	$[\min(0, \bar{y}_T - \bar{y}_S - t_\alpha\mathrm{se}),\ \max(0, \bar{y}_T - \bar{y}_S + t_\alpha\mathrm{se})]$
$CI_{2\alpha}$	$1 - 2\alpha$	$[\bar{y}_T - \bar{y}_S - t_\alpha\mathrm{se},\ \bar{y}_T - \bar{y}_S + t_\alpha\mathrm{se}]$

Here, CI_W is the so-called Westlake symmetric confidence interval with appropriate choices of $\alpha_1 + \alpha_2 = \alpha$ (Westlake, 1976); CI_L is derived from the confidence interval of $|\mu_T - \mu_S|$ (Liu, 1990); and CI_E is an expanded confidence interval derived by Hsu (1984) and Bofinger (1985, 1992). The last confidence interval, $CI_{2\alpha}$, is included because (8.2.1) is equivalent to the fact that confidence interval $CI_{2\alpha}$ falls within $(-\delta, \delta)$. Hence, although the use of $CI_{2\alpha}$ is operationally the same as the confidence interval approach, it is constructed based on the TOST approach, not the confidence interval approach.

8.2.2   Clarification of Confusion

The existence of two different approaches, namely, the TOST approach and the confidence interval approach, and the fact that the TOST approach is operationally the same as the confidence interval approach has caused some confusion in the pharmaceutical industry. We try to clarify this confusion in the following discussion.

Level $1 - \alpha$ Versus Level $1 - 2\alpha$

Note that confidence intervals CI_W, CI_L, and CI_E are of confidence level $1 - \alpha$, whereas confidence interval $CI_{2\alpha}$ is of confidence level $1 - 2\alpha$. Thus, there is confusion whether level $1 - \alpha$ or level $1 - 2\alpha$ should be used when applying the confidence interval approach in equivalence trials. The discussion in §8.2.1 or Theorem 4 in Berger and Hsu (1996) indicates that level $1 - \alpha$ should be used in the confidence interval approach. This is because the use of level $1 - \alpha$ guarantees that the corresponding test is of level α, whereas the use of level $1 - 2\alpha$ can only ensure that the corresponding test is of level 2α. When applying the approach of confidence interval to the problem of assessing average bioequivalence (in which the hypotheses of interest are the same as those in (8.1.1)), Berger and Hsu (1996) made the following conclusion:

> The misconception that size-α bioequivalence tests generally correspond to $100(1 - 2\alpha)\%$ confidence sets will be shown to lead to incorrect statistical practices, and should be abandoned.

However, a further problem arises. Why does the use of confidence interval $CI_{2\alpha}$ produce a level α test? To clarify this, we need to first understand the difference between the significance level and the size of a statistical test.

Significance Level Versus Size

Let T be a test procedure. The size of T is defined to be

$$\alpha_T = \sup_{P \text{ under } H_0} P(T \text{ rejects } H_0).$$

On the other hand, any $\alpha_1 \geq \alpha_T$ is called a significance level of T. Thus, a test of level α_1 is also of level α_2 for any $\alpha_2 > \alpha_1$ and it is possible that the test is of level α_0 that is smaller than α_1. The size of a test is its smallest possible level and any number larger than the size (and smaller than 1) is a significance level of the test. Thus, if α (e.g., 1% or 5%) is a desired level of significance and T is a given test procedure, then we must first ensure that $\alpha_T \leq \alpha$ (i.e., T is of level α) and then try to have $\alpha_T = \alpha$; otherwise T is too conservative.

We can now clarify the confusion about the level of the test obtained by using confidence interval $CI_{2\alpha}$. According to Theorem 4 in Berger and Hsu (1996), this test is of level 2α. However, since this test is the same as TOST test (§8.2.1), its size is actually equal to α (Berger and Hsu, 1996, Theorems 1 and 2). But the last conclusion cannot be reached using the confidence interval approach.

The previous discussion explains the difference between the TOST approach and the confidence interval approach. It also reveals a disadvantage of using the approach of confidence interval. That is, the test obtained using a level $1 - \alpha$ confidence interval may be too conservative in the sense that the size of the test may be much smaller than α. An immediate question is: What are the sizes of the tests obtained by using level $1 - \alpha$ confidence intervals CI_W, CI_L, and CI_E?

Comparisons

It can be verified that $\text{CI}_W \supset \text{CI}_L \supset \text{CI}_E \supset \text{CI}_{2\alpha}$. If the tests obtained by using these confidence intervals are T_W, T_L, T_E and $T_{2\alpha}$, respectively, then their sizes satisfy $\alpha_{T_W} \leq \alpha_{T_L} \leq \alpha_{T_E} \leq \alpha_{T_{2\alpha}}$. Since $T_{2\alpha}$ is the same as the TOST procedure whose size is α, $\alpha_{T_{2\alpha}} = \alpha$. Berger and Hsu (1996) showed that the size of T_E is also α, although CI_E is always wider than $\text{CI}_{2\alpha}$. Ghosh, Chan, and Biswas (2000) summarize the situations when CI_E and $\text{CI}_{2\alpha}$ reach the same conclusion, which are given below (see also Brown, Casella, and Hwang, 1995):

	$\text{CI}_{2\alpha}$	CI_E	$-\delta < L$	$U < \delta$	$\text{CI}_{2\alpha} = \text{CI}_E$
$L < 0 < U$	(L, U)	(L, U)	Yes	Yes	Yes
			Yes	No	No
			No	Yes	No
			No	No	No
$0 < L < U$	(L, U)	$(0, U)$	Yes	Yes	Yes
			Yes	No	No
$L < U < 0$	(L, U)	$(L, 0)$	Yes	Yes	Yes
			No	Yes	No

Here, L and U are the lower and upper limits of $\text{CI}_{2\alpha}$, respectively. Since T_W and T_L correspond to confidence intervals that are wider than CI_E, it is likely that their sizes are smaller than α.

It should be noted that the size of a test is not the only measure of its successfulness. The TOST procedure is of size α yet biased because the probability of rejection of the null hypothesis when it is false (power) may be lower than α. Berger and Hsu (1996) proposed a nearly unbiased and uniformly more powerful test than the TOST procedure. Brown, Hwang, and Munk (1997) provided an improved test that is unbiased and uniformly more powerful than the TOST procedure. These improved tests are, however, rather complicated as compared to the TOST procedure.

Conclusions

Based on the previous discussions, we reach the following conclusions.

1. The TOST procedure is a valid size α test for therapeutic equivalence. Although it can be improved, the TOST procedure is recommended because of its validity and simplicity.

2. The approach of using level $1 - \alpha$ confidence intervals produces level α tests, but the sizes of these tests may be smaller than α. The use of confidence interval CI_E results in a size α test.

3. The use of level $1 - 2\alpha$ confidence intervals generally does not ensure that the corresponding test be of level α, although the use of $\text{CI}_{2\alpha}$ is an exceptional case. To avoid confusion, it is strongly suggested that the approaches of confidence interval and TOST should be applied separately, although sometimes they are operationally equivalent.

8.2.3 Equivalence between Proportions

For testing noninferiority between proportions, we reject the null hypothesis if

$$Z = \frac{\hat{P}_T - \hat{P}_S + \delta}{\tilde{\sigma}} > z_\alpha,$$

where $\hat{P}_T$ and $\hat{P}_S$ are observed proportions (or response rates) of the test product and the standard therapy, respectively, and $\tilde{\sigma}$ is an estimate of the standard error of $\hat{P}_T - \hat{P}_S$. Large Z values favor the alternative hypothesis of noninferiority. Dunnett and Gent (1977) recommended estimating the variance of $\hat{P}_T - \hat{P}_S$ from fixed marginal totals. Blackwelder (1982) considered using the following observed variance:

$$\tilde{\sigma}_B^2 = \frac{1}{n_T}\hat{P}_T(1 - \hat{P}_T) + \frac{1}{n_S}\hat{P}_S(1 - \hat{P}_S),$$

where n_T and n_S are the sample sizes for the test group and the standard therapy group, respectively. Tu (1997) suggested using the following unbiased observed variance

$$\tilde{\sigma}_U^2 = \frac{1}{n_T - 1}\hat{P}_T(1 - \hat{P}_T) + \frac{1}{n_S - 1}\hat{P}_S(1 - \hat{P}_S).$$

Miettinen and Nurminen (1985) and Farrington and Manning (1990) recommend the following constrained maximum likelihood estimate (MLE), which can be derived under the null hypothesis:

$$\tilde{\sigma}_{RMLE}^2 = \frac{1}{n_T}\tilde{P}_T(1 - \tilde{P}_T) + \frac{1}{n_S}\tilde{P}_S(1 - \tilde{P}_S),$$

where $\tilde{P}_T$ and $\tilde{P}_S$ are the constrained MLE of P_T and P_S, which are derived under H_0, of the test product and the standard therapy, respectively.

For assessment of therapeutic equivalence between proportions, the method of confidence interval approach is commonly employed. Newcombe (1998) reviewed eleven methods for constructing confidence intervals for difference in proportions. These methods include simple asymptotic method with and without continuity correction (Fleiss, 1981), Beal's Haldane and Beal's Jeffreys-Perks methods (Beal, 1987), the method proposed by Mee (Mee, 1984), the method by Miettinen and Nurminen (Miettinen and Nurminen, 1985), true profile likelihood method and profile likelihood method based on either exact tail areas or mid-p tail areas (Miettinen and Nurminen, 1985), and methods based on the Wilson score method for the single proportion with and without continuity correction (Wilson, 1927). Based on a simulation study, it appears that the closely interrelated methods of Mee and Miettinen and Nurminen perform very well in terms of coverage probability and controlling the size and hence are recommended. Note that the discussion in §8.2.2 about the approach of confidence intervals can be directly applied to the problem of proportions.

8.3   Active Control Trials

In practice, it may not be ethical to conduct a placebo control study with very ill patients or patients with severe or life-threatening diseases (e.g., cancer or AIDS) to establish drug efficacy of a new drug. In this case, an active control trial is often considered as an alternative trial to evaluate the effectiveness and safety of the new drug by comparing it with an active control agent, which has been shown to be effective and safe for the intended disease. In recent years, the use of active control in clinical trials has become increasingly popular. Its foremost appeal over the placebo control is based on ethical considerations. Besides, it is often easier to enroll patients into a trial if they will be guaranteed an active treatment.

For a test drug product, the primary objective of an active control trial could be (i) to show that the test drug is equivalent to an active control agent, (ii) to demonstrate that the test drug is superior to the active control agent, or (iii) to establish the efficacy of the test drug. Statistical concepts and methods described in §8.1 are applicable to cases where objective (i) or (ii) is the main concern. For objective (iii), however, Pledger and Hall (1986) pointed out that an active control trial offers no *direct* evidence of effectiveness of the test drug. The only trial that will yield direct evidence of effectiveness of the test drug is a placebo control trial that compares the test drug with a placebo. In the following discussion we focus on the issue of establishment of the efficacy of the test drug in an active control trial.

8.3.1 Establishment of Drug Efficacy in Active Control Trials

In practice, since an active control is known to be an effective agent, it is often assumed that showing the two drug products are equivalent in an active control trial is to demonstrate that both drug products are effective. However, this assumption is not necessarily correct and can not be verified from the data obtained from the active control trial. Pledger and Hall (1986) compared the possible outcomes of an active control trial comparing a test drug product (denoted by T) and an active control agent (denoted by A) with a placebo control trial comparing T, A, and a placebo (denoted by P). Table 8.3.1 summarizes the comparison of the possible outcomes. It can be seen from Table 8.3.1 that the equivalence and superiority to the active control agent do not guarantee that the test drug product is effective. For example, showing equivalence between T and A may imply that T and A are both equally effective or equally ineffective. Even when A is known to be superior to P and equivalence between T and A are observed, it is still possible that T and P are equivalent, i.e., T is not effective. This is because $|\mu_T - \mu_A| < \delta$ and $\mu_A > \mu_P + \delta$ (see §8.1.2) do not imply $|\mu_T - \mu_P| > \delta$, where μ_T, μ_A, and μ_P are respectively the population means for T, A, and P. On the other hand, even when we observed that T is inferior to A, it is still possible that both A and T are superior to P and, thus, T is effective.

Table 8.3.1. Comparison of Possible Outcomes for an Active Control Trial and a Placebo Control Trial

Active Control Trial Outcome of T versus A	Placebo Control Trial Outcome of T versus A versus P
TA	TA>P; TAP, T>P; PTA, P>A; P>TA; TPA; TAP; PTA
AT	AT>P; ATP, A>P; PAT, P>T; P>AT; APT; ATP; PAT
T>A	T>AP; T>A>P; T>PA; TAP, T>A; TP>A; T>P>A; PT>A; P>T>A
A>T	A>TP; A>T>P; A>PT; ATP, A>T; AP>T; A>P>T; PA>T; P>A>T

T = test drug, A = active control, P = placebo.

Left to right order indicates decreasing improvement.

> denotes a statistically significant difference.

Source: Pledger and Hall (1986).

Hence, the interpretation of the results from active control trials is a critical issue. If the test drug is inferior, or even indistinguishable from a standard therapy, the results are not readily interpretable. In the absence of a placebo control, one does not know if the inferior test medicine has any efficacy at all. Similarly, equivalent performance may reflect simply a patient population that cannot distinguish between two treatments that differ considerably from each other, or between active drug and placebo.

When can we use an active control study for establishment of the efficacy of a test drug product? Temple (1983) recommended the following fundamental principle for active control trials.

> If we cannot be very certain that the positive control in a study would have beaten a placebo group, had one been present, the fundamental assumption of the positive control study cannot be made and that design must be considered inappropriate.

Under this fundamental principle, any condition in which large spontaneous or placebo responses occur, or in which there is great day-to-day variability, or in which effective drugs are not easily distinguished from placebo, should be considered a poor candidate for an active control study. Temple (1983) also indicated that active control trials may be served as primary evidence of effectiveness if the fundamental assumption of the active control is correct which usually cannot be verified. However, the following situations may be considered to support an active control study. These situations include the situation (i) where there is a retrospective review of known placebo control studies of the proposed active control to show that the drug regularly can be shown superior to a placebo, (ii) where active control trials are conducted utilizing a similar patient population and similar procedures (e.g., dose, dosage regimens, titration methods, response assessment methods, and control of concomitant therapy), and (iii) where there is an estimate of the effect size of the placebo response.

When an active control trial is used, for assessment of drug efficacy, the FDA indicates that there should be assessments of

1. the response of the active control agent in the present trial compared to previous studies of similar design that included comparison with placebo and

2. the ability of the study to have detected differences between the treatments of a defined size, e.g., by proving confidence limits for the difference between the test drug and active control and/or the power to detect a difference between the treatments of specified size.

Along this line, Pledger and Hall (1986) suggested that supplementary information, which is often obtained from previous trials conducted under a design similar in all important aspects such as patient population, dosage requirements, response assessment methods, and control of concomitant therapy, be provided.

8.3.2   Fleming's Approach

Fleming (1987, 1990) proposed a method for evaluation of efficacy in active control trials of oncologic drug products under the assumption that (i) it is not ethical to give placebo to patients, and (ii) the intent is to determine whether the test drug could replace the active control agent. The idea of Fleming's approach is to use the confidence interval of the efficacy of the test drug product to determine whether the test drug product has an improved therapeutic index over the active control agent and the placebo, assuming that supplementary information regarding the efficacy of the active control agent and the placebo is available. In the following discussion we illustrate Fleming's idea, assuming that the efficacy of the drug products can be assessed by comparing the population means μ_T, μ_A, and μ_P of the test drug product, the active control agent, and the placebo, respectively.

Let $\delta \geq 0$ be an equivalence limit (see §8.1.3), i.e., if $|\mu_T - \mu_A| \leq \delta$, then the test drug product and the active agent are considered to be equivalent. Let $(\underline{\mu}_T, \bar{\mu}_T)$ be a confidence interval for μ_T. Fleming's approach concludes that the test drug product is not inferior to the active control agent if $\underline{\mu}_T > \mu_A - \delta$ (assuming that a larger population mean indicates that the drug product is more effective) and that the test drug product is better than the placebo if $\underline{\mu}_T > \mu_P$. This procedure can be illustrated by Figure 8.3.1 with $\phi = \mu_P$, where part A of the figure indicates that the test drug product is not inferior to the active control agent and is better than the placebo, part B of the figure shows that the test drug product is inferior to the active control agent and but is better than the placebo, part C of the figure indicates that the test drug product is no inferior to the active control agent and but is not better than the placebo, and part D of the figure shows that the test drug product is inferior to the active control agent and is not better than the placebo.

Let $\delta' \geq 0$ be an equivalence limit for the test drug product and the placebo. Then, the previously described procedure should be modified by replacing μ_P by $\mu_P + \delta'$ (i.e., setting ϕ in Figure 8.3.1 to $\mu_P + \delta'$). Clearly, if $\delta' = 0$, then no modification is needed.

Although the values of δ and δ' can be determined by regulatory agencies, the values of μ_A and μ_P are assumed known in Fleming's approach. When μ_A and μ_P are unknown and are estimated using supplementary data, variation in estimating them has to be taken into account. From the active control trial, a confidence interval for μ_A can be obtained. Thus, one

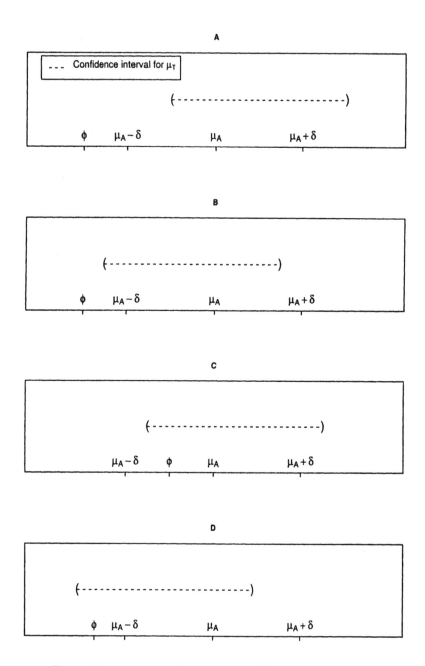

Figure 8.3.1. Graphical Presentation of Fleming's Method
of Comparing Drug Efficacy

might replace $\mu_A \pm \delta$ in Figure 8.3.1 by the confidence limits for μ_A. A better approach is, however, to consider a confidence interval of the difference $\mu_T - \mu_A$. That is, in Figure 8.3.1 we replace the confidence interval of μ_T by the confidence interval for $\mu_T - \mu_A$, μ_A by 0, and ϕ by the difference $\mu_P - \mu_A$ (assuming that $\mu_P - \mu_A$ is known). Similarly, we may replace the confidence interval of μ_T in Figure 8.3.1 by the confidence interval of the ratio μ_T/μ_A, μ_A by 1, and ϕ by the ratio μ_P/μ_A. When μ_P, $\mu_P - \mu_A$, or μ_P/μ_A is also unknown, however, the analysis should be based on some empirical results from a previous study of comparing the active control agent and placebo, which is discussed in the next three sections.

Example 8.3.1. To illustrate the use of Fleming's approach for assessment of clinical efficacy in active control trials, consider an example concerning the evaluation of an experimental therapeutic intervention (EXP) in delaying disease progression in treatment of patients with advanced breast cancer. The active control agent is a standard therapy (STD) currently available on the market. As indicated by Fleming (1990), the Cox proportional hazards regression analysis or log-rank test is usually performed to assess the relative efficacy of the EXP and STD using time to disease progression. These statistics focus on estimating the hazard ratio or relative risk of failures on the two treatments. The relative risk of failures on the two treatments is estimated to be 3.7 times higher with the EXP than with the STD (i.e., EXP/STD hazard ratio estimate is 3.7) and a 95(1.86, 7.45). Assume that δ in Figure 8.3.1 is chosen to be 0.1. Then, we conclude that the EXP is superior to the STD.

Since we do not have any information about the placebo treatment, in this example we cannot compare the EXP with the placebo.

8.4 Assessment of Drug Efficacy in Active Control Trials

Results from a previous study of comparing the active control agent and the placebo may be provided in different ways. In some situations, the original data from the previous trial are available. The related statistical methods for assessment of the efficacy of the test drug product are introduced in §8.5. If the result from a previous study is summarized in terms of a prior distribution of some relevant parameters, then a Bayesian approach can be applied (§8.6). In this section, we focus on the situation where only a confidence interval (for $\mu_A - \mu_P$, μ_A/μ_P, or μ_P) and some information regarding the previous study design (e.g., the sample sizes) are available.

8.4.1   Two-Group Parallel Design with Normally Distributed Data and a Common Variance

We first consider the simplest situation where a two-group parallel design is used in both the active control trial and the previous placebo control study and the data in both trials are normally distributed with a common variance. We always assume that data from the two trials are independent.

Let $\bar{y}_T$ and $\bar{y}_A$ be the sample means for the test drug product and the active control agent, respectively, based on the data from the active control trial, and let $\bar{x}_A$ and $\bar{x}_P$ be the sample means for the active control agent and the placebo, respectively, based on the data from the previous study. Let s_{yT}^2, s_{yA}^2, s_{xA}^2, and s_{xP}^2 be the sample variances corresponding to $\bar{y}_T$, $\bar{y}_A$, $\bar{x}_A$, and $\bar{x}_P$, respectively. Let n_T and n_A be the sample sizes for the test drug group and the active control group, respectively, in the active control study, and let m_A and m_P be the sample sizes for the active control group and the placebo group, respectively, in the previous study. Then a level $1 - 2\alpha$ confidence interval for $\mu_T - \mu_A$ has the following limits:

$$\bar{y}_T - \bar{y}_A \pm t_{1-\alpha;n_T+n_A-2}\hat{\sigma}_y\sqrt{\frac{1}{n_T} + \frac{1}{n_A}},$$

where

$$\hat{\sigma}_y^2 = \frac{(n_T - 1)s_{yT}^2 + (n_A - 1)s_{yA}^2}{n_T + n_A - 2}$$

and $t_{a;n_T+n_A-2}$ is the ath percentile of the central t-distribution with $n_T + n_A - 2$ degrees of freedom.

Suppose that the result from the previous placebo control study is given in terms of a confidence interval for $\mu_A - \mu_P$, (d_-, d_+), where

$$d_{\pm} = \bar{x}_A - \bar{x}_P \pm t_{1-\alpha;m_A+m_P-2}\hat{\sigma}_x\sqrt{\frac{1}{m_A} + \frac{1}{m_P}}$$

and

$$\hat{\sigma}_x^2 = \frac{(m_A - 1)s_{xA}^2 + (m_P - 1)s_{xP}^2}{m_A + m_P - 2}.$$

When m_A and m_P are known, values of $\bar{x}_A - \bar{x}_P$ and $\hat{\sigma}_x$ can be obtained using

$$\bar{x}_A - \bar{x}_P = \frac{d_- + d_+}{2} \tag{8.4.1}$$

and

$$\hat{\sigma}_x = \frac{d_+ - d_-}{2t_{1-\alpha;m_A+m_P-2}\sqrt{\frac{1}{m_A} + \frac{1}{m_P}}}. \tag{8.4.2}$$

If the result from the previous placebo control study is summarized in terms of $\bar{x}_A - \bar{x}_P$, an estimator of the relative efficacy $\mu_A - \mu_P$, and a two-sided p-value p, then $\hat{\sigma}_x^2$ can also be obtained according to

$$\hat{\sigma}_x = \frac{|\bar{x}_A - \bar{x}_P|}{t_{1-p/2;m_A+m_P-2}\sqrt{\frac{1}{m_A} + \frac{1}{m_P}}}. \qquad (8.4.3)$$

To study whether the test drug product is superior to the placebo, we need a confidence interval for $\mu_T - \mu_P$. Since

$$\mu_T - \mu_P = \mu_T - \mu_A + \mu_A - \mu_P,$$

a level $1 - 2\alpha$ confidence interval for $\mu_T - \mu_P$ has limits

$$\bar{y}_T - \bar{y}_A + \bar{x}_A - \bar{x}_P \pm t_{1-\alpha;n_T+n_A+m_A+m_P-4}\hat{\sigma}\sqrt{\frac{1}{n_T} + \frac{1}{n_A} + \frac{1}{m_A} + \frac{1}{m_P}}$$

where

$$\hat{\sigma}^2 = \frac{(n_T + n_A - 2)\hat{\sigma}_y^2 + (m_A + m_P - 2)\hat{\sigma}_x^2}{n_T + n_A + m_A + m_P - 4}. \qquad (8.4.4)$$

If $\delta' \geq 0$ is a prespecified difference of clinical importance, then the test drug product can be claimed to be superior to the placebo at level α if the lower limit of this confidence interval is larger than δ'. Note that these confidence limits can be computed using the data from the active control trial and the result from the previous study through (8.4.1)-(8.4.3).

If the result from the previous placebo control study is summarized in terms of level $1 - 2\alpha$ confidence intervals $(\hat{\mu}_{A-}, \hat{\mu}_{A+})$ and $(\hat{\mu}_{P-}, \hat{\mu}_{P+})$ for μ_A and μ_P, respectively, then

$$\bar{x}_P = \frac{\hat{\mu}_{P+} + \hat{\mu}_{P-}}{2}, \qquad (8.4.5)$$

$$s_{xA} = \frac{\sqrt{m_A}(\hat{\mu}_{A+} - \hat{\mu}_{A-})}{2t_{1-\alpha;m_A-1}}, \qquad (8.4.6)$$

and

$$s_{xP} = \frac{\sqrt{m_P}(\hat{\mu}_{P+} - \hat{\mu}_{P-})}{2t_{1-\alpha;m_P-1}}. \qquad (8.4.7)$$

A level $1 - \alpha$ confidence interval for $\mu_T - \mu_P$ has limits

$$\bar{y}_T - \bar{x}_P \pm t_{0.975;n_T+n_A+m_A+m_P-4}\hat{\sigma}\sqrt{\frac{1}{n_T} + \frac{1}{m_P}},$$

where $\hat{\sigma}^2$ is given by (8.4.4) with s_{xA} and s_{xP} computed according to (8.4.6) and (8.4.7).

8.4.2   Two-Group Parallel Design with Unequal Variances

The equal variance assumption in §8.4.1 is often questionable, especially when two different studies are involved. Without the equal variance and the normality assumptions, approximate confidence intervals can be obtained when all sample sizes are large. First, an approximate level $1-2\alpha$ confidence interval for $\mu_T - \mu_A$ has limits

$$\bar{y}_T - \bar{y}_A \pm z_{1-\alpha}\sqrt{\frac{s_{yT}^2}{n_T} + \frac{s_{yA}^2}{n_A}},$$

where z_a is the ath quantile of the standard normal distribution. If the result from the previous placebo control study is given by the confidence limits

$$d_\pm = \bar{x}_A - \bar{x}_P \pm z_{1-\alpha}\sqrt{\frac{s_{xA}^2}{m_A} + \frac{s_{xP}^2}{m_P}},$$

then $\bar{x}_A - \bar{x}_P$ can be obtained by (8.4.1) and

$$\frac{s_{xA}^2}{m_A} + \frac{s_{xP}^2}{m_P} = \frac{d_+ - d_-}{2z_{1-\alpha}}.$$

If the result from the previous placebo control study is summarized in terms of $\bar{x}_A - \bar{x}_P$ and a two-sided p-value p, then

$$\frac{s_{xA}^2}{m_A} + \frac{s_{xP}^2}{m_P} = \left(\frac{\bar{x}_A - \bar{x}_P}{z_{1-p/2}}\right)^2.$$

In any case, an approximate level $1 - 2\alpha$ confidence interval for $\mu_T - \mu_P$ has limits

$$\bar{y}_T - \bar{y}_A + \bar{x}_A - \bar{x}_P \pm z_{1-\alpha}\sqrt{\frac{s_{yT}^2}{n_T} + \frac{s_{yA}^2}{n_A} + \frac{s_{xA}^2}{m_A} + \frac{s_{xP}^2}{m_P}}.$$

Again, the test drug product can be claimed to be superior to the placebo if the lower limit of this confidence interval is larger than δ', a prespecified difference of clinical importance.

Finally, if the result from the previous placebo control study is summarized in terms of confidence intervals $(\hat{\mu}_{A-}, \hat{\mu}_{A+})$ and $(\hat{\mu}_{P-}, \hat{\mu}_{P+})$ for μ_A and μ_P, respectively, then an approximate level $1 - 2\alpha$ confidence interval for $\mu_T - \mu_P$ has limits

$$\bar{y}_T - \bar{x}_P \pm z_{1-\alpha}\sqrt{\frac{s_{yT}^2}{n_T} + \frac{s_{xP}^2}{m_P}},$$

where $\bar{x}_P$ is given by (8.4.5) and s_{xP} is given by (8.4.7).

8.4.3   The General Case

The idea in §8.4.1-8.4.2 can be applied to more complicated designs. In general, suppose that $\hat{\theta}_{T,A}$ is an estimator of $\theta_{T,A}$, the relative efficacy of the test drug product to the active control agent, and $s_{\hat{\theta}_{T,A}}$ is an estimated standard deviation of $\hat{\theta}_{T,A}$, based on the data from the active control trial. An approximate level $1 - 2\alpha$ confidence interval for $\theta_{T,A}$ is

$$\left(\hat{\theta}_{T,A} - z_{1-\alpha} s_{\hat{\theta}_{T,A}}, \ \hat{\theta}_{T,A} + z_{1-\alpha} s_{\hat{\theta}_{T,A}} \right).$$

Let $\theta_{A,P}$ be the relative efficacy of the active control to the placebo. Suppose that the result from the previous placebo control study is summarized in terms of a level $1 - 2\alpha$ confidence interval (d_-, d_+), which is constructed using the same method as that in the current study. Then, an estimator of $\theta_{A,P}$ is

$$\hat{\theta}_{A,P} = \frac{d_- + d_+}{2}$$

and an estimator of the standard deviation of $\hat{\theta}_{A,P}$ is

$$s_{\hat{\theta}_{A,P}} = \frac{d_+ - d_-}{2z_{1-\alpha}}.$$

Suppose that $\theta_{T,P}$, the relative efficacy of the test drug product to the placebo, is a function of $\theta_{T,A}$ and $\theta_{A,P}$, $g(\theta_{T,A}, \theta_{A,P})$ (e.g., the difference or the ratio of $\theta_{T,A}$ and $\theta_{A,P}$). Then, an approximate level $1 - 2\alpha$ confidence interval for $\theta_{T,P}$ has limits

$$g(\hat{\theta}_{T,A}, \hat{\theta}_{A,P}) \pm z_{1-\alpha} \sqrt{s^2_{\hat{\theta}_{T,A}} [h_1(\hat{\theta}_{T,A}, \hat{\theta}_{A,P})]^2 + s^2_{\hat{\theta}_{A,P}} [h_2(\hat{\theta}_{T,A}, \hat{\theta}_{A,P})]^2},$$

where

$$h_1(x,y) = \frac{\partial g(x,y)}{\partial x} \quad \text{and} \quad h_2(x,y) = \frac{\partial g(x,y)}{\partial y}.$$

As a specific example, we consider the situation where the ratio of population means is considered to be the measure of relative efficacy, i.e., $\theta_{T,A} = \mu_T / \mu_A$ and $\theta_{A,P} = \mu_A / \mu_P$. Then

$$\theta_{T,P} = \frac{\mu_T}{\mu_P} = \frac{\mu_T \mu_A}{\mu_A \mu_P} = \theta_{T,A} \theta_{A,P},$$

i.e., $g(x,y) = xy$, $h_1(x,y) = y$ and $h_2(x,y) = x$. Hence, an approximate level $1 - 2\alpha$ confidence interval for $\theta_{T,P} = \mu_T / \mu_P$ has limits

$$\hat{\theta}_{T,A} \hat{\theta}_{A,T} \pm z_{1-\alpha} \sqrt{s^2_{\hat{\theta}_{T,A}} \hat{\theta}^2_{A,P} + s^2_{\hat{\theta}_{A,P}} \hat{\theta}^2_{T,A}}. \tag{8.4.8}$$

For this special case, however, a better confidence interval for $\theta_{T,P} = \mu_T/\mu_P$ can be obtained using the fact that data from two studies are independent. Note that if X and Y are two independent random variables, then

$$\text{Var}(XY) = \text{Var}(X)\text{Var}(Y) + \text{Var}(X)(EY)^2 + \text{Var}(Y)(EX)^2.$$

Using this result, we obtain the following approximate level $1 - 2\alpha$ confidence limits for $\theta_{T,P} = \mu_T/\mu_P$:

$$\hat{\theta}_{T,A}\hat{\theta}_{A,T} \pm z_{1-\alpha}\sqrt{s^2_{\hat{\theta}_{T,A}}\hat{\theta}^2_{A,P} + s^2_{\hat{\theta}_{A,P}}\hat{\theta}^2_{T,A} + s^2_{\hat{\theta}_{T,A}}s^2_{\hat{\theta}_{A,P}}}.$$

The difference between these confidence limits and those in (8.4.8) is a high-order correction term $s^2_{\hat{\theta}_{T,A}} s^2_{\hat{\theta}_{A,P}}$.

8.5 Active Control Equivalence Trials

When the original data of the previous placebo control trial are available, we can combine them with the data from the active control trial. The combined data set is almost the same as that from an *active control equivalence trial* proposed by Huque and Dubey (1990) and Pledger and Hall (1986), which is a three-treatment trial with the test drug, active control and placebo control as the treatments. The only difference may be that the combined data set from two trials may not satisfy the equal variance assumption. In this section, we introduce some statistical methods for active control equivalence trials. These methods can be directly applied to the analysis of the combined data from an active control trial and a previous placebo control trial.

8.5.1 Active Control Equivalence Trials

An active control equivalence trial is a three-group parallel design in which n_T patients receive the test drug treatment, n_A patients receive the active control treatment (or a reference drug treatment), and n_P patients receive the placebo treatment. Let μ_T, μ_A, and μ_P be the population means of the test drug, the active control, and the placebo control, respectively. For the purpose of showing that the test drug product and the active control agent are equivalent and both of them are superior to the placebo, the following hypotheses are of interest:

$$H_0 : \mu_T - \mu_A \le -\delta \text{ or } \mu_T - \mu_A \ge \delta$$
$$\text{or } \mu_T \le \mu_P + \delta' \text{ or } \mu_A \le \mu_P + \delta' \tag{8.5.1}$$

versus

$$H_1 : -\delta < \mu_T - \mu_A < \delta \text{ and}$$
$$\mu_T > \mu_P + \delta' \text{ and } \mu_A > \mu_P + \delta', \tag{8.5.2}$$

where δ and δ' are a prespecified equivalence limits. Note that the hypothesis in (8.5.1) is the union of the null hypotheses in the following four one-sided hypothesis testing problems:

$$H_0 : \mu_T - \mu_A \leq -\delta \quad \text{versus} \quad H_1 : \mu_T - \mu_A > -\delta, \tag{8.5.3}$$

$$H_0 : \mu_T - \mu_A \geq \delta \quad \text{versus} \quad H_1 : \mu_T - \mu_A < \delta, \tag{8.5.4}$$

$$H_0 : \mu_T \leq \mu_P + \delta' \quad \text{versus} \quad H_1 : \mu_T > \mu_P + \delta', \tag{8.5.5}$$

and

$$H_0 : \mu_A \leq \mu_P + \delta' \quad \text{versus} \quad H_1 : \mu_A > \mu_P + \delta'. \tag{8.5.6}$$

The first two one-sided hypothesis testing problems, (8.5.3) and (8.5.4), focus on the assessment of equivalence in efficacy between the test drug product and the active control agent, whereas hypothesis testing problems (8.5.5) and (8.5.6) assess the superiority in effectiveness of the test drug product and active control agent as compared to the placebo.

The proposed procedure in Huque and Dubey (1990) and Pledger and Hall (1986) is to test all four one-sided hypothesis testing problems (8.5.3)-(8.5.6). If all four one-sided null hypotheses in (8.5.3)-(8.5.6) are rejected at the α level of significance, then we reject H_0 in (8.5.1), i.e., we conclude that the efficacy of the test drug product and the active control agent are equivalent and they are superior to the placebo, at the α level of significance. Note that this test is an intersection-union test described in Berger and Hsu (1996).

Let $\bar{y}_T$, $\bar{y}_A$, and $\bar{y}_P$ be the sample means from patients receiving the test drug, the active control, and the placebo control, respectively, and let $se_{T,A}$, $se_{T,P}$, and $se_{A,P}$ be the usual estimators of the standard deviations of $\bar{y}_T - \bar{y}_A$, $\bar{y}_T - \bar{y}_P$, and $\bar{y}_A - \bar{y}_P$, respectively. Then, the null hypothesis H_0 in (8.5.1) is rejected if and only if

$$\bar{y}_T - \bar{y}_A + \delta > q_{\alpha,1} se_{T,A},$$

$$\bar{y}_T - \bar{y}_A - \delta < q_{\alpha,1} se_{T,A},$$

$$\bar{y}_T - \bar{y}_P - \delta' > q_{\alpha,2} se_{T,P}$$

and

$$\bar{y}_A - \bar{y}_P - \delta' > q_{\alpha,3} se_{A,P}$$

hold, where $q_{\alpha,k}$'s are percentiles depending on n_T, n_A, n_P, and the assumption on the distributions of the observations. If data are normally distributed and the variances for patients in all groups are the same, then $q_{\alpha,k}$'s are percentiles of central t-distributions with appropriate degrees of freedom. In such a case, all four one-sided tests are of size α. Hence, using Theorem 2 in Berger and Hsu (1996), we can show that the corresponding intersection-union test is of size α. If variances from different groups are different but all sample sizes n_T, n_A, and n_P are large, then $q_{\alpha,k}$'s can be chosen to be the upper α quantile of the standard normal distribution and the corresponding intersection-union test can be shown to have asymptotic size α.

The approach of confidence set described in §8.2.1 can also be applied to construct a level α test for hypotheses in (8.5.1) and (8.5.2). For this purpose, we rewrite the hypothesis H_1 in (8.5.2) as

$$H_1 : \mu_T - \mu_P > \delta' \text{ and } \mu_A - \mu_P > \delta'$$
$$\text{and } -\delta < (\mu_T - \mu_P) - (\mu_A - \mu_P) < \delta,$$

which is the shadowed area in the two-dimensional space with coordinates $\mu_A - \mu_P$ and $\mu_T - \mu_P$ (Figure 8.5.1). Let C be a level $1 - \alpha$ confidence region for $\mu_A - \mu_P$ and $\mu_T - \mu_P$. Then, a level α test rejects H_0 in (8.5.1) if C is entirely within the shadowed area in Figure 8.5.1. For example, part A of Figure 8.5.1 shows the situation where we reject H_0, whereas part B of Figure 8.5.1 shows the situation where H_0 can not be rejected.

As we discussed in §8.2.2, however, the confidence set approach may produce a too conservative test in the sense that its size is much smaller than α. Tests better than the intersection-union test and those based on the confidence set approach may be derived using the approach of Berger and Hsu (1996).

8.5.2   Active Control and Placebo Control Trials

Consider now the situation where we have data from a current active control trial and data from a previous placebo control trial that compares the same active control agent with the placebo control. If the hypotheses of interest are the same as those in (8.5.1) and (8.5.2), then the methods in §8.5.1 can be applied, except that procedures requiring equal variance assumption over all groups should not be used due to the fact that data from two different trials may have different variances. If $\bar{y}_A$ in §8.5.1 is calculated based on data from both trials, the unequal variances issue should also be appropriately addressed.

In this situation the hypotheses of interest may be different from those in (8.5.1) and (8.5.2). For example, if we would like to establish the therapeutic equivalence between the test drug and the active control agent and the therapeutic superiority of the test drug over the placebo control, then

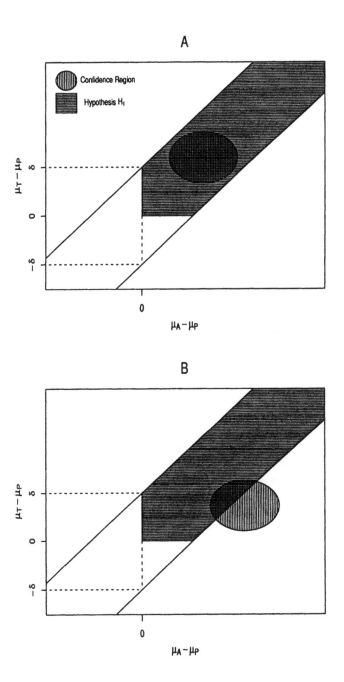

Figure 8.5.1. Graphical Presentation of Hypothesis H_1
and A Confidence Region

we may consider H_0 to be the union of three H_0's in (8.5.3)-(8.5.5). Under the assumptions described in §8.5.1, an intersection-union test of size α rejects this H_0 if and only if

$$\bar{y}_T - \bar{y}_A + \delta > q_{\alpha,1}\mathrm{se}_{T,A},$$

$$\bar{y}_T - \bar{y}_A - \delta < q_{\alpha,1}\mathrm{se}_{T,A}$$

and

$$\bar{y}_T - \bar{y}_P - \delta' > q_{\alpha,2}\mathrm{se}_{T,P}.$$

For certain types of hypotheses, statistical testing can be performed using the methods described in §8.4, i.e., using some summary statistics but not the original data from the previous placebo control trial. When the original data from the previous placebo control trial are available, however, more accurate statistical analysis may be possible and more complicated hypotheses can be tested.

Example 8.5.1. A clinical trial was conducted to compare a test compound (a doxorubicin liposome injection) versus doxorubicin injection (a standard doxorubicin as an active control) in patients with metastatic breast cancer. A total of 216 patients participated in this trial. One of the primary objectives of this trial was to demonstrate that the efficacy of the test compound is equivalent to the efficacy of the standard doxorubicin and is superior to no treatment. In addition to the response rate (i.e., complete response plus partial response), one of the primary efficacy endpoints of interest is the duration of survival, which was determined for all patients, including patients that are discontinued from the study, from the time of entry into the study until the time of death. For illustration purpose, partial survival data (20 subjects in each treatment group) are given in Table 8.5.1, which yields

$$\bar{y}_T - \bar{y}_A = 76.6 \quad \text{and} \quad \mathrm{se}_{T,A} = 165.2.$$

From the historical database at respective investigator sites, we obtain that $\bar{y}_P = 179.5$ with estimated standard error 40.1. Thus,

$$\bar{y}_T - \bar{y}_P = 491.5 \quad \text{and} \quad \mathrm{se}_{T,A} = 136.0.$$

When $\alpha = 0.05$, $q_{\alpha,1} = q_{\alpha,2} \approx 1.645$. With $\delta = \delta' = 50$, we conclude that the efficacy of the test compound is equivalent to the efficacy of the standard doxorubicin and is superior to no treatment.

Table 8.5.1. List of Survival Data (Day)

Active control	Test compound
828	1529
321	819
209	179
1839	1894
1413	452
399	794
1212	345
1025	779
872	150
294	191
301	597
793	102
672	1531
104	1894
526	324
274	219
476	253
356	885
255	658
808	969

8.6 A Bayesian Approach for Active Control Trials

If the results from previous placebo control trial are summarized in terms of a prior distribution on some relevant parameters, then a Bayesian approach can be applied to analyzing data from the current active control trial.

8.6.1 Balanced Design with Known Variance

We first introduce the result in Simon (1999) for the case where $n_T = n_A = n$ observations are obtained respectively from a test drug product and an active control agent and data are independent and normally distributed with a known variance σ^2. Let $\bar{y}_T$ and $\bar{y}_A$ be respectively the sample means of the test drug group and the active control group. Let μ_T, μ_A, and μ_P be the population means for the test drug product, active control agent, and placebo, respectively. Simon (1999) showed that, if the prior of

$$\phi = \begin{pmatrix} \mu_P \\ \mu_A - \mu_P \\ \mu_T - \mu_P \end{pmatrix}$$

is the following multivariate normal

$$N\left(\begin{pmatrix} u_1 \\ u_2 \\ u_3 \end{pmatrix}, \begin{pmatrix} \sigma_1^2 & 0 & 0 \\ 0 & \sigma_2^2 & 0 \\ 0 & 0 & \sigma_3^2 \end{pmatrix} \right)$$

with known constants u_k and σ_k^2, then the posterior distribution of ϕ is multivariate normal with mean vector

$$\frac{1}{c}\begin{pmatrix} r_1(1+r_2)(1+r_3)u_1 + r_2(1+r_3)(\bar{y}_A - u_2) + r_3(1+r_2)(\bar{y}_T - u_3) \\ r_2[r_3 + (1+r_1)(1+r_3)]u_2 + r_1(1+r_3)(\bar{y}_A - u_1) + r_3(\bar{y}_A - \bar{y}_T + u_3) \\ r_3[r_2 + (1+r_1)(1+r_2)]u_3 + r_1(1+r_2)(\bar{y}_T - u_1) + r_2(\bar{y}_T - \bar{y}_A + u_2) \end{pmatrix}$$

and covariance matrix

$$\frac{\sigma^2}{nc}\begin{pmatrix} (1+r_2)(1+r_3) & -(1+r_3) & -(1+r_2) \\ -(1+r_3) & r_3 + (1+r_1)(1+r_3) & 1 \\ -(1+r_2) & 1 & r_2 + (1+r_1)(1+r_2) \end{pmatrix},$$

where $r_k = \sigma^2/(n\sigma_k^2)$, $k = 1, 2, 3$, and $c = r_1(1+r_2)(1+r_3) + r_2(1+r_3) + r_3(1+r_2)$. The effect of the test drug product can be assessed using this posterior distribution. For example, if therapeutic noninferiority of the test drug with respect to the placebo is tested, then the posterior probability of $\mu_T - \mu_P > -\delta$ is $\Phi((\delta+\eta)/\sqrt{v})$, where Φ is the standard normal distribution function,

$$\eta = \frac{r_3[r_2 + (1+r_1)(1+r_2)]u_3 + r_1(1+r_2)(\bar{y}_T - u_1) + r_2(\bar{y}_T - \bar{y}_A + u_2)}{r_1(1+r_2)(1+r_3) + r_2(1+r_3) + r_3(1+r_2)},$$

and

$$v = \frac{\sigma^2[r_2 + (1+r_1)(1+r_2)]}{n[r_1(1+r_2)(1+r_3) + r_2(1+r_3) + r_3(1+r_2)]}.$$

Under the Bayesian approach, the null hypothesis that $\mu_T - \mu_P \leq -\delta$ can be rejected if $\Phi((\delta + \eta)/\sqrt{v}) > \xi$ (a given value). Similarly, hypothesis H_0 in (8.5.1) can be rejected if the posterior probability of the shadowed area in Figure 8.5.1A is larger than ξ.

Simon (1999) discussed the use of noninformative priors in cases where prior information (about u_k's and σ_k^2's) is not available. A noninformative prior can be obtained by letting one or two of σ_k^2's tend to infinity. The posterior distribution can be obtained by setting the corresponding r_k's to 0. For example, if the prior for $\mu_T - \mu_P$ is noninformative, then the posterior distribution is multivariate normal with mean

$$\frac{1}{r_1(1+r_2)+r_2} \begin{pmatrix} r_1(1+r_2)u_1 + r_2(\bar{y}_A - u_2) \\ r_2(1+r_1)u_2 + r_1(\bar{y}_A - u_1) \\ r_1(1+r_2)(\bar{y}_T - u_1) + r_2(\bar{y}_T - \bar{y}_A + u_2) \end{pmatrix}$$

and covariance matrix

$$\frac{\sigma^2}{n[r_1(1+r_2)+r_2]} \begin{pmatrix} 1+r_2 & -1 & -(1+r_2) \\ -1 & 1+r_1 & 1 \\ -(1+r_2) & 1 & r_2 + (1+r_1)(1+r_2) \end{pmatrix}.$$

If the prior for $\mu_A - \mu_P$ is also noninformative, then the posterior distribution is multivariate normal with mean

$$\begin{pmatrix} u_1 \\ \bar{y}_A - u_1 \\ \bar{y}_T - u_1 \end{pmatrix}$$

and covariance matrix

$$\frac{\sigma^2}{nr_1} \begin{pmatrix} 1 & -1 & -1 \\ -1 & 1+r_1 & 1 \\ -1 & 1 & 1+r_1 \end{pmatrix}.$$

However, the posterior distribution is degenerate if the prior distributions for all three components of ϕ are noninformative.

8.6.2 Unbalanced Design with Unknown Variance

We now consider the case where n_T and n_A are not the same and σ^2 is unknown. Consider the following noninformative prior density for ϕ and σ^2:

$$\pi(\phi, \sigma^2) = \frac{1}{\sigma^2} \frac{1}{\sqrt{2\pi\sigma}} e^{-(\mu_P - u_1)^2/(2\sigma^2)},$$

where u_1 is a known prior mean of μ_P. Note that this prior is noninformative for $\mu_T - \mu_P$, $\mu_A - \mu_P$, and σ^2 and is slightly different from the noninformative prior in §8.6.1. A straightforward calculation shows that the posterior density of ϕ and $\tau = \sigma^{-2}$ is

$$p_1(\mu_A - \mu_P|\mu_P, \tau, W)p_2(\mu_T - \mu_P|\mu_P, \tau, W)p_3(\mu_P|\tau, W)p_4(\tau|W),$$

where $W = (\bar{y}_A, \bar{y}_T, s_A^2, s_T^2)$, s_A^2 and s_T^2 are the sample variance of the test group and active control group, respectively, $p_1(\mu_A - \mu_P | \mu_P, \tau, W)$ is the density of $N(\bar{y}_A - \mu_P, \sigma^2/n_A)$, $p_2(\mu_T - \mu_P | \mu_P, \tau, W)$ is the density of $N(\bar{y}_T - \mu_P, \sigma^2/n_T)$, $p_3(\mu_P | \tau, W)$ is the density of $N(u_1, \sigma^2)$, and $p_4(\tau | W)$ is the density of the gamma distribution with shape parameter $(n_A + n_T - 2)/2$ and scale parameter $2[(n_A - 1)s_A^2 + (n_T - 1)s_T^2]^{-1}$. The posterior probability of $\mu_T - \mu_P > \delta$ can be calculated as

$$
\begin{aligned}
P(\mu_T - \mu_P > \delta | W) &= E\left[P\left(\mu_T - \mu_P > \delta \middle| \mu_P, \tau, W\right) \middle| W\right] \\
&= E\left[\Phi\left(\frac{\bar{y}_T - \mu_P - \delta}{\sigma/\sqrt{n_T}}\right) \middle| W\right] \\
&= E\left\{E\left[\Phi\left(\frac{\bar{y}_T - \mu_P - \delta}{\sigma/\sqrt{n_T}}\right) \middle| \tau, W\right] \middle| W\right\} \\
&= E\left\{E\left[P\left(\sigma Z/\sqrt{n_T} + \mu_P \le \bar{y}_T - \delta\right) \middle| \tau, W\right] \middle| W\right\} \\
&= E\left\{P\left(\sigma Z/\sqrt{n_T} + \mu_P \le \bar{y}_T - \delta \middle| \tau, W\right) \middle| W\right\} \\
&= E\left\{\Phi\left(\frac{\bar{y}_T - u_1 - \delta}{\sigma\sqrt{1 + n_T^{-1}}}\right) \middle| W\right\} \\
&= \int_0^\infty \Phi\left(\frac{\bar{y}_T - u_1 - \delta}{\sigma\sqrt{1 + n_T^{-1}}}\right) p_4(\tau | W) d\tau,
\end{aligned}
$$

where Z denotes a standard normal random variable independent of μ_P. The last integral has to be evaluated using numerical methods. Testing for therapeutic noninferiority can be carried out by comparing this posterior probability with a given level ξ. Other hypotheses can be tested similarly.

Example 8.6.1. Using the data in Example 8.5.1 (Table 8.5.1) and $u_1 = 179.5$ (historical information), we obtained the posterior probability

$$P(\mu_T - \mu_P > \delta | W) = 0.7929,$$

where δ is chosen to be 50.

8.7   Discussion

Since the ethical concern regarding the inclusion of a concurrent placebo control in active control equivalence trials, Huque and Dubey (1990) have explored the possibility of designing a group sequential trial by performing interim analyses for the purpose of stopping placebo arm with continuation of the test and reference active control. However, in order to stop the placebo group early based on results from interim analyses, the randomization codes of all three groups must be broken to reveal the treatment assignment of each patient. As a result, bias will be unavoidably introduced into subsequent assessment between the test and active control and consequently, the primary goal for an unbiased evaluation of the equivalence between the two drugs may be in serious jeopardy.

For binary data, the sample size determination and equivalence limits depend upon not only the assumed reference response rate but also the overall response rate (Huque and Dubey, 1990). It should be noted that the observed reference and overall response rates might differ from the assumed rates used for sample size determination at the planning stage of the trial. In addition, they may be different from one interim look to another. It is, however, not clear whether the same prespecified equivalence limit should be used for all interim analyses. Durrleman and Simon (1990) and Jennison and Turnball (1993) provide some thoughtful considerations in design, conduct, monitoring and analysis of sequential active control equivalence trials. However, their methodology did not cover the joint evaluation of the equivalence and superiority in efficacy of active drugs as compared to the placebo.

Chapter 9

Analysis of Incomplete Data

In practice, despite a thoughtful and well-written study protocol, the data set from a clinical trial is often incomplete. The possible causes for incomplete data could be the duration of study, the nature of the disease, the efficacy and adverse effects of the drug under study, intercurrent illness, accidents, patient refusal or moving, and administrative reasons unrelated to the study. In many clinical trials, the proportion of missing values could be as high as 40% of the whole set of data. There are two types of incomplete data according to Diggle, Liang, and Zeger (1994). The first type is dropout, which occurs when patients withdraw or discontinue prematurely from a trial at any time before its planned completion. Missing values other than dropouts are referred to as intermittent missing values, which is the second type of incomplete data.

A key to the analysis of incomplete data is whether or not the mechanism of missing values is statistically related to the primary response variable under study, or roughly speaking, whether or not the population (of the primary response variable) of patients with missing values is different from the population of patients without missing values. A precise study of this issue is given in §9.1. If the mechanism of missing values is independent of the primary response variable, then a valid statistical analysis can be carried out by simply conditioning on the observed incomplete data. The main concerns in this case are (i) whether an appreciable rate of missing affects the statistical power of the tests for treatment effects; and (ii) whether information provided by auxiliary variables can be used to improve the statistical power. These issues are considered in §9.2-9.4. It is considerably more difficult to analyze incomplete data when the mechanism of missing values is related to the primary response variable, although a solution can be found by data transformation in some cases (§9.4.3). In the last two sections, we consider longitudinal data (repeated measurements) when the mechanism of missing is related to the primary response variable. §9.5 focuses on the analysis of last observations in intention-to-treat analyses, whereas §9.6 discusses the analyses of longitudinal data.

9.1 Mechanism of Missing Values

Let y be the primary response variable of a patient in a clinical study. Suppose that there is a vector of covariates related to the patients that do not have any missing values. For example, in a study with a parallel-group design for comparing a treatments, the indicator variable of different treatments can be considered as a covariate. Other covariates include demographics (e.g., age, sex, and race), baseline patient characteristics (e.g., disease status and medical history), and study centers in a multicenter trial. Let x and z denote different vectors of covariates. Let r be the indicator of whether y is observed, i.e., $r = 1$ if y is not missing and $r = 0$ if y is missing.

Statistical methods of analyzing incomplete data depend upon whether or not the following assumption holds:

$$P(r = 1|y, x, z) = P(r = 1|z), \qquad (9.1.1)$$

where the left hand side of equation (9.1.1) is the conditional probability of observing y, given the values of y, x and z, whereas the right hand side of equation (9.1.1) is the conditional probability of observing y, given z. If assumption (9.1.1) holds, then the probability of observing y is independent of y and the covariate x, conditional on the observed covariate z. Under this assumption, whether or not y is missing may still be treatment-related; for example, z is an indicator for treatment and/or center. When z is the treatment indicator under a parallel-group design, assumption (9.1.1) means that the probability of missing depends on the treatment, but within a treatment, it is a constant for all patients. For many clinical trials, this is a reasonable assumption.

The mechanism of missing values is said to be *noninformative* with respect to y and x if assumption (9.1.1) holds and *informative* if assumption (9.1.1) does not hold. Note that noninformative missingness is very similar to the concept of missing at random as described in Little and Rubin (1987). A special case of (9.1.1) is

$$P(r = 1|y, x, z) = P(r = 1), \qquad (9.1.2)$$

i.e., the probability of observing y depends on neither the primary response variable nor covariates. The mechanism of missing values satisfying (9.1.2) is said to be completely random (Little and Rubin, 1987), but it rarely occurs in practice.

If the mechanism of missing values is noninformative, then the statistical analysis can be carried out by conditioning on the observed incomplete data. This can be justified as follows. Let $f(a|b)$ be the conditional probability density (either discrete or continuous) of a, given b, e.g., $f(y|x, z, r = 1)$ is the conditional probability density of y, given x, z and $r = 1$. Regardless of whether (9.1.1) holds, we have

$$f(y|x, z, r = 1) = \frac{P(r = 1|y, x, z)f(y|x, z)}{P(r = 1|x, z)}. \tag{9.1.3}$$

If assumption (9.1.1) holds, then $P(r = 1|x, z) = P(r = 1|z)$ and it follows from (9.1.3) that

$$f(y|x, z, r = 1) = f(y|x, z).$$

Similarly,

$$f(y|x, z, r = 0) = f(y|x, z).$$

In other words, given x and z, the population of patients with missing values and the population of patients without missing values are the same. Conclusions drawn from statistical inference on $f(y|x, z, r = 1)$ based on observed data (i.e,. y values with $r = 1$) can be applied to $f(y|x, z, r = 0)$ and $f(y|x, z)$, since they are the same.

Under assumption (9.1.1), some statistical methods designed for the case of no missing data are still valid when they are applied to incomplete data (with suitable sample size adjustments), although statistical efficiency (power) is reduced when the incomplete data set has a much smaller size than the complete data set. For example, consider the parallel-group design for the comparison of a treatments, where z is the indicator of the treatment group. If there is no missing value, a test of treatment difference can be derived from the one-way analysis of variance (ANOVA) with sample size $n_1 + \cdots + n_a$, where n_i is the number of selected patients in treatment group i, $i = 1, ..., a$. When there are missing values and assumption (9.1.1) holds, we can still apply the same test procedure but use the incomplete data set which has size $m_1 + \cdots + m_a$, where m_i is the number of patients in group i whose y values are not missing. Although the significance level of the test remains unchanged, the power of the test decreases because $m_i \leq n_i$ for all i (see §9.2).

If the mechanism of missing values is informative, then $f(y|x, z, r = 1) \neq f(y|x, z, r = 0)$ and the inference based on the completers would be biased. Making statistical inference is very difficult, since no information about $f(y|x, z, r = 0)$ is provided by the data. Under some parametric or semiparametric model assumptions, analysis of incomplete data with informative missingness can be carried out by using the likelihood approach. For example, we may consider parametric models

$$P(r = 1|y, x) = \psi(y, x, \beta)$$

and

$$f(y|x) = \phi(y, x, \theta),$$

where ψ and ϕ are known functions and β and θ are unknown parameter vectors. The likelihood is then

$$\prod_{j:r_j=1} \psi(y_j, x_j, \beta)\phi(y_j, x_j, \theta) \prod_{j:r_j=0} \left[1 - \int \psi(y, x_j, \beta)\phi(y, x_j, \theta) dy \right].$$

An empirical likelihood for the case where $f(y|x)$ is nonparametric is introduced in Qin, Leung, and Shao (2002).

However, the required sample size for an efficient statistical analysis based on this type of likelihood is usually very large. Also, the required computation could be very intensive.

The FDA and ICH guidelines on clinical reports both indicate that despite the difficulty, the possible effects of dropouts and missing values on magnitude and direction of bias must be explored as fully as possible. That is to say, before any analyses of efficacy endpoints, at various intervals during the study the frequency, reasons, and time to dropouts and missing values should also be compared between treatment groups. Their impact on the trial's efficacy has to be fully explored and understood, and only after the missingness mechanism has been identified can appropriate statistical methods be employed for the analysis (Diggle, 1989; Ridout and Morgan, 1991).

9.2 The Power of ANOVA Tests

As discussed in §9.1, the test for treatment effects derived from the ANOVA under a parallel-group design can be applied to analyzing incomplete data if the missingness is noninformative. However, the power of the ANOVA test decreases as the proportion of missing values increases. In practice, sample sizes are usually selected to account for possible loss in power due to missing data. In this section, we illustrate how to address this issue with tests derived from the one-way ANOVA. Results for tests derived from k-way ANOVA with a $k \geq 2$ can be similarly obtained.

Let $a \geq 2$ be the number of treatments under study and y_{ij} be the response value of the jth patient in the ith treatment group, $j = 1, ..., n_i$,

$i = 1, ..., a$. Here, n_i is the original sample size in the ith treatment group. Usually n_i's are chosen to be the same. But, in some situations different n_i's are desirable (see §6.2.4), which will be discussed later. Assume that y_{ij}'s are independently distributed as $N(\mu_i, \sigma^2)$. If there is no missing value, then the null hypothesis $H_0 : \mu_1 = \cdots = \mu_a$ is rejected at the 5% level of significance if $T > F_{0.95;a-1,n-a}$, where $F_{0.95;a-1,n-a}$ is the 95th percentile of the F-distribution with $a - 1$ and $n - a$ degrees of freedom, $n = n_1 + \cdots + n_a$,

$$T = \frac{\text{SST}/(a - 1)}{\text{SSE}/(n - a)},$$

$\text{SST} = \sum_{i=1}^{a} n_i(\bar{y}_i - \bar{y})^2$, $\text{SSE} = \sum_{i=1}^{a} \sum_{j=1}^{n_i} (y_{ij} - \bar{y}_i)^2$, $\bar{y}_i$ is the sample mean based on the data in the ith group, and $\bar{y}$ is the overall sample mean. The power of this test is given by

$$1 - \mathcal{F}_{a-1,n-a}(F_{0.95;a-1,n-a}|\theta),$$

where $\mathcal{F}_{a-1,n-a}(\cdot|\theta)$ is the the noncentral F-distribution function with $a-1$ and $n - a$ degrees of freedom and the noncentrality parameter

$$\theta = \sum_{i=1}^{a} \frac{n_i(\mu_i - \bar{\mu})^2}{\sigma^2}$$

and $\bar{\mu} = \sum_{i=1}^{a} n_i \mu_i / n$.

Suppose that there are missing values and assumption (9.1.1) holds with $x \equiv 1$ and z being the indicator of treatment groups, i.e., $z = i$ for a patient in group i, $i = 1, ..., a$. Let $m_i \leq n_i$ be the number of observed y_{ij}'s in the ith treatment group, $i = 1, ..., a$, and $m = m_1 + \cdots + m_a$. Let T_m be the same as T but based on observed incomplete data. Under the noninformative missingness assumption, the test that rejects H_0 if $T_m > F_{0.95;a-1,m-a}$ is still a test with the 5% level of significance. If we start with sample sizes m_i instead of n_i and there is no missing value, then it seems that we have the same test procedure. But the difference is that m_i's are random in the presence of missing values. Conditioning on m_i's, we obtain the power

$$1 - \mathcal{F}_{a-1,m-a}(F_{0.95;a-1,m-a}|\theta_m),$$

where θ_m is the same as θ with n_i's replaced by m_i's. Let $m = (m_1, ..., m_a)$ and $\mu = (\mu_1, ..., \mu_a)$. Then the conditional power is a function of m and μ/σ.

Under the noninformative missingness assumption, m_i has the binomial distribution with size n_i and mean $p_i n_i$, where $p_i = P(r = 1|z = i)$, i.e., the probability of observing the y value for patients in group i. Let $p = (p_1, ..., p_a)$ and $n = (n_1, ..., n_a)$. The unconditional power is then

$$E[1 - \mathcal{F}_{a-1,m-a}(F_{0.95;a-1,m-a}|\theta_m)], \tag{9.2.1}$$

where the expectation E is with respect to m. With given μ/σ, p and n, the power given by (9.2.1) can be evaluated numerically. Table 9.2.1 lists values of the power given by (9.2.1) for $a = 2$ and some values of $n_1 = n_2 = n$, $(\mu_1 - \mu_2)/\sigma$, p_1, and p_2. The results in Table 9.2.1 shows us the effect of missing values. When $n = 20$ and $(\mu_1 - \mu_2)/\sigma = 0.89$, for example, the power is 78.31% when there is no missing values, but the power reduces to 61.33% when each group has about 30% missing values $(p_1 = p_2 = 70\%)$.

When n_i's are large, we may consider some approximations to simplify the computation of the power. First, $\mathcal{F}_{a-1,m-a}(\cdot|\theta_m)$ can be approximated by $\tilde{\mathcal{F}}_{a-1}(\cdot|\theta_m)$, the distribution function of $(a-1)^{-1}$ times a noncentral chi-square random variable with $a - 1$ degrees of freedom and the noncentrality parameter θ_m. Then, when n_i's are large and all p_i's are positive,

$$E[1 - \mathcal{F}_{a-1,m-a}(F_{0.95;a-1,m-a}|\theta_m)] \approx E[1 - \tilde{\mathcal{F}}_{a-1}(F_{0.95;a-1,m-a}|\theta_m)],$$

which can be further approximated by

$$1 - \tilde{\mathcal{F}}_{a-1}(\tilde{F}_{0.95;a-1}|E\theta_m) \approx 1 - \tilde{\mathcal{F}}_{a-1}(\tilde{F}_{0.95;a-1}|\tilde{\theta}), \qquad (9.2.2)$$

where $\tilde{F}_{0.95;a-1}$ be the 95th percentile of $\tilde{\mathcal{F}}_{a-1}(\cdot|0)$,

$$\tilde{\theta} = \sum_{i=1}^{a} \frac{p_i n_i (\mu_i - \tilde{\mu})^2}{\sigma^2} \qquad (9.2.3)$$

and $\tilde{\mu} = \sum_{i=1}^{a} p_i n_i \mu_i / \sum_{i=1}^{a} p_i n_i$. Note that $\tilde{\mathcal{F}}_{a-1}(\tilde{F}_{0.95;a-1}|\tilde{\theta})$ can be easily computed when $p_i n_i$ and μ_i/σ, $i = 1, ..., a$, are given. Table 9.2.2 gives values of the approximate power given by (9.2.2) for the same values of a, $n_1 = n_2 = n$, $(\mu_1 - \mu_2)/\sigma$, p_1, and p_2 in Table 9.2.1. Comparing the results in Tables 9.2.1 and 9.2.2, we find that the approximation (9.2.2) is better when n is larger, and is adequate when $n = 30$.

Formula (9.2.2) can also be used in selecting sample sizes n_i's to account for the power loss due to missing values. Suppose that we have some initial values of μ_i/σ and p_i, $i = 1, ..., a$. Using formulas (9.2.2) and (9.2.3), we can obtain numerical solutions $n_1, ..., n_a$ satisfying

$$1 - \tilde{\mathcal{F}}_{a-1}(\tilde{F}_{0.95;a-1}|\tilde{\theta}) = \beta,$$

where β is a desired level of power (e.g., 80%).

In the important special case of comparing $a = 2$ treatments, a more explicit solution for sample sizes can be obtained. When $a = 2$, $\tilde{\theta}$ reduces to

$$\frac{(\mu_1 - \mu_2)^2}{\sigma^2} \bigg/ \left(\frac{1}{p_1 n_1} + \frac{1}{p_2 n_2} \right). \qquad (9.2.4)$$

Table 9.2.1. Values of Power (9.2.1) Approximated by 10,000 Simulations

n	$\frac{\mu_1-\mu_2}{\sigma}$	p_1	p_2 1.0	0.9	0.8	0.7	0.6	0.5
10	1.26	1.0	.7595	.7315	.6978	.6583	.6087	.5514
		0.9		.7042	.6720	.6334	.5861	.5308
		0.8			.6405	.6012	.5592	.5049
		0.7				.5675	.5238	.4735
		0.6					.4855	.4383
		0.5						.3963
	1.45	1.0	.8655	.8425	.8125	.7754	.7247	.6654
		0.9		.8178	.7879	.7505	.7024	.6432
		0.8			.7579	.7196	.6738	.6167
		0.7				.6850	.6400	.5828
		0.6					.5955	.5409
		0.5						.4909
20	0.89	1.0	.7831	.7588	.7291	.6932	.6483	.5937
		0.9		.7349	.7062	.6717	.6280	.5757
		0.8			.6779	.6447	.6039	.5542
		0.7				.6133	.5758	.5291
		0.6					.5397	.4964
		0.5						.4575
	1.03	1.0	.8876	.8683	.8443	.8123	.7726	.7159
		0.9		.8487	.8243	.7923	.7514	.6995
		0.8			.7998	.7680	.7280	.6768
		0.7				.7374	.6987	.6490
		0.6					.6611	.6156
		0.5						.5703
30	0.73	1.0	.7940	.7704	.7424	.7076	.6648	.6106
		0.9		.7479	.7207	.6863	.6460	.5919
		0.8			.6936	.6616	.6225	.5719
		0.7				.6312	.5937	.5478
		0.6					.5604	.5183
		0.5						.4800
	0.84	1.0	.8923	.8744	.8513	.8219	.7827	.7306
		0.9		.8559	.8332	.8032	.7646	.7123
		0.8			.8100	.7801	.7416	.6922
		0.7				.7512	.7147	.6658
		0.6					.6790	.6345
		0.5						.5916

Table 9.2.2. Values of Approximate Power (9.2.2)

n	$\frac{\mu_1-\mu_2}{\sigma}$	p_1	p_2					
			1.0	0.9	0.8	0.7	0.6	0.5
10	1.26	1.0	.8044	.7830	.7569	.7247	.6844	.6333
		0.9		.7620	.7367	.7055	.6667	.6175
		0.8			.7123	.6825	.6455	.5988
		0.7				.6544	.6198	.5761
		0.6					.5880	.5481
		0.5						.5129
	1.45	1.0	.9001	.8841	.8637	.8370	.8018	.7541
		0.9		.8678	.8471	.8205	.7856	.7388
		0.8			.8264	.8000	.7657	.7202
		0.7				.7742	.7410	.6972
		0.6					.7094	.6681
		0.5						.6303
20	0.89	1.0	.8036	.7821	.7560	.7238	.6835	.6323
		0.9		.7612	.7358	.7046	.6657	.6166
		0.8			.7114	.6815	.6445	.5979
		0.7				.6535	.6188	.5752
		0.6					.5871	.5472
		0.5						.5121
	1.03	1.0	.9027	.8869	.8667	.8403	.8053	.7579
		0.9		.8708	.8503	.8239	.7892	.7427
		0.8			.8298	.8036	.7695	.7241
		0.7				.7779	.7448	.7012
		0.6					.7133	.6721
		0.5						.6343
30	0.73	1.0	.8071	.7858	.7598	.7277	.6874	.6363
		0.9		.7649	.7396	.7085	.6697	.6206
		0.8			.7153	.6855	.6485	.6018
		0.7				.6575	.6228	.5790
		0.6					.5910	.5510
		0.5						.5157
	0.84	1.0	.9021	.8862	.8659	.8395	.8044	.7569
		0.9		.8700	.8495	.8231	.7883	.7417
		0.8			.8289	.8027	.7685	.7231
		0.7				.7770	.7438	.7001
		0.6					.7123	.6710
		0.5						.6333

Since $\tilde{\mathcal{F}}_{a-1}(\cdot|\theta)$ is a decreasing function of θ, the power is maximized if $\frac{1}{p_1 n_1}+\frac{1}{p_2 n_2}$ reaches its minimum. Suppose that the total sample size n_1+n_2 is fixed. Then, the power reaches its maximum if

$$\frac{n_1}{n_2} = \frac{\sqrt{p_2}}{\sqrt{p_1}}. \qquad (9.2.5)$$

In other words, if the ratio $\rho = p_1/p_2$ is known, then the sample size allocation should be made according to $n_2 = \sqrt{\rho}n_1$ to achieve the highest power. Note that the use of equal sample sizes $n_1 = n_2$ is a good idea only when the ratio $\rho = 1$. Let ξ_β be the solution of

$$\tilde{\mathcal{F}}_{a-1}(\tilde{F}_{0.95;a-1}|\xi_\beta) = 1 - \beta.$$

Then, it follows from (9.2.2), (9.2.4), and (9.2.5) that the optimal sample sizes are given by

$$n_1 = \frac{\sigma^2 \xi_\beta}{(\mu_1 - \mu_2)^2}\left(\frac{1}{p_1} + \frac{1}{\sqrt{p_1 p_2}}\right)$$

and

$$n_2 = \frac{\sigma^2 \xi_\beta}{(\mu_1 - \mu_2)^2}\left(\frac{1}{p_2} + \frac{1}{\sqrt{p_1 p_2}}\right).$$

9.3 Imputation for Missing Data

When auxiliary variables are available, they can be used to make up part of loss due to missing values. One approach of using auxiliary data is to perform imputation. In this section we consider a method of imputation under a parallel-group design for comparing $a = 2$ treatments. Assume that x is a vector of auxiliary variables (e.g., observations from demographics and baseline patient characteristics) and that

$$P(r = 1|y, x, i) = P(r = 1|i), \qquad i = 1, 2,$$

i.e., the mechanism of missing value is noninformative with respect to y and x. Hence, statistical inference can be made by conditioning on m_i's. Throughout this section, all probability distributions are conditional on m_i's. The auxiliary variables and y are assumed to be related according to the following linear regression model:

$$y_{ij} = \alpha_i + \beta_i' x_{ij} + e_{ij}, \qquad j = 1, ..., n_i, i = 1, 2, \qquad (9.3.1)$$

where e_{ij}'s are independent random variables distributed as $N(0, \sigma_{ei}^2)$, e_{ij}'s and x_{ij}'s are independent, and α_i, β_i, and σ_{ei}^2 are unknown parameters depending on $i = 1, 2$. Furthermore, x_{ij}'s are assumed to be independent and normally distributed.

In the case of no missing values,

$$\bar{y}_1 - \bar{y}_2 \sim N\left(\mu_1 - \mu_2, \ \frac{\sigma_1^2}{n_1} + \frac{\sigma_2^2}{n_2}\right),$$

where

$$\mu_i = E(y_{ij}) = \alpha_i + \beta_i' E(x_{ij})$$

and

$$\sigma_i^2 = \sigma_{ei}^2 + \beta_i' \mathrm{Var}(x_{ij})\beta_i.$$

Since σ_1^2 and σ_2^2 are unlikely the same, testing treatment effect can be carried out using the following large sample approximation:

$$\frac{\bar{y}_1 - \bar{y}_2}{\sqrt{\frac{s_1^2}{n_1} + \frac{s_2^2}{n_2}}} \sim N(0, 1),$$

where s_i^2 is the sample variance based on y_{ij}, $j = 1, ..., n_i$.

Assume that x_{ij}'s are all observed. For notation simplicity, assume that y_{ij}, $j = 1, ..., m_i$, are observed and y_{ij}, $j = m_i + 1, ..., n_i$, are missing. If we don't use auxiliary data, then the inference can be made based on

$$\tilde{y}_1 - \tilde{y}_2 \sim N\left(\mu_1 - \mu_2, \ \frac{\sigma_1^2}{m_1} + \frac{\sigma_2^2}{m_2}\right),$$

where $\tilde{y}_i$ is the sample mean based on y_{ij}, $j = 1, ..., m_i$. Under model (9.3.1), a missing value y_{ij} can be imputed by its predicted value obtained from the fitted regression model using observed y values, i.e., y_{ij} with $j \geq m_i + 1$ are imputed by

$$y_{ij}^* = \hat{\alpha}_i + \hat{\beta}_i' x_{ij},$$

where

$$\hat{\beta}_i = M_i^{-1} \sum_{j=1}^{m_i} (x_{ij} - \tilde{x}_i) y_{ij},$$

$$\hat{\alpha}_i = \tilde{y}_i - \hat{\beta}_i' \tilde{x}_i,$$

$\tilde{x}_i$ is the sample mean based on x_{ij}, $j = 1, ..., m_i$, and

$$M_i = \sum_{j=1}^{m_i} (x_{ij} - \tilde{x}_i)(x_{ij} - \tilde{x}_i)'.$$

By treating imputed values as observed data, we obtain the following sample mean

$$\bar{y}_i^* = \frac{1}{n_i}\left(\sum_{j=1}^{m_i} y_{ij} + \sum_{j=m_i+1}^{n_i} y_{ij}^*\right)$$
$$= \tilde{y}_i + \hat{\beta}_i'(\bar{x}_i - \tilde{x}_i)$$
$$= \sum_{j=1}^{m_i}\left(\frac{1}{m_i} + c_{ij}\right) y_{ij},$$

where $\bar{x}_i$ is the sample mean based on x_{ij}, $j = 1, ..., n_i$, and

$$c_{ij} = (x_{ij} - \tilde{x}_i)' M_i^{-1}(\bar{x}_i - \tilde{x}_i).$$

To calculate the expected value and variance of $\bar{y}_i^*$, let E_y and Var_y be the conditional mean and variance, respectively, given all x values. Under model (9.3.1) and the noninformative missingness assumption,

$$E_y(\bar{y}_i^*) = \alpha_i + \beta_i'\bar{x}_i$$

and

$$\text{Var}_y(\bar{y}_i^*) = \sigma_{ei}^2\left(\frac{1}{m_i} + \sum_{j=1}^{m_i} c_{ij}^2\right)$$
$$= \sigma_{ei}^2\left[\frac{1}{m_i} + (\bar{x}_i - \tilde{x}_i)' M_i^{-1}(\bar{x}_i - \tilde{x}_i)\right].$$

Thus,

$$E(\bar{y}_i^*) = \alpha_i + \beta_i' E(\bar{x}_i) = \mu_i,$$

i.e., $\bar{y}_i^*$ is an unbiased estimator of the mean μ_i of treatment i. Conditioning on m_i's, we have

$$\text{Var}(\bar{y}_i^*) = \text{Var}[E_y(\bar{y}_i^*)] + E[\text{Var}_y(\bar{y}_i^*)]$$
$$= \beta_i'\text{Var}(\bar{x}_i)\beta_i + \sigma_{ei}^2\left\{\frac{1}{m_i} + E[(\bar{x}_i - \tilde{x}_i)' M_i^{-1}(\bar{x}_i - \tilde{x}_i)]\right\}.$$

When $n_i \to \infty$,

$$E[(\bar{x}_i - \tilde{x}_i)' M_i^{-1}(\bar{x}_i - \tilde{x}_i)] = O(n_i^{-2})$$

and, hence,

$$\text{Var}(\bar{y}_i^*) = \frac{\beta_i'\text{Var}(x_{ij})\beta_i}{n_i} + \frac{\sigma_{ei}^2}{m_i} + O\left(\frac{1}{n_i^2}\right).$$

This leads to two conclusions. First, when n_i is large, $\bar{y}_i^*$ is approximately normal. Second, the variance of $\bar{y}_i^*$ is nearly

$$\frac{\sigma_i^2 - \sigma_{ei}^2}{n_i} + \frac{\sigma_{ei}^2}{m_i} = \frac{\sigma_i^2}{n_i} + \frac{(n_i - m_i)\sigma_{ei}^2}{m_i n_i} < \frac{\sigma_i^2}{m_i}.$$

Therefore, $\bar{y}_i^*$ is asymptotically more efficient than $\tilde{y}_i$, the estimator of μ_i without imputation. If σ_{ei}^2 is much smaller than $\beta_i'\mathrm{Var}(x_{ij})\beta_i$, then the efficiency of $\bar{y}_i^*$ is close to that of $\bar{y}_i$, the estimator of μ_i based on the complete data set.

From the theory of least squares, an unbiased estimator of σ_{ei}^2 is

$$\hat{\sigma}_{ei}^2 = \frac{1}{m_i - k} \sum_{j=1}^{m_i} (y_{ij} - \hat{\alpha}_i - \hat{\beta}_i' x_{ij})^2,$$

where k is 1 plus the dimension of x. Let S_{xi} be the sample variance-covariance matrix based on x_{ij}, $j = 1, ..., n_i$. Then, testing for the treatment effect can be carried out based on the following approximation:

$$\frac{\bar{y}_1^* - \bar{y}_2^*}{\sqrt{v^*}} \sim N(0, 1),$$

where

$$v^* = \sum_{i=1}^{2} \left(\frac{\hat{\beta}_i' S_{xi} \hat{\beta}_i}{n_i} + \frac{\hat{\sigma}_{ei}^2}{m_i} \right).$$

9.4   Crossover Designs

As discussed in Chapter 5, crossover designs are commonly employed for assessment of bioequivalence between drug products. However, when a crossover experiment is conducted, subjects may withdraw from the study especially when they have to be confined in the pharmacology unit or hospital during the conduct of the trial. Discontinuation is most likely to occur for higher-order crossover designs with more than two dosing periods. In what follows we will discuss dropouts and/or missing values for 2×2, 2×3, and 2×4 crossover designs, respectively. We still assume noninformative missingness, although in many cases such assumption is not needed (see the discussion in §9.4.3).

9.4.1   Estimation of Treatment Effect

Consider the 2×2 crossover design in which n_1 patients receive treatment 1 at the first period and treatment 2 at the second period and n_2 patients receive treatment 2 at the first period and treatment 1 at the second period. The 2×2 crossover design can be used to test the effect between two treatments or to assess the average bioequivalence between a test product and a reference product (see §5.3.1). When there are dropouts and/or missing values, analysis can be done based on data from patients who have data for all periods. In this case, patients having data for only one period are excluded from the analysis. The loss in power due to missing values can be analyzed using the same method described in §9.2.

Similarly, when a crossover design with more than two periods is used, analysis can be done based on data from patients who have data for all periods. However, data from patients who have completed at least two periods of study may be used to increase the efficiency.

Consider the 2×3 crossover design described in §5.4.1 in which n_1 subjects in sequence 1 receive two treatments (A and B) at three periods in the order of ABA, while n_2 subjects in sequence 2 receive treatments at three periods in the order of BAB. Let y_{ijk} be the response of the ith patient in the kth sequence at the jth period. Assume that y_{ijk}'s follow model (5.2.3) with $l = A, B$, and

$$W_{ljk} = P_j + Q_k + C_{jk}, \tag{9.4.1}$$

where P_j is the jth period effect $(P_1 + 2P_2 + P_3 = 0)$, Q_k is the kth sequence effect $(Q_1 + Q_2 = 0)$, and C_{jk}'s are effect of interaction $(C_{jk} = C$ when $(j, k) = (1, 1)$ or $(3, 2)$; $C_{jk} = -C$ when $(j, k) = (3, 1)$ or $(1, 2)$; and $C_{jk} = 0$ when $(j, k) = (2, 1)$ or $(2, 2)$). Without loss of generality, it is assumed that in the kth sequence, the first m_{1k} subjects have data for all three periods; the next m_{2k} subjects have data for periods 1 and 2; the next m_{3k} subjects have data for periods 2 and 3; and the last m_{4k} subjects have data for periods 1 and 3, where $m_{1k} + m_{2k} + m_{3k} + m_{4k} = m_k \le n_k$ (subjects having data for only one period have to be excluded). Chow and Shao (1997) proposed to consider the within subject differences

$$
\begin{aligned}
d_{i11} &= \tfrac{1}{2}(y_{i11} + y_{i31}) - y_{i21} & 1 &\le i \le m_{11}, \\
d_{i21} &= y_{i11} - y_{i21} & m_{11} + 1 &\le i \le m_{11} + m_{21}, \\
d_{i31} &= y_{i21} - y_{i31} & m_{11} + m_{21} + 1 &\le i \le m_{11} + m_{21} + m_{31}, \\
d_{i41} &= y_{i11} - y_{i31} & m_{11} + m_{21} + m_{31} + 1 &\le i \le m_1, \\
d_{i12} &= \tfrac{1}{2}(y_{i12} + y_{i32}) - y_{i22} & 1 &\le i \le m_{12}, \\
d_{i22} &= y_{i12} - y_{i22} & m_{12} + 1 &\le i \le m_{12} + m_{22}, \\
d_{i32} &= y_{i22} - y_{i32} & m_{12} + m_{22} + 1 &\le i \le m_{12} + m_{22} + m_{32}, \\
d_{i42} &= y_{i12} - y_{i32} & m_{12} + m_{22} + m_{32} + 1 &\le i \le m_2.
\end{aligned}
$$

Under (9.4.1),

$$d_{i11} = \tfrac{1}{2}(P_1 - 2P_2 + P_3) + F_A - F_B + S_{i1A} - S_{i1B} + \tfrac{1}{2}(e_{i11} + e_{i31}) - e_{i21},$$
$$d_{i21} = P_1 - P_2 + F_A - F_B + C + S_{i1A} - S_{i1B} + e_{i11} - e_{i12},$$
$$d_{i31} = P_2 - P_3 + F_B - F_A + C + S_{i1B} - S_{i1A} + e_{i21} - e_{i31},$$
$$d_{i41} = P_1 - P_3 + 2C + e_{i11} - e_{i31},$$
$$d_{i12} = \tfrac{1}{2}(P_1 - 2P_2 + P_3) + F_B - F_A + S_{i1B} - S_{i1A} + \tfrac{1}{2}(e_{i12} + e_{i32}) - e_{i22},$$
$$d_{i22} = P_1 - P_2 + F_B - F_A - C + S_{i2B} - S_{i2A} + e_{2i1} - e_{2i2},$$
$$d_{i32} = P_2 - P_3 + F_A - F_B - C + S_{i2A} - S_{i2B} + e_{i22} - e_{i32},$$
$$d_{i42} = P_1 - P_3 - 2C + e_{i12} - e_{i32}.$$

Let d be the vector of these differences (arranged according to the order of the subjects). Under the assumption of noninformative missingness,

$$d \sim N(Z\theta, \, \Sigma),$$

where

$$\theta' = (P_1 - P_2, P_2 - P_3, F_A - F_B, C),$$

$$Z = \begin{pmatrix}
1_{m_{11}} \otimes (\; \tfrac{1}{2} \;\; \tfrac{1}{2} \;\; 1 \;\; 0 \;) \\
1_{m_{21}} \otimes (\; 1 \;\; 0 \;\; 1 \;\; 1 \;) \\
1_{m_{31}} \otimes (\; 0 \;\; 1 \;\; -1 \;\; 1 \;) \\
1_{m_{41}} \otimes (\; 1 \;\; 1 \;\; 0 \;\; 2 \;) \\
1_{m_{12}} \otimes (\; \tfrac{1}{2} \;\; \tfrac{1}{2} \;\; -1 \;\; 0 \;) \\
1_{m_{22}} \otimes (\; 1 \;\; 0 \;\; -1 \;\; -1 \;) \\
1_{m_{32}} \otimes (\; 0 \;\; 1 \;\; 1 \;\; -1 \;) \\
1_{m_{42}} \otimes (\; 1 \;\; 1 \;\; 0 \;\; -2 \;)
\end{pmatrix},$$

1_m is the m-dimensional vector of ones, $\otimes$ is the Kronecker product, and Σ is the variance-covariance matrix of d. Thus, an unbiased estimator of θ is the least squares estimator

$$\hat{\theta} = (Z'Z)^{-1}Z'd \sim N\left(\theta, (Z'Z)^{-1}Z'\Sigma Z(Z'Z)^{-1}\right).$$

Let σ_{WA}^2 be the variance of e_{ijk} corresponding to the y_{ijk} under treatment A, σ_{WB}^2 be the variance of e_{ijk} corresponding to the y_{ijk} under treatment B, σ_D^2 be the variance of $S_{ikA} - S_{ikB}$, and

$$\sigma_{a,b}^2 = \sigma_D^2 + a\sigma_{WA}^2 + b\sigma_{WB}^2.$$

Then

$$\Sigma = \begin{pmatrix}
\sigma_{0.5,1}^2 I_{m_{11}} & & & & & \\
& \sigma_{1,1}^2 I_{m_{21}+m_{31}} & & & & \\
& & 2\sigma_{WA}^2 I_{m_{41}} & & & \\
& & & \sigma_{1,0.5}^2 I_{m_{21}} & & \\
& & & & \sigma_{1,1}^2 I_{m_{22}+m_{32}} & \\
& & & & & 2\sigma_{WB}^2 I_{m_{42}}
\end{pmatrix},$$

where I_m is the identity matrix of order m. Then an estimator of the variance-covariance matrix of $\hat{\theta}$ can be obtained by replacing $\sigma_{1,1}^2$, $\sigma_{0.5,1}^2$, $\sigma_{1,0.5}^2$, σ_{WA}^2, and σ_{WB}^2 in Σ with their estimators. Let s_{djk}^2 be the sample variance based on d_{ijk}, $i = 1, ..., m_{jk}$. Then, unbiased estimators of $\sigma_{0.5,1}^2$, $\sigma_{1,0.5}^2$, and $\sigma_{1,1}^2$ are, respectively,

$$s_{d11}^2 \sim \frac{\sigma_{0.5,1}^2 \chi_{m_{11}-1}^2}{m_{11} - 1},$$

$$s_{d12}^2 \sim \frac{\sigma_{1,0.5}^2 \chi_{m_{12}-1}^2}{m_{12} - 1},$$

and

$$\frac{1}{m_*} \sum_{k=1}^{2} \sum_{j=2}^{3} (m_{jk} - 1) s_{djk}^2 \sim \frac{\sigma_{1,1}^2 \chi_{m_*}^2}{m_*},$$

where

$$m_* = \sum_{k=1}^{2} \sum_{j=2}^{3} (m_{jk} - 1).$$

Let s_{d5k}^2 be the sample variance based on $y_{i1k} - y_{i3k}$, $i = 1, ..., m_{1k}$. Then, unbiased estimator of σ_{WA}^2 and σ_{WB}^2 are, respectively,

$$\frac{(m_{41} - 1)s_{d41}^2 + (m_{11} - 1)s_{d51}^2}{2(m_{41} - 1 + m_{11} - 1)} \sim \frac{\sigma_{WA}^2 \chi_{m_{41}-1+m_{11}-1}^2}{m_{41} - 1 + m_{11} - 1}$$

and

$$\frac{(m_{42} - 1)s_{d42}^2 + (m_{12} - 1)s_{d52}^2}{2(m_{42} - 1 + m_{12} - 1)} \sim \frac{\sigma_{WB}^2 \chi_{m_{42}-1+m_{12}-1}^2}{m_{42} - 1 + m_{12} - 1}.$$

When $m_{jk} = 0$, an adjustment should be made by setting $m_{jk} - 1$ in the previous formulas to 0. For example, if missing values are always due to dropout, then if $y_{ij_0 k}$ is missing, then so are y_{ijk}'s with $j > j_0$. Therefore, $m_{3k} = m_{4k} = 0$, $k = 1, 2$.

The discussion for the 2×4 crossover design described in §5.2 is similar, although it is more complicated. We only consider dropouts. Suppose that in the kth sequence, the first m_{1k} patients have data for all four periods, the next m_{2k} patients have data for the first three periods, and the last m_{3k} patients have data for the first two periods, where $m_{1k} + m_{2k} + m_{3k} = m_k \leq n_k$. Let y_{ijk} be the response of the ith patient in the kth sequence at the jth period. Assume that y_{ijk}'s follow model (5.2.3) with $l = A, B$.

Define

$$
\begin{aligned}
d_{i11} &= \tfrac{1}{2}(y_{i11} + y_{i31}) - \tfrac{1}{2}(y_{i21} + y_{i41}), & 1 \le i \le m_{11}, \\
d_{i21} &= \tfrac{1}{2}(y_{i11} + y_{i31}) - y_{i21}, & m_{11}+1 \le i \le m_{11}+m_{21}, \\
d_{i31} &= y_{i11} - y_{i21}, & m_{11}+m_{21}+1 \le i \le m_1, \\
d_{i12} &= \tfrac{1}{2}(y_{i12} + y_{i32}) - \tfrac{1}{2}(y_{i22} + y_{i42}), & 1 \le i \le m_{12}, \\
d_{i22} &= \tfrac{1}{2}(y_{i12} + y_{i32}) - y_{i22}, & m_{12}+1 \le i \le m_{12}+m_{22}, \\
d_{i32} &= y_{i12} - y_{i22}, & m_{12}+m_{22}+1 \le i \le m_2.
\end{aligned}
$$

Let d be the vector of these differences. Then

$$ d \sim N(Z\theta, \Sigma), $$

where

$$ \theta' = (F_A - F_B, W_{11} - W_{21}, W_{31} - W_{21}, W_{31} - W_{41}, W_{12} - W_{22}, W_{32} - W_{22}), $$

$$
Z = \begin{pmatrix}
\mathbf{1}_{m_{11}} \otimes \begin{pmatrix} 1 & \tfrac{1}{2} & 0 & \tfrac{1}{2} & 0 & 0 \end{pmatrix} \\
\mathbf{1}_{m_{21}} \otimes \begin{pmatrix} 1 & \tfrac{1}{2} & \tfrac{1}{2} & 0 & 0 & 0 \end{pmatrix} \\
\mathbf{1}_{m_{31}} \otimes \begin{pmatrix} 1 & 1 & 0 & 0 & 0 & 0 \end{pmatrix} \\
\mathbf{1}_{m_{12}} \otimes \begin{pmatrix} -1 & \tfrac{1}{2} & 0 & \tfrac{1}{2} & 0 & 0 \end{pmatrix} \\
\mathbf{1}_{m_{22}} \otimes \begin{pmatrix} -1 & 0 & 0 & 0 & \tfrac{1}{2} & \tfrac{1}{2} \end{pmatrix} \\
\mathbf{1}_{m_{32}} \otimes \begin{pmatrix} -1 & 0 & 0 & 0 & 1 & 0 \end{pmatrix}
\end{pmatrix},
$$

and

$$
\Sigma = \begin{pmatrix}
\sigma^2_{0.5,0.5} I_{m_{11}} & & & & & \\
& \sigma^2_{0.5,1} I_{m_{21}} & & & 0 & \\
& & \sigma^2_{1,1} I_{m_{31}} & & & \\
& & & \sigma^2_{0.5,0.5} I_{m_{12}} & & \\
& 0 & & & \sigma^2_{1,0.5} I_{m_{22}} & \\
& & & & & \sigma^2_{1,1} I_{m_{32}}
\end{pmatrix}.
$$

Estimators of $\sigma^2_{a,b}$ can be obtained using sample variances based on d_{ijk}'s.

9.4.2   Assessing Individual Bioequivalence

In its 1999 and 2001 guidances, the FDA recommends a 2×4 crossover design or a 2×3 crossover design be used for assessment of individual bioequivalence (IBE). Potential dropouts at the third or fourth dosing period is a concern. Although analysis can be done using data from subjects who have data from all periods, the loss in power may be substantial when the dropout rate is high.

As discussed in §9.4.1, the efficiency in estimating the drug effect $\delta = F_T - F_R$ can be increased by making use of partially completed data (i.e., data from subjects who completed at least two periods of the study). For testing IBE, in addition to the drug effect, several variance components need to be estimated (see §5.3.2). In this section we address the issue of estimating variance components using partially completed data under the 2×4 crossover design described in §5.2. Note that for a 2×3 crossover design (either the standard 2×3 crossover design described in §5.4.1 or the 2×3 extra-reference design described in §5.4.2), partially completed data (i.e., data from patients who completed two periods of the study) are not useful in estimating variance components.

Suppose that in the kth sequence, the first m_{1k} patients have data for all four periods, the next m_{2k} patients have partially completed data from the first three periods, and the last m_{3k} patients have partially completed data from the first two periods, where $m_{1k}+m_{2k}+m_{3k} = m_k \leq n_k$. For assessing IBE, independent estimators of $\sigma_{0.5,0.5}^2$, σ_{WT}^2, and σ_{WR}^2 are required (see §5.3.2). Let $\hat{\sigma}_{0.5,0.5}^2$, $\hat{\sigma}_{WT}^2$, and $\hat{\sigma}_{WR}^2$ be the estimators of $\sigma_{0.5,0.5}^2$, σ_{WT}^2, and σ_{WR}^2, respectively, given in §5.3.2 but based on data from the subjects who have data for all four periods (i.e., n_k should be replaced by m_{1k}, $k = 1, 2$). For $k = 1, 2$, let s_{dk}^2 be the sample variance based on $y_{i1k} - y_{i3k}$, $i = m_{1k} + 1, ..., m_{1k} + m_{2k}$. Then an improved estimator of σ_{WT}^2 is

$$\tilde{\sigma}_{WT}^2 = \frac{(m_{21} - 1)s_{d1}^2/2 + (m_{11} + m_{12} - 2)\hat{\sigma}_{WT}^2}{m_{21} + m_{11} + m_{12} - 3}$$
$$\sim \frac{\sigma_{0.5,0.5}^2 \chi_{m_{21}+m_{11}+m_{12}-3}^2}{m_{21} + m_{11} + m_{12} - 3},$$

and an improved estimator of σ_{WR}^2 is

$$\tilde{\sigma}_{WR}^2 = \frac{(m_{22} - 1)s_{d2}^2/2 + (m_{11} + m_{12} - 2)\hat{\sigma}_{WR}^2}{m_{22} + m_{11} + m_{12} - 3}$$
$$\sim \frac{\sigma_{0.5,0.5}^2 \chi_{m_{22}+m_{11}+m_{12}-3}^2}{m_{22} + m_{11} + m_{12} - 3}.$$

These estimators of variance components and the estimator of δ are still independent and, thus, the procedure in §5.3.2 can still be applied.

9.4.3 Handling Informative Missingness by Transformation

When there are repeated values from each patient (e.g., when a crossover design is used), missingness is often related to the response values through a random subject effect and, therefore, analysis can be carried out after a suitable data transformation. Suppose that the response vector y follows the following model:

$$y = Z\theta + Hr + e, \tag{9.4.2}$$

where θ is a vector of treatment effects and other covariate effects (such as time effects), r is a vector of random subject effects, e is a vector of random measurement errors, and Z and H are fixed matrices of appropriate orders. Assume further that

$$Hr = H_1 r_1 + H_2 r_2 \qquad (9.4.3)$$

and that the probability of whether a response value is missing depends on components of r_1, not r_2 and e, where H_1 and H_2 are fixed matrices. If there exists a matrix A such that $AH_1 = 0$, then the missing mechanism is independent of the transformed data

$$Ay = AZ\theta + AH_2 r_2 + Ae. \qquad (9.4.4)$$

Thus, assessing θ can be done by using model (9.4.4) and the procedures applicable for the case of noninformative missingness.

One example of (9.4.2) is the crossover designs where r is the vector of random subject effects S_{ikl}'s in (5.2.1) or (5.2.3). Assume that

$$S_{ikl} = r_{ik} + r_{ilk}$$

and that the missing mechanism depends only on r_{ik}'s. Then (9.4.3) holds with r_1 being the vector of r_{ik}'s and the transformation A corresponds to taking differences of data from the same patient. Since the results in §9.4.1-9.4.2 are based on such differences, they are still valid when missingness is informative but the missingness mechanism depends on r_{ik}'s only.

9.5   Analysis of Last Observations

In clinical trials, data are often collected over a period of time (multiple visits) from participated patients. Data of this type are called longitudinal data or repeated measurements. Longitudinal data analysis refers to the analysis of data over time under certain statistical models (see §9.6). In many situations, however, analyses are based on data from the last time point (the end of the study) or change-of-efficacy measurements from baseline to the last time point. In this section we focus on the analysis of last observations when some patients dropped out prior to the end of the study. According to Heyting, Tolboom, and Essers (1992), dropout in a multiple-visit study is often informative, i.e., the population of patients who completed the study is different from the population of patients who dropped out.

9.5.1   Intention-to-Treat Analysis

Intention-to-treat (ITT) analysis is usually considered as the primary analysis in most randomized clinical trials testing new drug products (see FDA,

1988; ICH, 1998b; Knickerbocker, 2000). An ITT analysis is referred to as an analysis conducted according to the ITT principle, which requires that any comparison among treatment groups in a randomized clinical trial is based on results for all subjects in the treatment groups to which they were randomly assigned. The ITT principle implies that (i) the analysis should include all randomized subjects and (ii) compliance with this principle would necessitate complete follow-up of all randomized subjects for study outcomes (ICH, 1998b). It, however, should be noted that in practice, it may be difficult to achieve this ITT *ideal* of including all randomized subjects due to protocol violations. Basically, there are two types of major protocol violations. One is violation of entry eligibility (inclusion/exclusion criteria) and the other is the violation after randomization. Commonly seen protocol violations after randomization include (i) error in treatment assignment, (ii) the use of excluded medications, (iii) poor compliance, (iv) loss to follow-up, (v) missing data, and (vi) other violations such as errors due to miscommunication. The violations of the protocol that occur after randomization may have an impact on the data and conclusion if their occurrence is related to the treatment assignment. Therefore, it is suggested that the data from such subjects should be included in the analysis according to the ITT principle.

The ICH guideline classifies the analysis sets as either the full analysis set or per protocol analysis sets. The full analysis set is referred to as the analysis set that is as complete as possible and as close as possible to the ITT ideal of including all randomized subjects. In many clinical trials, the full analysis set includes all randomized subjects who had at least one evaluation post randomization (for efficacy) or took at least one dose of trial medication (for safety). The full analysis set is also known as the ITT analysis set. In practice, an ITT analysis can best reflect medical practice, i.e., the observed clinical results are valid and applicable to the target patient population under the randomization scheme. A per protocol analysis set is a subset of the ITT analysis set, which may be characterized by (i) the completion of a certain prespecified minimal exposure to the treatment regimen, (ii) the availability of measurements of the primary variable(s), and (iii) the absence of any major protocol violations including violation of entry criteria (ICH, 1998b). For example, a per protocol analysis set may be (i) all subjects with any observations or with a certain minimum number of observations, (ii) all subjects completing the study (completer's analysis), (iii) all subjects with an observation during a particular time window, or (iv) all subjects with a specified degree of compliance (Chow and Liu, 1998). Analyses based on these subgroups are usually referred to as evaluable, per protocol, or protocol correct analyses. Both the FDA and ICH guidelines indicate that if the results obtained based on the ITT analysis set are substantially different from those from the per protocol analysis set, comparability of treatment groups in both analysis sets should be examined and any other reasons for such differences should be discussed.

The target patient populations of a per protocol analysis and an ITT analysis are different when dropout is informative, which can be explained as follows. Suppose that in a 3-week clinical study of a drug product, the efficacy of the drug product is evaluated from n patients at weeks 1, 2, and 3, and that n_1 patients dropped out after week 1, n_2·patients dropped out after week 2, and $n_3 = n - n_1 - n_2$ patients completed the study. The target population of an intention-to-treat analysis is the population of all randomized patients, which consists of three subpopulations: the subpopulation of patients who are on therapy for one week, the subpopulation of patients who are on therapy for two weeks, and the subpopulation of patients who are on therapy for three weeks (the estimated proportions of the three subpopulations are n_1/n, n_2/n, and n_3/n, respectively). The target population of a per protocol analysis of completers, however, is the last subpopulation. If dropout is informative, then these subpopulations are different and conclusions drawn from a per protocol analysis of completers may be very different from those based on an ITT analysis.

9.5.2   Last Observation Carry-Forward

In an ITT analysis, the last observations for patients who dropped out are referred to as the last observations prior to dropout. As a popular and simple ITT analysis, the last observation carry-forward (LOCF) analysis carries forward the last observation to the last time point for each patient who dropped out and performs an analysis by treating carried-forward data as observed data at the last time point. Although the LOCF analysis has a long history of application and it is well-known that treating carried-forward data as observed data may not preserve the size of the tests for treatment effects when dropout is informative (Ting, 2000), a systematic study of merits and limitations of the LOCF analysis is not available until recently Shao and Zhong (2001) established some statistical properties for the LOCF ANOVA test.

Consider a typical parallel-group design for comparing $a \geq 2$ treatments. A total of n patients are randomly assigned to a treatment groups, where the ith treatment group has n_i patients, $i = 1, ..., a$. Suppose that patients are evaluated at s time points (visits). Let μ_{is} be the mean of the response under treatment i at the last visit. If there is no dropout, then the last observation analysis applies a typical one-way ANOVA to test the null hypothesis

$$H_0 : \mu_{1s} = \cdots = \mu_{as}, \tag{9.5.1}$$

using the last observations from all patients.

Suppose that in the ith group, n_{ij} patients drop out after the jth visit. Note that n_{ij} is random but $\sum_{j=1}^{s} n_{ij} = n_i$. When there are dropouts, what should the null hypothesis of no treatment effect be? Clearly, using hypothesis (9.5.1) corresponds to the per protocol analysis of completers.

Under the ITT analysis, the patient population under treatment i consists of s subpopulations, where the jth subpopulation is the population of patients who are on therapy and drop out after the jth visit (the subpopulation with $j = s$ is the population of completers). Let μ_{ij} be the mean of the jth subpopulation under treatment i. The global mean of the patient population under treatment i is then

$$\mu_i = \sum_{j=1}^{s} p_{ij}\mu_{ij},$$

where $p_{ij} = E(n_{ij}/n_i)$ is the true proportion of patients in the jth subpopulation under treatment i. If we use the global mean as the measure of treatment effect, then the null hypothesis of no treatment effect should be

$$H_0 : \mu_1 = \cdots = \mu_a. \tag{9.5.2}$$

If dropout is informative, then the hypotheses in (9.5.1) and (9.5.2) are different.

Let us now introduce the LOCF test. Under treatment i, let y_{ijk} denote the last observed response for subject k in the group of patients dropping out after visit j ($k = 1, ..., n_{ij}$). The LOCF analysis treats y_{ijk} as the unobserved y_{isk} when $j < s$ and applies the usual ANOVA test. That is, the LOCF analysis concludes that there is a treatment effect if and only if

$$\frac{\text{MSTR}}{\text{MSE}} > F_{1-\alpha;a-1,n-a},$$

where $F_{1-\alpha;a-1,n-a}$ is the $(1-\alpha)$th quantile of the F-distribution with $a-1$ and $n-a$ degrees of freedom, α is a given nominal size,

$$\text{MSTR} = \frac{1}{a-1} \sum_{i=1}^{a} n_i(\bar{y}_{i..} - \bar{y}_{...})^2,$$

$$\text{MSE} = \frac{1}{n-a} \sum_{i=1}^{a} \sum_{j=1}^{s} \sum_{k=1}^{n_{ij}} (y_{ijk} - \bar{y}_{i..})^2,$$

$$\bar{y}_{i..} = \frac{1}{n_i} \sum_{j=1}^{s} \sum_{k=1}^{n_{ij}} y_{ijk},$$

and

$$\bar{y}_{...} = \frac{1}{n} \sum_{i=1}^{a} \sum_{j=1}^{s} \sum_{k=1}^{n_{ij}} y_{ijk}.$$

What is the null hypothesis that this LOCF test rejects when dropout is informative? Since a large MSTR/MSE rejects the null hypothesis and MSTR is large when the difference among $\bar{y}_{i..}$ (an unbiased estimator of μ_i), $i = 1, ..., a$, is large, it is reasonable to say that the null hypothesis for the LOCF test is the H_0 given in (9.5.2). However, treating y_{ijk} as the unobserved y_{isk} makes one think that the LOCF test preassumes that $\mu_{ij} = \mu_{is} = \mu_i$ for all j (i.e., dropout is noninformative). Indeed, if $\mu_{ij} = \mu_i$ for all j, then the size of the LOCF test is exactly equal to α when y_{ijk}'s are independent and normally distributed with a constant variance σ^2 and approximately equal to α when the normality assumption is removed but n_i's are large for all i. But, what is the behavior of the LOCF test when $\mu_{ij} = \mu_i$ is not true (i.e., dropout is informative)?

The following are the main findings in Shao and Zhong (2001).

1. In the special case of $a = 2$, the asymptotic size ($n_i \to \infty$) of the LOCF test when H_0 in (9.5.2) is used as the null hypothesis is $\leq \alpha$ if and only if

$$\lim \left(\frac{n_2 \tau_1^2}{n} + \frac{n_1 \tau_2^2}{n} \right) \leq \lim \left(\frac{n_1 \tau_1^2}{n} + \frac{n_2 \tau_2^2}{n} \right) \qquad (9.5.3)$$

where

$$\tau_i^2 = \sum_{j=1}^{s} p_{ij} (\mu_{ij} - \mu_i)^2. \qquad (9.5.4)$$

If $\lim \frac{n_1}{n} = \lim \frac{n_2}{n}$ (n_1 and n_2 are nearly the same), then the equality in (9.5.3) holds and the asymptotic size of the LOCF test is α, regardless of whether dropout is informative or not and whether the variances of data from two treatment groups are the same or not. When $\lim \frac{n_1}{n} \neq \lim \frac{n_2}{n}$, the asymptotic size of the LOCF test is not α, unless $\tau_1^2 = \tau_2^2$ (the only practical situation in which this occurs is when $\tau_1^2 = \tau_2^2 = 0$, i.e., $\mu_{ij} = \mu_i$ for all j and dropout is noninformative).

2. When $a = 2$, $\tau_1^2 \neq \tau_2^2$ and $n_1 \neq n_2$, the LOCF test has an asymptotic size smaller than α if

$$(n_2 - n_1)\tau_1^2 < (n_2 - n_1)\tau_2^2 \qquad (9.5.5)$$

or larger than α if $<$ in (9.5.5) is replaced by $>$. If treatment 1 is the placebo, then often $n_1 < n_2$ and $\tau_1^2 < \tau_2^2$ (i.e., the variation among

μ_{2j}'s is larger than that among μ_{1j}'s) and, thus, (9.5.5) holds and the LOCF test is too conservative in the sense that its size is too small. Note that if the size of a test is unnecessarily small, the power of detecting treatment effects is unnecessarily low.

3. When $a \geq 3$, the asymptotic size of the LOCF test when H_0 in (9.5.2) is used as the null hypothesis is generally not α except for some special cases (e.g., $\tau_1^2 = \cdots = \tau_a^2 = 0$).

9.5.3   Analysis of Last Observations

Since the LOCF test is incorrect in terms of its asymptotic size when $a \geq 3$ or $a = 2$ but $n_1 \neq n_2$, Shao and Zhong (2001) proposed an asymptotically valid test procedure for H_0 in (9.5.2), using the last observations from patients randomized to the study. The difference between this last observation analysis and the LOCF analysis is that, for patients who drop out, their last observations are not *carried forward*; instead, y_{ijk}'s are poststratified according to j.

The poststratified sample mean under treatment i is

$$\hat{\mu}_i = \sum_{j=1}^{s} \frac{n_{ij}}{n_i} \bar{y}_{ij.} = \frac{1}{n_i} \sum_{j=1}^{s} \sum_{k=1}^{n_{ij}} y_{ijk} = \bar{y}_{i..},$$

where n_{ij}/n_i is the poststratification weight and $\bar{y}_{ij.} = n_{ij}^{-1} \sum_{k=1}^{n_{ij}} y_{ijk}$ is the sample mean of the jth stratum. For independent y_{ijk}'s, it can be shown that $\hat{\mu}_i$ is an unbiased estimator of μ_i and the variance of $\hat{\mu}_i$ is

$$V_i = \frac{1}{n_i} \left(\sum_{j=1}^{s} p_{ij} \sigma_{ij}^2 + \tau_i^2 \right),$$

where $\sigma_{ij}^2 = \mathrm{Var}(y_{ijk})$. An approximately unbiased estimator of V_i is

$$\hat{V}_i = \frac{1}{n_i(n_i - 1)} \sum_{j=1}^{s} \sum_{k=1}^{n_{ij}} (y_{ijk} - \bar{y}_{i..})^2.$$

Let

$$T = \sum_{i=1}^{a} \frac{1}{\hat{V}_i} \left(\bar{y}_{i..} - \frac{\sum_{i=1}^{a} \bar{y}_{i..}/\hat{V}_i}{\sum_{i=1}^{a} 1/\hat{V}_i} \right)^2. \tag{9.5.6}$$

Then, a test of hypothesis H_0 in (9.5.2) with asymptotic size α (when all n_i's are large) rejects H_0 if and only if $T > \chi_{1-\alpha;a-1}^2$, where $\chi_{1-\alpha;a-1}^2$ is the $(1 - \alpha)$th quantile of the chi-square distribution with $a - 1$ degrees of freedom. This test is referred to as the χ^2-test.

In the special case of $a = 2$, T in (9.5.6) becomes

$$T = \frac{(\bar{y}_{1..} - \bar{y}_{2..})^2}{\hat{V}_1 + \hat{V}_2},$$

i.e., χ^2-test is simply the same as the two sample t-test with unequal variances of $\bar{y}_{1..}$ and $\bar{y}_{2..}$ estimated by $\hat{V}_1$ and $\hat{V}_2$, respectively. When $a = 2$ and $n_1 = n_2$, a straightforward calculation shows that $T = \frac{\text{MSTR}}{\text{MSE}}$, which is the LOCF test statistic.

If $\sigma_{ij}^2 = \sigma^2$ for all i, j, then $V_i = \frac{\sigma^2 + \tau_i^2}{n_i}$ and $\hat{V}_i$ can be replaced by a combined estimator

$$\tilde{V}_i = \frac{(n_i - s)\hat{\sigma}^2}{n_i(n_i - 1)} + \frac{1}{n_i(n_i - 1)} \sum_{j=1}^{s} n_{ij}(\bar{y}_{ij.} - \bar{y}_{i..})^2,$$

where

$$\hat{\sigma}^2 = \frac{1}{n - as} \sum_{i=1}^{a} \sum_{j=1}^{s} \sum_{k=1}^{n_{ij}} (y_{ijk} - \bar{y}_{ij.})^2.$$

A simulation study was conducted in Shao and Zhong (2001) to investigate the finite sample performance of the LOCF test and the χ^2-test, in the case where $s = 3$ and $a = 2$. The performance of each test was evaluated by its type I error probability (approximated by 2,000 simulations) with H_0 in (9.5.2) being the null hypothesis. The α value was chosen to be 5%. The subpopulations were normal with the following subpopulation parameters.

	Treatment $i = 1$ (placebo)			Treatment $i = 2$ (drug)		
	$j = 1$	$j = 2$	$j = 3$	$j = 1$	$j = 2$	$j = 3$
p_{ij}	0.20	0.20	0.60	0.15	0.15	0.70
μ_{ij}	25	24	21	40	32	16.6
σ_{ij}^2	100	100	100	100	100	100
μ_i			22.4			22.4
τ_i^2			3.04			84.1

Note that the global means μ_1 and μ_2 are the same but μ_{ij}'s are different so that τ_1^2 and τ_2^2 given by formula (9.5.4) are not 0 and very different (i.e., dropout is informative).

Sample sizes $n = n_1 + n_2 = 30, 40, 50, 60, 70, 80, 90, 100$, and 160 were considered. For each sample size n, $n_1 = 30\%$ of n, 40% of n, 50% of n (i.e., $n_1 = n_2$), 60% of n, and 70% of n were considered. Under each combination of sample sizes, simulation results based on 2,000 runs are given in Table 9.5.1. The results in Table 9.5.1 can be summarized as follows.

Table 9.5.1. Type I Error Probabilities of the LOCF Test
and χ^2-Test (Based on 2,000 simulations)

$n_1 + n_2$	$n_1 = 30\%$ of $n_1 + n_2$		$n_1 = 60\%$ of $n_1 + n_2$	
	LOCF test	χ^2-test	LOCF test	χ^2-test
30	0.0235	0.0545	0.0480	0.0445
40	0.0275	0.0600	0.0555	0.0510
50	0.0260	0.0490	0.0610	0.0555
60	0.0320	0.0530	0.0680	0.0590
70	0.0290	0.0550	0.0575	0.0510
80	0.0295	0.0540	0.0660	0.0555
90	0.0350	0.0600	0.0635	0.0530
100	0.0280	0.0525	0.0565	0.0495
160	0.0285 .	0.0540	0.0600	0.0485
	$n_1 = 40\%$ of $n_1 + n_2$		$n_1 = 70\%$ of $n_1 + n_2$	
	LOCF test	χ^2-test	LOCF test	χ^2-test
30	0.0275	0.0490	0.0610	0.0450
40	0.0390	0.0570	0.0690	0.0555
50	0.0415	0.0560	0.0675	0.0515
60	0.0395	0.0590	0.0740	0.0535
70	0.0405	0.0515	0.0695	0.0470
80	0.0340	0.0500	0.0740	0.0520
90	0.0400	0.0590	0.0685	0.0395
100	0.0335	0.0450	0.0735	0.0505
160	0.0430	0.0590	0.0755	0.0480
	$n_1 = n_2$			
	LOCF test	χ^2-test		
30	0.0430	0.0520		
40	0.0465	0.0535		
50	0.0535	0.0580		
60	0.0515	0.0565		
70	0.0520	0.0560		
80	0.0485	0.0520		
90	0.0525	0.0550		
100	0.0475	0.0495		
160	0.0460	0.0460		

1. As the asymptotic results in §9.5.2 indicated, the type I error probability of the LOCF test is close to $\alpha = 5\%$ when $n_1 = n_2$, but is considerably smaller (or larger) than α when $n_1 = 30\%$ of n ($n_1 = 70\%$ of n).

2. The type I error probability of the χ^2-test is within $\alpha \pm 0.01$, regardless of whether n_i's are equal or not.

3. According to the previous discussion, the LOCF test statistic and T in (9.5.6) are the same when $n_1 = n_2$. But the results in Table 9.5.1 for the case of $n_1 = n_2$ are different, because of the fact that in the LOCF test, $F_{1-\alpha;1,n-2}$ is used as the critical value, whereas the χ^2-test uses $\chi^2_{1-\alpha;1}$ as the critical value. It can be seen from Table 9.5.1 that the difference becomes negligible when $n > 100$.

9.6 Analysis of Longitudinal Data

Instead of analyzing the last observations, an analysis of longitudinal data makes inference using the whole data set. It should be noted that an analysis of longitudinal data may not make much sense in clinical trials unless some model assumptions are imposed. For example, if a drug is for the treatment of chronic disease, then frequently the treatment effect is only seen at the end or near the end of study; thus, if the mean drug effects in visits prior to the last visit are not related to the mean drug effect of the last visit, then an analysis of longitudinal data does not offer any more insight than the analysis of data from the last visit. Hence, in clinical trials, an longitudinal analysis (under an assumed model) is often a supplementary analysis included in submissions to relevant agencies such as the FDA. Models on the mean drug effects are usually established using some covariates that are related to the main response variable, such as time points, ethnic factors, demographics, and baseline characteristics/responses.

When there is no missing value or missing is noninformative (§9.1), analyses of longitudinal data are summarized in many statistical textbooks, e.g., Diggle, Liang, and Zeger (1994). A common statistical software is SAS procedure MIXED. When missing is informative, however, there is no standard procedure. In what follows we introduce two approaches of analyzing longitudinal data with informatively missing data.

9.6.1 Selection Models

Let y_{ijk} be the response for subject k under treatment i at the jth visit, where $i = 1, ..., a$, $j = 1, ..., s$, and $k = 1, ..., n_i$ when there is no missing value. That is, when there is no missing value, under treatment i, every subject has s observations. Let $r_{ijk} = 1$ when y_{ijk} is observed and $r_{ijk} = 0$ when y_{ijk} is missing. The type of missing values can be either dropout or intermittent. For subject k under treatment i, let y_{ik} be the vector of y-values, r_{ik} be the vector of r-values, and x_{ik} be a matrix of covariates (such as the visit times associated with the kth subject). Also, let b_{ik} be a vector of random effects associated with the kth subject under treatment i. Then, the joint probability density of (y_{ik}, r_{ik}, b_{ik}), conditional on the covariates x_{ik}, can be written as

$$f_i(y_{ik}, r_{ik}, b_{ik}|x_{ik}) = g_i(y_{ik}|b_{ik}, x_{ik})h_i(b_{ik}|x_{ik})m_i(r_{ik}|y_{ik}, b_{ik}, x_{ik}),$$

where g_i, h_i and m_i are probability density functions. This model is called a selection model (Wu and Carroll, 1988). Typically, g_i and h_i are continuous probability densities (such as normal densities) and m_i is a discrete probability density.

When all densities are parametric (i.e., they are known densities up to some unknown parameters), a likelihood based on respondents can be obtained by using functions $f_i(y_{ik}, r_{ik}, b_{ik}|x_{ik})$ and integrating out the random effects b_{ik} and unobserved parts of y_{ik}'s. Although in principle all unknown parameters can be estimated by maximizing the likelihood based on respondents, the numerical implementation of the maximization procedure is usually very difficult, since the integration over the random effects is usually intractable (even when g_i and h_i are normal densities). Thus, the application of this approach is limited without imposing some further conditions.

9.6.2 The Method of Grouping

A method of grouping is introduced in Park, Palta, Shao, and Shen (2002). This method is simple to implement and does not require a very specific assumption on the missing mechanism (the probability density m_i in §9.6.1). We introduce this method in the following special case where

$$y_{ijk} = \alpha_i + \beta_i'x_{ijk} + b_{\alpha ik} + b_{\beta ik}'x_{ijk} + \epsilon_{ijk}, \tag{9.6.7}$$

α_i and β_i are unknown parameters, x_{ijk} is a vector of observed covariates for the jth visit of the kth subject under treatment i, $(b_{\alpha ik}, b_{\beta ik})$ is the subject random effect, ϵ_{ijk} is the random measurement error, ϵ_{ijk}'s and $(b_{\alpha ik}, b_{\beta ik})$'s are independent, and $E(\epsilon_{ijk}) = 0$ and $E(b_{\alpha ik}, b_{\beta ik}) = (0, 0)$. A reasonable assumption in this setting is that ϵ_{ijk}'s are identically distributed and are independent of r_{ijk}'s (the response indicators).

Consider the case where the type of missingness is dropout. Let $m_{ik} = \sum_{j=1}^{s} r_{ijk}$ be the number of responses from subject k under treatment i.

If $m_{ik} = l$, then the corresponding subject dropped out after the lth visit unless $l = s$ (in which case the subject is a completer). Under model (9.6.7),

$$E(y_{ijk}|m_{ik} = l) = [\alpha_i + E(b_{\alpha ik}|m_{ik} = l)] + [\beta_i + E(b_{\beta ik}|m_{ik} = l)]'x_{ijk}.$$

Let $\alpha_{il} = \alpha_i + E(b_{\alpha ik}|m_{ik} = l)$ and $\beta_{il} = \beta_i + E(b_{\beta ik}|m_{ik} = l)$. Given $m_{ik} = l$ (i.e., all subjects dropped out after visit l), the observed responses follow the following model:

$$y_{ijkl} = \alpha_{il} + \beta_{il}'x_{ijk} + \epsilon_{ijkl}, \qquad (9.6.8)$$

where y_{ijkl} is y_{ijk} when $m_{ik} = l$ and ϵ_{ijkl}'s are some independent and identically distributed random variables with mean 0. Suppose that model (9.6.8) is fitted (e.g., using MIXED in SAS) for each l based on data in group l. Let the resulting estimators of α_{il} and β_{il} be $\hat{\alpha}_{il}$ and $\hat{\beta}_{il}$, respectively. Given l, $\hat{\alpha}_{il}$ and $\hat{\beta}_{il}$ are respectively consistent estimators of α_{il} and β_{il}. Let $p_{il} = P(m_{ik} = l)$, which can be consistently estimated by $\hat{p}_{il}$ = the observed proportion of subjects with $m_{ik} = l$ under treatment i. Then, a consistent estimator of α_i is $\sum_l \hat{p}_{il}\hat{\alpha}_{il}$, since

$$\sum_l p_{il}\alpha_{il} = \alpha_i + \sum_l p_{il}E(b_{\alpha ik}|m_{ik} = l) = \alpha_i + E(b_{\alpha ik}) = \alpha_i.$$

Similarly, a consistent estimator of β_i is $\sum_l \hat{p}_{il}\hat{\beta}_{il}$. Furthermore, it is shown in Park (2001) that $\sqrt{n_i}[(\hat{\alpha}_i, \hat{\beta}_i')' - (\alpha_i, \beta_i')']$ is asymptotically normal with mean 0 and covariance matrix

$$\Sigma_i = \sum_l p_{il} \left[\Sigma_{il} + \begin{pmatrix} \alpha_{il}^2 & \alpha_{il}\beta_{il}' \\ \alpha_{il}\beta_{il} & \beta_{il}\beta_{il}' \end{pmatrix} \right] - \begin{pmatrix} \alpha_i^2 & \alpha_i\beta_i' \\ \alpha_i\beta_i & \beta_i\beta_i' \end{pmatrix},$$

where n_i is the number of subjects under treatment i and Σ_{il} is the covariance matrix of $(\hat{\alpha}_{il}, \hat{\beta}_{il}')'$, given l, which can be estimated by $\hat{\Sigma}_{il}$ obtained, for example, using MIXED in SAS under model (9.6.8) with data in the lth group. An estimated Σ_i can be obtained by replacing Σ_{il}, α_{il} and β_{il} by $\hat{\Sigma}_{il}$, $\hat{\alpha}_{il}$ and $\hat{\beta}_{il}$, respectively. Thus, drug effects can be assessed by making inference on the parameters α_i and β_i, $i = 1, ..., a$.

Typical covariates include time points, ethnic factors, demographics, and baseline characteristics/responses. For the described analysis of longitudinal data with dropouts, the use of covariates closely related to y_{ijk}'s is important. For example, if time points are the only covariates and at the first visit, $x_{i1k} = 0$ for all subjects, then in group 1, β_{i1} is not estimable and, thus, the described procedure does not work.

When there are intermittent missing values, the previously described grouping method can still be applied. But the lth group may be constructed using some statistic other than m_{ik}. More details can be found in Park (2001).

Chapter 10

Meta-Analysis

Meta-analysis is a systematic reviewing strategy for addressing research questions that is especially useful when (i) results from several independent studies disagree with regard to direction of treatment effects, (ii) sample sizes are individually too small to detect an effect, or (iii) a large trial is too costly and time-consuming to perform (L'Abbe et al., 1987). As indicated in Dubey (1988), the primary concerns for performing a meta-analysis from a regulatory perspective include publication (or selection) bias and treatment-by-study interaction (a precise description of treatment-by-study interaction is given in §10.1.2 and §10.1.4). Thus, it is suggested that meta-analysis should be avoided in uncombinable studies (i.e., there is a significant treatment-by-study interaction). If there is a significant treatment-by-study interaction, statistical inference based on combining all studies could be biased. In this chapter we focus on meta-analysis for the purpose of assessing whether there is treatment-by-study interaction and/or increasing the power for an overall assessment of the treatment effect.

In clinical research and development, a multicenter trial can be viewed as a special case of a meta-analysis when each center is treated as a study. Statistical methods for meta-analysis are, of course, applicable to analysis of data from a multicenter trial. Unlike a multicenter trial, however, the study protocols, inclusion/exclusion criteria, patient populations, dosages and routes of administration, trial procedure, and duration may be different from study to study in a meta-analysis. This means that it is more likely to have study-to-study variation and/or treatment-by-study interaction in a meta-analysis than in a multicenter trial. Hence, knowing how to assess and handle these variations is important when performing a meta-analysis.

In §10.1-10.3, we consider meta-analyses for combining independent studies that are designed to study the same drug products. In particular, we concentrate on the comparison of the treatment difference of two drug products (one of which may be a placebo or standard therapy). In §10.1, we review some existing statistical methods for meta-analysis and introduce the concept of treatment-by-study interaction. Recent developments in assessing treatment-by-study interaction are introduced in §10.2. Section 10.3 describes some recently developed statistical tests for treatment difference. Sections 10.4-10.5 are devoted to meta-analysis in which each study investigates the treatment difference between a test drug and a standard therapy that is common to all studies, where all test drug products are different. An example is a study of bioequivalence among a brand-name drug and several generic copies. The last section contains a discussion.

10.1   Traditional Approaches

Methodology for combining findings from independent research studies has a long history. Early examples can be found in replicated astronomical and physical measurements, agricultural experiments, and social science studies (Hedges and Olkin, 1985). DerSimonian and Laird (1986) considered some statistical methods for meta-analysis in clinical trials. In this section we introduce some traditional statistical methods in meta-analysis.

We assume that there are $H \geq 2$ independent studies (clinical trials) and each study is designed to investigate the same drug products, e.g., a test drug product and a standard therapy (or placebo treatment). The extension to the case where each study investigates the same $a \geq 3$ drug treatments is straightforward.

10.1.1   The Approach of p-Values

The classical method for combining results is the approach of p-values proposed by Tippett (1931). Suppose that in the hth study, the objective is to test hypotheses

$$H_{0h} : \theta_h = 0 \quad \text{versus} \quad H_{1h} : \theta_h \neq 0, \tag{10.1.1}$$

where θ_h is defined to be the mean treatment difference (between a test drug product and a standard therapy or a placebo) in the hth study, $h = 1, ..., H$. Let p_h be the observed p-value for testing hypotheses (10.1.1) calculated based on the data from the hth study. For simplicity, assume that data from each study are continuous so that under H_{0h}, the p-value p_h has a uniform distribution on the interval $(0, 1)$, $h = 1, ..., H$. Since p_h's are independent, a test of significance level $\alpha \in (0, 1)$ for testing the null hypothesis

$$H_0 : \theta_h = 0, \quad h = 1, ..., H, \tag{10.1.2}$$

rejects the null hypothesis H_0 if

$$\min_{1 \le h \le H} p_{(h)} < 1 - (1-\alpha)^{1/H}.$$

Although this test procedure is very simple, it may not be useful in clinical trials since the alternative hypothesis for the null hypothesis in (10.1.2),

$$H_1 = H_{01} \cup \cdots \cup H_{0H} = \{\text{at least one } \theta_h \ne 0\},$$

is too big. When H_0 in (10.1.2) is rejected, one does not know whether $\theta_h \ne 0$ for all h, or there is only one $\theta_h \ne 0$; that is, one does not have a strong evidence that overall, the test drug product is different from the standard therapy, although one may conclude that the test drug product is different from the standard therapy in some studies.

10.1.2 Treatment-by-Study Interaction

As suggested by the FDA, we may want to test whether there is a treatment-by-study interaction before combining data and performing an analysis. Consider the following decomposition of the mean treatment difference θ_h:

$$\theta_h = \theta + \Delta_h, \quad h = 1, ..., H, \tag{10.1.3}$$

where θ is a *main effect* of drug treatment difference and Δ_h's are the effects of *treatment-by-study interaction*. If Δ_h's are treated as fixed effects, then the usual restriction of $\Delta_1 + \cdots + \Delta_H = 0$ should be imposed and θ is simply the average of θ_h's. If Δ_h's are random effects, then they are assumed to be independent and identically distributed with mean 0 and variance σ_Δ^2. Decomposition (10.1.3) can be derived from the following general model. Let μ_{ih} be the population mean of the ith drug treatment in study h, where $i = 0$ for a standard therapy or a placebo control and $i = 1$ for the test drug product. Under the usual two-way additive model,

$$\mu_{ih} = \mu + \alpha_i + \beta_h + \gamma_{ih},$$

where α_i is the main effect of drug treatment i, β_h is the main effect of study h, γ_{ih} is the interaction between drug treatment i and study h, and μ is the overall population mean. Then,

$$\theta_h = \mu_{1h} - \mu_{0h} = \alpha_1 - \alpha_0 + \gamma_{1h} - \gamma_{0h}$$

and (10.1.3) holds with $\theta = \alpha_1 - \alpha_0$ and $\Delta_h = \gamma_{1h} - \gamma_{0h}$.

Under the random effects model for Δ_h's, DerSimonian and Laird (1986) proposed the following test for the null hypothesis $\sigma_\Delta^2 = 0$ (i.e., there is no treatment-by-study interaction) versus the alternative $\sigma_\Delta^2 \neq 0$. Let

$$\bar{\theta}_w = \sum_{h=1}^{H} w_h \hat{\theta}_h \left/ \sum_{h=1}^{H} w_h \right. \tag{10.1.4}$$

and

$$Q_w = \sum_{h=1}^{H} w_h (\hat{\theta}_h - \bar{\theta}_w)^2,$$

where $\hat{\theta}_h$ is the estimator of θ_h based on the data from the hth study and w_h's are some statistics. The most popular choice of w_h is the inverse of an estimator of the variance of $\hat{\theta}_h$. Under the null hypothesis that $\sigma_\Delta^2 = 0$, Q_w is asymptotically (as the number of observations increases to infinity for each study) distributed as the central chi-square distribution with $k - 1$ degrees of freedom. Thus, DerSimonian and Laird's test rejects the null hypothesis that $\sigma_\Delta^2 = 0$ if Q is larger than a percentile of the the central chi-square distribution with $k - 1$ degrees of freedom.

DerSimonian and Laird's test can also be applied when Δ_h's are fixed effects, in which case the null hypothesis is $\Delta_h = 0$ for all h (no treatment-by-study interaction).

Under either the fixed or random effects model, DerSimonian and Laird's test provides no strong statistical evidence when the null hypothesis is not rejected (i.e., there is no treatment-by-study interaction). From a pharmaceutical company's viewpoint, it is more interesting to provide a strong statistical evidence that there is no treatment-by-study interaction so that analyzing the main effect of treatment difference is meaningful. Further discussions of this issue are given in §10.1.4 and §10.2.

10.1.3   The Average Treatment Difference

When there is no treatment-by-study interaction, the efficacy of the drug product can be assessed through hypothesis testing concerning the average treatment difference θ defined in (10.1.3). Data from all independent studies can be combined to provide an overall and perhaps more powerful assessment of the drug efficacy. If $\Delta_h = 0$ for all h, θ can be estimated by either $\bar{\theta}_w$ in (10.1.4) or the unweighted estimator

$$\bar{\theta} = \frac{1}{H} \sum_{h=1}^{H} \hat{\theta}_h.$$

Both estimators are asymptotically unbiased and consistent. A test for the null hypothesis $\theta = 0$ (or $\theta \leq 0$) can be constructed using a t-type statistic based on $\bar{\theta}_w$ or $\bar{\theta}$.

When Δ_h's are fixed effects and some of them are not 0, $\bar{\theta}_w$ is a biased estimator of θ but $\bar{\theta}$ is still unbiased. When Δ_h's are random effects with mean 0, both $\bar{\theta}_w$ and $\bar{\theta}$ are (asymptotically) unbiased. Testing for $\theta = 0$ (or $\theta \leq 0$) can be carried out using the combined data and a t-type statistic based on an asymptotically unbiased estimator of θ.

When effects of treatment-by-study interaction are nonzero, however, it is possible that the drug product is effective ($\theta_h > 0$) for some h's but not effective ($\theta_h \leq 0$) for other h's. In such a case testing a single hypothesis of $\theta = 0$ or $\theta \leq 0$ is not enough, since the results from different studies are inconsistent and θ is only a measure of the drug effect average over all studies.

10.1.4   Quantitative and Qualitative Interactions

If some θ_h's are positive and some θ_h's are negative, then we say that there is a *qualitative* treatment-by-study interaction. On the other hand, if all θ_h's have the same sign, then we say that there is a *quantitative* treatment-by-study interaction. This definition is the same as the definition of quantitative and qualitative treatment-by-center interactions in multicenter studies (Gail and Simon, 1985; Chow and Liu, 1998). For the case of $H = 2$, Figure 10.1.1 illustrates three different situations of no interaction, part (a), quantitative interaction, part (b), and qualitative interaction, part (c), between treatment and study.

A quantitative interaction between treatment and study indicates that the treatment differences are in the same direction across studies but the magnitude differs from study to study, while a qualitative treatment-by-study interaction reveals that substantial treatment differences occur in different directions in different studies. Thus, in the presence of a quantitative treatment-by-study interaction, it is easy to assess and interpret the overall treatment difference. In the presence of a qualitative treatment-by-study interaction, however, it is even hard (if not impossible) to define a measure of the overall treatment difference.

Gail and Simon (1985) proposed a test for qualitative interaction in multicenter trials, which can also be applied in meta-analysis to test the null hypothesis

H_0 : there is no qualitative treatment-by-study interaction   (10.1.5)

versus the alternative hypothesis

H_1 : there is qualitative treatment-by-study interaction.   (10.1.6)

Let $\hat{\theta}_h$ be the estimator of the treatment difference in the hth study and s_h

(a) No Interaction

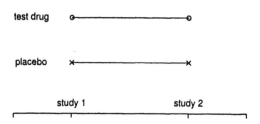

(b) Quantitative Interaction

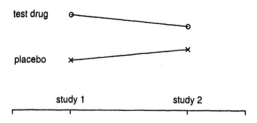

(c) Qualitative Interaction

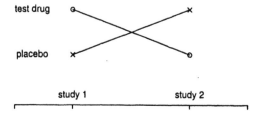

Figure 10.1.1. Treatment-by-Study Interaction

be an estimated standard deviation of $\hat{\theta}_h$, $h = 1, ..., H$. Define

$$Q^- = \sum_{h=1}^{H} \frac{\hat{\theta}_h^2}{s_h^2} I(\hat{\theta}_h < 0)$$

and

$$Q^+ = \sum_{h=1}^{H} \frac{\hat{\theta}_h^2}{s_h^2} I(\hat{\theta}_h > 0),$$

where $I(\cdot)$ is the indicator function. Gail and Simon's test rejects the null hypothesis H_0 in (10.1.5) when

$$\min(Q^-, Q^+) > c,$$

where c is the critical value provided in Table 1 of Gail and Simon (1985).

If Gail and Simon's test rejects the null hypothesis H_0 in (10.1.5), then no conclusion about the overall treatment difference can be made. If Gail and Simon's test does not reject the null hypothesis H_0 in (10.1.5), then we do not have a strong evidence to conclude whether the treatment-by-study interaction is qualitative or quantitative (since we do not have any control on the type II error rate of the test) and, thus, even if we draw a conclusion about the overall treatment difference by assuming there is only quantitative treatment-by-study interaction, the result does not have any statistical assurance. From this point of view, Gail and Simon's test is not useful in assessing the overall effect of treatment difference. What we need is a statistical test with H_1 in (10.1.6) being the null hypothesis and H_0 in (10.1.5) being the alternative hypothesis so that if we reject the hypothesis that there is a qualitative treatment-by-study interaction, we can assess the treatment difference with some statistical assurance. This is studied in the next two sections.

10.2 Testing of No Qualitative Interaction

As we discussed in the previous section, it is of interest for the purpose of assessing drug treatment difference to verify that there is no qualitative interaction, i.e., to perform a statistical test with the null hypothesis being the hypothesis that there is a qualitative treatment-by-study interaction.

10.2.1 Intersection-Union Tests

Let θ_h be the population treatment difference in the hth study, $h = 1, ..., H$. Then, one may specify the hypothesis (of having qualitative treatment-by-study interaction) as

$$H_0 : \theta_h\text{'s do not have the same sign}$$

and the alternative hypothesis (of no qualitative treatment-by-study inter-action) as

$$H_1 : \theta_h > 0 \text{ for all } h \quad \text{or} \quad \theta_h < 0 \text{ for all } h. \tag{10.2.1}$$

In view of the discussion in §8.1, however, an effect less than an equiv-alence limit δ in absolute value can be treated as 0 and, thus, it may be more practical to form the alternative hypothesis of no (serious) qualitative treatment-by-study interaction as

$$H_1(\delta) : \theta_h > -\delta \text{ for all } h \quad \text{or} \quad \theta_h < \delta \text{ for all } h \tag{10.2.2}$$

with an equivalence limit $\delta > 0$ and the null hypothesis as

$$H_0(\delta) : H_1(\delta) \text{ does not hold.}$$

The idea is that when there is a small negligible qualitative treatment-by-study interaction, it can be treated as if there is no qualitative treatment-by-study interaction in the assessment of drug treatment difference. For example, if $\theta_h > -\delta$ for all h, then θ_h is either positive or nearly 0 and the drug treatment difference can be assessed using the average of θ_h's.

Graphical illustrations of H_1 and $H_1(\delta)$ in the case of $H = 2$ are given in Figure 10.2.1.

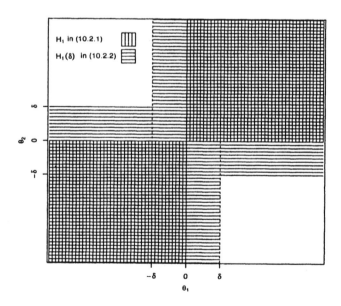

Figure 10.2.1. Regions of Hypotheses (10.2.1) and (10.2.2)

Note that $H_1(\delta)$ in (10.2.2) is a union of

$$H_1^-(\delta) : \theta_h > -\delta \text{ for all } h \qquad (10.2.3)$$

and

$$H_1^+(\delta) : \theta_h < \delta \text{ for all } h, \qquad (10.2.4)$$

which are intersections of hypotheses of the form $\theta_h > -\delta$ (or $\theta_h < \delta$). Thus, the approach of intersection-union (Berger and Hsu, 1996; see also §8.2) can be applied.

Consider the situation where the estimator of the treatment difference in the hth study, $\hat{\theta}_h$, is a difference of the sample means from a two group parallel design with normally distributed responses having variance σ_h^2, $h = 1, ..., H$. Let v_h be the usual unbiased estimator (based on sample variances) of the variance of $\hat{\theta}_h$. Let us first focus on the hypothesis in (10.2.3), which is an intersection of $H_{1h}^-(\delta) : \theta_h > -\delta$, $h = 1, ..., H$. For a fixed h, the usual size α test for $H_{1h}^-(\delta)$ rejects the null hypothesis $H_{0h}^-(\delta)$ if and only if

$$\hat{\theta}_h - t_{1-\alpha;m_h}\sqrt{v_h} > -\delta, \qquad (10.2.5)$$

where m_h is the degrees of freedom of v_h and $t_{1-\alpha;m_h}$ is the $1 - \alpha$ quantile of the t-distribution with m_h degrees of freedom. Consequently, the intersection-union test for $H_1^-(\delta)$ in (10.2.3) rejects its null hypothesis if and only if (10.2.5) holds for all h. This test is actually of size α (Cheng, 2002).

Applying the previous argument to hypothesis (10.2.4), we obtain a size α intersection-union test that rejects the null hypothesis corresponding to $H_1^+(\delta)$ if and only if

$$\hat{\theta}_h + t_{1-\alpha;m_h}\sqrt{v_h} < \delta \qquad (10.2.6)$$

for all h. Then, by Bonferroni's inequality, a level 2α test that rejects the null hypothesis corresponding to the alternative hypothesis in (10.2.2) if and only if either (10.2.5) holds for all h or (10.2.6) holds for all h.

In this situation we may modify the hypothesis in (10.2.2) to

$$H_1(\delta) : \frac{\theta_h}{\sigma_h} > -\delta \text{ for all } h \quad \text{or} \quad \frac{\theta_h}{\sigma_h} < \delta \text{ for all } h. \qquad (10.2.7)$$

That is, the equivalence limit δ in (10.2.7) is selected with respect to a relative measure θ_h/σ_h. It follows from the previous argument and a result in Shao (1999, Example 6.17) that a level 2α test that rejects the null hypothesis corresponding to $H_1(\delta)$ in (10.2.7) if and only if either

$$\frac{\hat{\theta}_h}{\sqrt{v_h}} > t_{1-\alpha;m_h}(-m_h\delta) \text{ for all } h$$

or

$$\frac{\hat{\theta}_h}{\sqrt{v_h}} < t_{1-\alpha;m_h}(m_h\delta) \quad \text{for all } h,$$

where $t_{1-\alpha;m_h}(u)$ is the $1-\alpha$ quantile of the noncentral t-distribution with m_h degrees of freedom and noncentrality parameter u.

10.2.2 An Aggregated Test

The intersection-union tests described in §10.2.1 are adequate when H is small, but may be much too conservative when H is moderate or large. For example, the power of the intersection-union test for $H_1^-(\delta)$ in (10.2.3), which rejects its null hypothesis if and only if (10.2.5) holds for all h, is equal to

$$\prod_{h=1}^{H} P\left(\hat{\theta}_h - t_{1-\alpha;m_h}\sqrt{v_h} > -\delta\right),$$

which is equal to $(0.8)^H$ if, for every h, the test defined by (10.2.5) has power 80%. When $H = 2$, $(0.8)^H = 0.64$. But $(0.8)^H = 0.3277$ when $H = 5$.

This problem of the intersection-union tests is from the fact that when H is moderate or large, the hypothesis $H_1(\delta)$ given by (10.2.2) is too restrictive. An aggregated measure on the qualitative treatment-by-study interaction is desired when H is not small.

Consider the situation where the estimator of the treatment difference $\hat{\theta}_h$ is a difference of the sample means from a two group parallel design in the hth study, $h = 1, ..., H$. Using the notation in (10.1.3), we find that the hypothesis of no treatment-by-study interaction, i.e., $\Delta_h = 0$ for all h, is equivalent to $\sum_{h=1}^{H} \Delta_h^2 = 0$. Thus, we may use $\sum_{h=1}^{H} \Delta_h^2$ to assess qualitative treatment-by-study interaction and define the hypothesis of no qualitative treatment-by-study interaction as $\sum_{h=1}^{H} \Delta_h^2 < \delta^2$, where δ is an equivalence limit. However, when the population variances $\sigma_1^2, ..., \sigma_H^2$ are different, it may be more suitable to use $\sum_{h=1}^{H}(\Delta_h - \tilde{\Delta})^2/\sigma_h^2$ to assess qualitative treatment-by-study interaction, where $\tilde{\Delta} = (\sum_{h=1}^{H}\sigma_h^{-2}\Delta_h)/(\sum_{h=1}^{H}\sigma_h^{-2})$. This leads to the following hypothesis of no qualitative treatment-by-study interaction:

$$H_1(\delta) : \frac{1}{H}\sum_{h=1}^{H}\frac{(\Delta_h - \tilde{\Delta})^2}{\sigma_h^2} < \delta^2. \tag{10.2.8}$$

When $H = 2$, the hypotheses in (10.2.2) and (10.2.8) are displayed in Figure 10.2.2. It is clear that the hypothesis in (10.2.8) is more restrictive than that in (10.2.2). When H is not small, however, the hypothesis in (10.2.8) is much less restrictive than the hypothesis in (10.2.2).

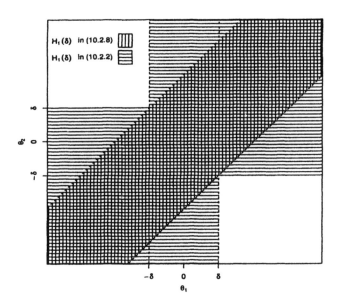

Figure 10.2.2. Regions of Hypotheses (10.2.2) and (10.2.8)

When σ_h^2's are equal, it is possible to derive a test of exactly size α for testing hypothesis (10.2.8) (Cheng, 2002). When σ_h^2's are unequal, we have to use tests that have asymptotic size (or level) α. It is shown in Cheng (2002) that rejecting the null hypothesis corresponding to $H_1(\delta)$ in (10.2.8) if and only if

$$\sum_{h=1}^{H} \frac{(\ddot{\theta}_h - \tilde{\theta})^2}{\hat{\sigma}_h^2} \leq (H-1)\delta^2 - 2z_\alpha \delta \sqrt{\frac{H-1}{n^*}}$$

produces a test of asymptotic size α for testing the hypothesis in (10.2.8), where z_α is the αth quantile of the standard normal distribution, $\hat{\sigma}_h^2$ is a consistent estimator of σ_h^2 for every h, $n_* = \lambda N$, $N = \sum_{i,h} n_{ih}$, n_{ih} is the sample size of the ith treatment in study h, and

$$n_{ih}/N \to \lambda \quad \text{for all } i, h, \quad 0 < \lambda < 1 \tag{10.2.9}$$

is assumed. Note that assumption (10.2.9) means that sample sizes n_{ih}'s in all studies are almost the same, which may be true when sample sizes are planned to be the same but are different due to administrative reasons. Some tests for the cases where assumption (10.2.9) does not satisfy can be found in Cheng (2002).

10.3   Assessing Drug Efficacy

The main problem of the p-value approach described in §10.1.1 is the use
of the null hypothesis given in (10.1.2). Mathematically, it can be shown
that the null hypothesis H_0 in (10.1.2) is equivalent to

$$H_0 : \theta = 0 \quad \text{and} \quad \Delta_h = 0, \ h = 1, ..., H,$$

i.e., not only the main effect θ is 0, but also all study effects are 0, where
Δ_h's are fixed effects defined in (10.1.3) and $\Delta_1 + \cdots + \Delta_H = 0$. This
is certainly not the null hypothesis we should focus on, because the null
hypothesis should be the opposite of the hypothesis we would like to verify
(with a strong statistical evidence). In this section we introduce some hypotheses of interest in assessing drug treatment difference in meta-analysis
and some recently developed statistical tests for these hypotheses.

10.3.1   Simultaneous Tests

To establish the effectiveness of the drug product, one may want to verify the hypothesis that the test drug is simultaneously noninferior to the
standard therapy,

$$H_1 : \theta_h > -\delta \ \text{ for all } h, \tag{10.3.1}$$

or the hypothesis that the test drug is simultaneously superior to the standard therapy,

$$H_1 : \theta_h > \delta \ \text{ for all } h, \tag{10.3.2}$$

or the hypothesis that the test drug is nonequivalent to the standard therapy simultaneously,

$$H_1 : \theta_h > \delta \ \text{ for all } h \quad \text{or} \quad \theta_h < -\delta \ \text{ for all } h, \tag{10.3.3}$$

where δ is 0 or a given positive equivalence limit. The corresponding null
hypothesis is the complement of H_1. Figure 10.3.1 shows the hypotheses in
(10.3.1)-(10.3.3) for the case of $H = 2$.

Note that the hypothesis given by (10.3.1) is exactly the same as that
in (10.2.3). Hence, the test procedure developed in §10.2 can be used for
this hypothesis. For the hypothesis in (10.3.2), the size α intersection-union
test rejects the corresponding null hypothesis if and only if

$$\hat{\theta}_h - t_{1-\alpha;m_h} s_h > \delta \ \text{ for all } h.$$

Finally, the intersection-union approach and Bonferroni's inequality lead to
a level 2α test for (10.3.3) which rejects the null hypothesis corresponding
to H_1 in (10.3.3) if and only if either

$$\hat{\theta}_h - t_{1-\alpha;m_h} s_h > \delta \ \text{ for all } h$$

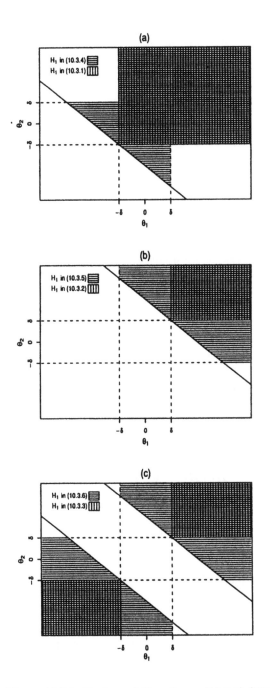

Figure 10.3.1. Regions of Hypotheses (10.3.1)-(10.3.6)
when $H_1(\delta)$ is defined by (10.2.2)

or

$$\hat{\theta}_h + t_{1-\alpha;m_h} s_h < -\delta \quad \text{for all } h.$$

10.3.2   Two-Step Tests

If the hypothesis H_1 in (10.2.1) or $H_1(\delta)$ in (10.2.2) is concluded in a test of no qualitative treatment-by-study interaction (see §10.2) with a given significance level, then the overall drug treatment effect can be evaluated by assessing the average treatment difference $\theta = H^{-1} \sum_{h=1}^{H} \theta_h$, where θ_h is the population treatment difference in the hth study. Testing procedures using t-type statistics described in §10.1.3 can be used to test the null hypothesis such as $\theta \leq -\delta$ (a noninferiority test), $\theta \leq \delta$ (a superiority test), or $|\theta| \leq \delta$ (a nonequivalence test) with a equivalence limit δ.

Under this approach, the overall test for drug efficacy is a two-step test. In the first step, a test of no qualitative treatment-by-study interaction (§10.2) with a significance level α is performed. If the result is significant (e.g., $H_1(\delta)$ in (10.2.2) or (10.2.8) is concluded), then a test for the average treatment effect with a significant level α is carried out. The treatment effect is significant if and only if both null hypotheses in two steps are rejected. The overall significance level of this two-step test is α, since this two-step test is a intersection-union test described in Theorem 2 of Berger and Hsu (1996). The alternative hypothesis H_1 of the two-step test is the intersection of the two alternative hypotheses in two steps; that is,

$$H_1 : H_1(\delta) \text{ holds and } \theta > -\delta \tag{10.3.4}$$

for testing of noninferiority, where $H_1(\delta)$ is given by (10.2.2) and θ is the average of θ_h's;

$$H_1 : H_1(\delta) \text{ holds and } \theta > \delta \tag{10.3.5}$$

for testing of superiority; and

$$H_1 : H_1(\delta) \text{ holds and } |\theta| > \delta \tag{10.3.6}$$

for testing of nonequivalence.

Figure 10.3.1 includes the regions of the alternative hypotheses given in (10.3.4)-(10.3.6) for the two-step test when $H = 2$ and $H_1(\delta)$ is defined by (10.2.2). Comparing the regions in Figure 10.3.1, we conclude that the region defined by the alternative hypothesis in simultaneous testing is contained in the alternative hypothesis in the two-step test. Thus, simultaneous testing is more conservative than two-step testing when the intersection-union test described in §10.2.1 is used in step 1.

Figure 10.3.2 displays the regions of the alternative hypotheses given in (10.3.4)-(10.3.6) for the two-step test when $H = 2$ and $H_1(\delta)$ is defined by

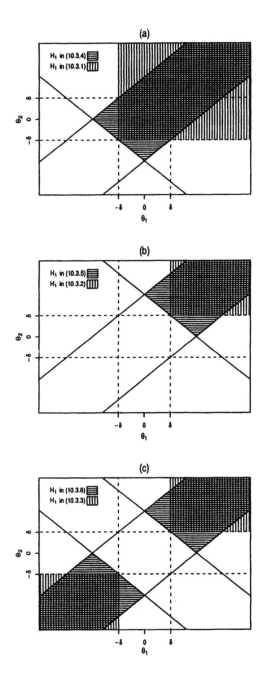

Figure 10.3.2. Regions of Hypotheses (10.3.1)-(10.3.6)
when $H_1(\delta)$ is defined by (10.2.8)

(10.2.8), and the regions of the alternative hypotheses in (10.3.1)-(10.3.3) for simultaneous testing. For $H = 2$, the region defined by the alternative hypothesis in simultaneous testing is not contained in the alternative hypothesis in the two-step test. When H is not small, however, simultaneous testing is more conservative than two-step testing when the aggregated test described in §10.2.2 is used in step 1.

10.3.3   Evaluation of Equivalence

In some situations it is of interest to verify whether a test drug product is equivalent to a standard therapy (see §8.2). If we adopt the simultaneous testing approach in §10.3.2, then the null hypothesis is the complement of the following alternative hypothesis

$$H_1 : |\theta_h| < \delta \ \text{ for all } h, \tag{10.3.7}$$

where δ is a equivalence limit. If the two-step test approach in §10.3.1 is considered, then the alternative hypothesis is

$$H_1 : H_1(\delta) \text{ in } (10.2.2) \text{ holds and } |\theta| < \delta \tag{10.3.8}$$

when the intersection-union approach in §10.2.1 is used, or

$$H_1 : H_1(\delta) \text{ in } (10.2.8) \text{ holds and } |\theta| < \delta \tag{10.3.9}$$

when the aggregated testing approach in §10.2.2 is used, where θ is the average of θ_h's. When $H = 2$, the regions defined by H_1 in (10.3.7) and (10.3.8) are compared in part (a) of Figure 10.3.3 and the regions defined by H_1 in (10.3.8) and (10.3.9) are compared in part (b) of Figure 10.3.3.

   The hypothesis in (10.3.7) can be tested using the intersection-union approach, i.e., the null hypothesis corresponding to H_1 in (10.3.7) is rejected if and only if

$$-\delta < \hat{\theta}_h - t_{1-\alpha;m_h} s_h \quad \text{and} \quad \hat{\theta}_h + t_{1-\alpha;m_h} s_h < \delta, \quad h = 1, ..., H,$$

where $t_{1-\alpha;m_h}$ is the $(1-\alpha)$th quantile of the t-distribution with m_h degrees of freedom. According to Theorem 2 in Berger and Hsu (1996), the size of this test is α. However, this test is too conservative if H is not small.

   The hypothesis in (10.3.8) or (10.3.9) can be tested using the two-step test described in §10.3.2, i.e., the null hypothesis corresponding to H_1 in (10.3.8) or (10.3.9) is rejected if and only if no qualitative treatment-by-study interaction is concluded and the null hypothesis $|\theta| \geq \delta$ is rejected. When H is not small, the hypothesis in (10.3.9) should be considered and the aggregated test in §10.2.2 should be used in step 1.

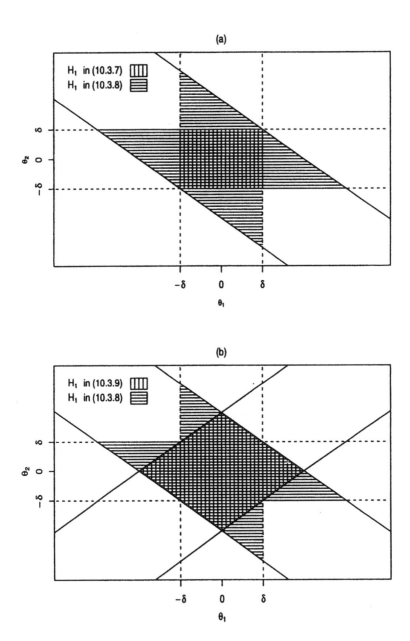

Figure 10.3.3. Regions of Hypotheses (10.3.7)-(10.3.9)

10.4   Multiple Products

In this section and the next section, we consider a meta-analysis involving H studies that compare H different test drug products with a common standard therapy. Sometimes it is also of interest to compare two or several test drug products. Some general discussions are presented in this section. Applications in bioequivalence studies are discussed in §10.5.

10.4.1   Parallel Designs

Suppose that in study h, a parallel design is used to compare a test drug product h and a standard therapy, $h = 1, ..., H$, where the standard therapy is the same for all H studies. Let y_{hij} be the jth observation under treatment i in study h, where $j = 1, ..., n_{hi}$ for some sample size n_{hi}, $i = 0$ (standard therapy) or 1 (test drug treatment), and $h = 1, ..., H$. Assume that y_{hij}'s are independent and the population means are given by

$$\mu_0 = E(y_{h0j}) \quad j = 1, ..., n_{h0}, \ h = 1, ..., H,$$

and

$$\mu_h = E(y_{h1j}) \quad j = 1, ..., n_{h1}, \ h = 1, ..., H.$$

Define

$$
\begin{aligned}
z_{hj} &= y_{h1j}, \quad j = 1, ..., n_{h1}, \ h = 1, ..., H, \\
z_{0j} &= y_{10j}, \quad j = 1, ..., n_{10}, \\
z_{0(n_{10}+j)} &= y_{10j}, \quad j = 1, ..., n_{20}, \\
z_{0(n_{10}+n_{20}+j)} &= y_{20j}, \quad j = 1, ..., n_{30}, \\
&\cdots\cdots\cdots \quad \cdots\cdots\cdots \quad \cdots\cdots\cdots \\
z_{0(n_{10}+\cdots+n_{(H-1)0}+j)} &= y_{20j}, \quad j = 1, ..., n_{H0}.
\end{aligned}
$$

Then, the combined data set

$$\{z_{hj} : j = 1, ..., n_h, h = 0, 1, ..., H\},$$

where $n_h = n_{h1}$ and $n_0 = n_{10} + \cdots + n_{H0}$, is the same as that from a one-way analysis of variance model.

Consider first the simple case where $\text{Var}(z_{hj}) = \sigma^2$ is a constant. Then the usual ANOVA test can be applied to assess the treatment differences $\mu_h - \mu_0$ for all h and $\mu_h - \mu_g$ for all pairs of h and g with $h < g$. By combining data from H studies, we not only obtain a more accurate estimator of μ_0, but also a more accurate estimator of σ^2.

In meta-analysis, it is likely that the variance of z_{hj} vary with h (the study). Without the equal variance assumption, we may use the following asymptotic (large n_h's) confidence intervals for $\mu_h - \mu_g$:

$$\left(\bar{z}_h - \bar{z}_g - z_{0.975}\sqrt{\frac{s_h^2}{n_h} + \frac{s_g^2}{n_g}}, \quad \bar{z}_h - \bar{z}_g - z_{0.975}\sqrt{\frac{s_h^2}{n_h} + \frac{s_g^2}{n_g}} \right),$$

where $\bar{z}_h$ and s_h^2 are the sample mean and sample variance, respectively, based on z_{hj}, $j = 1, ..., n_h$, and $z_{0.975}$ is the 97.5th percentile of the standard normal distribution.

10.4.2   Crossover Designs

Crossover designs are widely used in bioequivalence studies. Suppose that in study h, a 2×2 crossover design is used to compare a test drug product h and a standard therapy, $h = 1, ..., H$, where the standard therapy is the same for all H studies. Let y_{hijk} be the ith observation in period j, sequence k, and study h, where $i = 1, ..., n_{kh}$, $j = 1, 2$, $k = 1, 2$, and $h = 1, ..., H$. Within study h, y_{hijk}'s follow a model similar to that in (5.2.3) with an additional subscript, h, being added to all parameters, i.e.,

$$y_{ijkh} = \mu_{lh} + W_{ljkh} + S_{iklh} + e_{ijkh}, \quad l = T, R, \quad \quad (10.4.1)$$

and the variance components are σ_{TTh}^2, σ_{BTh}^2, σ_{WTh}^2, σ_{Dh}^2, etc. However, when $l = R$ (standard therapy or reference formulation), the parameters do not vary with h, i.e., $\mu_{Rh} = \mu_R$ for all h, $\sigma_{BRh}^2 = \sigma_{BR}^2$, and $\sigma_{WRh}^2 = \sigma_{WR}^2$ for all h.

Unlike the situation with a parallel design, combining data under standard therapy from H independent studies with the same crossover design does not always lead to a more efficient statistical procedure, because data within a study are usually positively correlated and, thus, analyzing each individual data set may be more efficient when the between-subject variation is much larger than the within-subject variation. We illustrate this issue by considering the estimation of the treatment effect $\delta_h = \mu_{Th} - \mu_R$ or $\delta_h - \delta_g = \mu_{Th} - \mu_{Tg}$, $h \neq g$.

The best unbiased estimator of μ_R based on the H independent data sets is

$$\hat{\mu}_R = \sum_{h=1}^{H} \frac{\bar{y}_{21h} + \bar{y}_{12h}}{2c_h} \Big/ \sum_{h=1}^{H} \frac{1}{c_h},$$

where $\bar{y}_{jkh}$ is the sample mean based on y_{ijkh}, $i = 1, ..., n_{kh}$ and $c_h = (n_{1h}^{-1} + n_{2h}^{-1})/4$. Thus, an unbiased estimator of δ_h based on the meta-analysis (combined data) is

$$\tilde{\delta}_h = \frac{\bar{y}_{11h} + \bar{y}_{22h}}{2} - \hat{\mu}_R,$$

whereas the estimator of δ_h based on data from study h only is given by (5.3.2), i.e.,

$$\hat{\delta}_h = \frac{\bar{y}_{11h} + \bar{y}_{22h} - \bar{y}_{12h} - \bar{y}_{21h}}{2}.$$

Chow and Shao (1999) showed that $\tilde{\delta}_h$ is not always better than $\hat{\delta}_h$. In fact,

$$\text{Var}(\hat{\delta}_h) - \text{Var}(\tilde{\delta}_h) = (c_h - C_H)(\sigma_{TR}^2 - 2\rho_h \sigma_{BTh} \sigma_{BR}),$$

where $C_H = (\sum_{h=1}^{H} c_h^{-1})^{-1} \leq c_h$. That is, combining data sets leads to a more efficient estimator of δ_h if and only if the total variance of the reference formulation is larger than two times of the covariance between the two observations from the same subject.

Chow and Shao (1999) also proposed a test procedure to determine whether a meta-analysis provides a better estimator of δ_h. Let $n_{0h} = \min\{n_{1h}, n_{2h}\}$, $x_{i1h} = y_{i11h} - y_{i12h} + y_{i21h} - y_{i22h}$, $x_{i2h} = y_{i11h} + y_{i22h}$, s_{xjh}^2 be the sample variance based on $x_{ijh}, i = 1, ..., n_{0h}, j = 1, 2$. Then $F_h = s_{x1h}^2 / s_{x2h}^2$ has the F-distribution with degrees of freedom $n_{0h} - 1$ and $n_{0h} - 1$ when $\sigma_{TR}^2 = 2\rho_h \sigma_{BTh} \sigma_{BR}$. Thus, an exact size α test rejects the hypothesis that $\text{Var}(\hat{\delta}_h) \leq \text{Var}(\tilde{\delta}_h)$ when F_h is larger than the upper α quantile of the F-distribution with degrees of freedom $n_{0h} - 1$ and $n_{0h} - 1$.

Consider now the estimation of $\delta_h - \delta_g = \mu_h - \mu_g$, $h \neq g$. Note that an estimator of $\delta_h - \delta_g$ based on data from studies h and g is $\hat{\delta}_h - \hat{\delta}_g$, whereas an estimator based on the meta-analysis is

$$\tilde{\delta}_h - \tilde{\delta}_g = \frac{\bar{y}_{11h} + \bar{y}_{22h}}{2} - \frac{\bar{y}_{11g} + \bar{y}_{22g}}{2},$$

since the meta-analysis uses $\hat{\mu}_R$ as a common estimator for μ_R. These two estimators are unbiased and normally distributed with variances

$$\text{Var}(\hat{\delta}_h - \hat{\delta}_g) = c_h \sigma_{1,1,h}^2 + c_g \sigma_{1,1,g}^2$$

and

$$\text{Var}(\tilde{\delta}_h - \tilde{\delta}_g) = c_h \sigma_{TTh}^2 + c_g \sigma_{TTg}^2,$$

where $\sigma_{1,1,h}^2 = \sigma_{Dh}^2 + \sigma_{WTh}^2 + \sigma_{WR}^2$. Confidence intervals for $\delta_h - \delta_g$ can be obtained by estimating the variance components by sample variances.

Example 10.4.1. We consider PK responses from three independent bioequivalence studies. Data from study 1 and study 2 are listed in Table 10.4.1 and data from study 3 are given by Table 5.3.1. In each study, the standard 2×2 crossover design was used to assess bioequivalence between a test formulation and a reference formulation. The same reference formulation was used for all three studies.

Table 10.4.1. PK Responses from Bioequivalence Studies

	Sequence 1		Sequence 2	
	Period 1	Period 2	Period 1	Period 2
Study 1	4.7715	4.6025	4.6445	4.6104
	4.6557	4.5414	4.7719	4.5316
	4.6107	4.5170	4.6804	4.9791
	4.5566	4.7277	4.9572	4.4743
	4.6165	4.6979	4.4570	4.7782
	4.6446	4.7441	4.8333	4.7906
	4.5156	4.4945	4.8327	4.6732
	4.7461	4.8767	4.6009	4.4802
	4.5275	4.8566	4.7402	4.7901
	4.5848	4.6482	4.4748	4.7378
	4.4630	4.6441	4.8065	4.4383
	4.6954	4.7787	4.4772	4.3670
Study 2	4.6974	4.4814	4.4902	4.6058
	4.6818	4.9480	4.7208	4.7824
	4.5329	4.4697	4.8940	4.9102
	4.9905	4.5137	4.6753	4.9106
	4.7481	4.7476	4.6354	4.8466
	4.7420	4.6282	4.6973	4.8401
	4.5469	4.6518	4.6558	4.6844
	4.9154	4.3600	4.6164	4.8815
	4.7344	4.8155	4.6977	4.8506
	4.6322	4.6847	4.5732	4.9825
	4.6611	4.5936	4.6282	4.8060
	4.9243	4.7327	4.8046	4.9338

Table 10.4.2. Approximate 90% Confidence Intervals (Example 10.4.1)

	Meta-analysis	Non-meta-analysis
Test 1 vs reference	$(-0.0892, 0.0217)^*$	$(-0.1291, 0.0152)^*$
Test 2 vs reference	$(0.0760, 0.1734)^*$	$(0.0656, 0.1949)^*$
Test 3 vs reference	$(-0.0296, 0.1109)^*$	$(-0.0342, 0.0949)^*$
Test 1 vs test 2	$(-0.2468, -0.0701)$	$(-0.3366, -0.0379)$
Test 1 vs test 3	$(-0.1605, 0.0117)^*$	$(-0.2610, 0.0305)$
Test 2 vs test 3	$(-0.0110, 0.1790)^*$	$(-0.0818, 0.2258)$

*Intervals contained in $(-0.223, 0.223)$ (for assessing ABE)

The ratio F_h proposed by Chow and Shao (1999) for study 1, 2, and 3 are $F_1 = 1.918$, $F_2 = 1.19$, and $F_3 = 1.915$. This indicates that the meta-analysis should provide better results, although the difference may not be substantial.

Approximate 90% confidence intervals for population difference between each test formulation and the reference formulation or between two test formulations are given in Table 10.4.2. For each case, two intervals are given, one is based on the meta-analysis and the other is based on data within a particular study (non-meta-analysis). In all cases, intervals obtained from the meta-analysis are shorter.

10.5 Bioequivalence Studies

When a brand-name drug is going off patent, there may exist several generic copies of the same drug. Although each generic copy is demonstrated to be bioequivalent to the brand-name drug, current regulation does not indicate that under what conditions one generic copy can be used as a substitute for another generic copy. In this section we address this issue through a meta-analysis by combining data from H independent *in vivo* bioequivalence studies. A meta-analysis by combining data from all H studies provides not only a way to assess bioequivalence between two generic copies, but also a possibly more efficient bioequivalence test between each generic copy and the brand-name drug.

Assume that the H independent *in vivo* bioequivalence studies use one of the designs described in §5.2-5.4. Each study compares a generic drug (test formulation) with the same brand-name drug (reference formulation). Thus, data from the brand-name drug in different studies are from the same population, whereas data from generic drugs may have different populations. We assume the general model given by (10.4.1), which is the same as those in §5.2-5.4 except that an additional subscript, h, is added to indicate different studies. Since data from the reference formulation are from the same population, μ_R, σ_{BR}^2, and σ_{WR}^2 do not vary with h.

10.5.1 Meta-Analysis for ABE

For assessing the ABE (see §5.3.1), the construction of a confidence interval for $\delta_h = \mu_{Th} - mu_R$ is the key issue. Thus, the results in §10.4.2 (Chow and Shao, 1999) can be applied.

For testing the ABE between the hth test formulation and the reference formulation based on data from the standard 2×2 crossover design, a meta-analysis produces the following 90% confidence interval limits:

$$\tilde{\delta}_h \pm t_{0.95;n_{1h}+n_{2h}-2} \frac{\hat{\sigma}_{TTh}}{2} \sqrt{\frac{1}{n_{1h}} + \frac{1}{n_{2h}}},$$

where

$$\hat{\sigma}_{TTh}^2 = \frac{(n_{1h}-1)s_{11h}^2 + (n_{2h}-1)s_{22h}^2}{n_{1h}+n_{2h}-2}$$

and s_{jkh}^2 is the sample variance based on $\{y_{ijkh}, i=1,...,n_{kh}\}$. Without applying meta-analysis, a confidence interval for δ_h can be obtained using the data from study h and the method described in §5.3.1.

Two test formulations, h and g, are considered to be ABE if a 90% confidence interval for $\mu_{Th} - \mu_{Tg} = \delta_h - \delta_g$ is within (δ_L, δ_U), where δ_L and δ_U are ABE limits given in §5.3.1. It follows from the results in §10.4.2 that a 90% confidence interval for $\delta_h - \delta_g$ using meta-analysis has limits

$$\tilde{\delta}_h - \tilde{\delta}_g \pm t_{0.95;n_{1h}+n_{2h}-2} \sqrt{c_h \hat{\sigma}_{TTh}^2 + c_g \hat{\sigma}_{TTg}^2}$$

and a 90% confidence interval for $\delta_h - \delta_g$ using non-meta-analysis has limits

$$\hat{\delta}_h - \hat{\delta}_g \pm t_{0.95;n_{1h}+n_{2h}-2} \sqrt{c_h \hat{\sigma}_{1,1,h}^2 + c_g \hat{\sigma}_{1,1,g}^2},$$

where $\hat{\sigma}_{1,1,h}^2$ is the same as that in (5.3.4) but based on the data from study h.

Example 10.5.1. We consider the data in Example 10.4.1 again, which lead to confidence intervals given in Table 10.4.2. Some conclusions can be made from the results in Table 10.4.2. First, ABE can be claimed between each test formulation and the reference formulation, in terms of either meta-analysis or non-meta-analysis. Second, from the non-meta-analysis, ABE between any two test formulations cannot be claimed, because none of the confidence intervals is within (δ_L, δ_U). Finally, according to the results from the meta-analysis, we can claim ABE between test formulations 1 and 3 and between test formulations 2 and 3. However, ABE between test formulations 1 and 2 cannot be claimed. Note that when we cannot claim bioequivalence based on one statistical procedure, it is possible that a more powerful (efficient) statistical procedure reaches a different conclusion. In this example, the results indicate that the meta-analysis is more efficient than the non-meta-analysis.

10.5.2   Meta-Analysis for PBE

The design and model for the PBE are the same as those for the ABE. Hence, we can use the same notation as in §10.5.1.

Consider first the PBE between test formulation h and the reference formulation. In addition to the estimation of δ_h, estimation of variance components σ^2_{TTh} and σ^2_{TR} is required for the PBE. While δ_h and σ^2_{TTh} can be estimated by $\hat{\delta}$ and $\hat{\sigma}^2_{TTh}$, which are the same as $\hat{\delta}$ and $\hat{\sigma}^2_{TT}$ in §5.5 but are based on data from study h, a better estimator of σ^2_{TR} can be obtained from the meta-analysis. Combining data from the H studies, σ^2_{TR} can be estimated by

$$\hat{\sigma}^2_{TR} = a_h \hat{\sigma}^2_{TRh} + (1 - a_h)\tilde{\sigma}^2_{TRh}, \qquad (10.5.1)$$

where $a_h = (n_{1h} + n_{2h} - 2)/n_H$, $n_H = \sum_{h=1}^{H}(n_{1h} + n_{2h} - 2)$,

$$\hat{\sigma}^2_{TRh} = \frac{1}{n_{1h} + n_{2h} - 2}\left[\sum_{i=1}^{n_{1h}}(y_{i21h} - \bar{y}_{21h})^2 + \sum_{i=1}^{n_{2h}}(y_{i12h} - \bar{y}_{12h})^2\right]$$

is the same as $\hat{\sigma}^2_{TR}$ in §5.5 but based on data in study h, and

$$\tilde{\sigma}^2_{TRh} = \frac{1}{n_H(1 - a_h)}\sum_{g \neq h}\left[\sum_{i=1}^{n_{1g}}(y_{i21g} - \bar{y}_{21g})^2 + \sum_{i=1}^{n_{2g}}(y_{i12g} - \bar{y}_{12g})^2\right]$$

is an unbiased estimator of σ^2_{TR} based on data from studies other than study h. As a result, the PBE between test formulation h and the reference formulation can be tested using the procedure in §5.5.1 with $\hat{\sigma}^2_{TR}$ defined by (10.5.1) and with V replaced by

$$\left(2\hat{\delta}_h, 1, -ba_h, -b(1 - a_h)\right) C \left(2\hat{\delta}_h, 1, -ba_h, -b(1 - a_h)\right)',$$

where $b = 1 + \theta_{PBE}$ if reference-scaled criterion is used and $b = 1$ if constant-scaled criterion is used,

$$C = \begin{pmatrix} C_h & 0 \\ 0 & \frac{2(1-a_h)^2 \tilde{\sigma}^2_{TRh}}{n_H - (n_{1h} + n_{2h} - 2)} \end{pmatrix},$$

and C_h is the same as C in (5.5.2) but based on data in study h.

Now, consider the PBE between two test formulations, h and g. We define the following PBE parameter similar to that in (5.1.1):

$$\theta_{h,g} = \begin{cases} \dfrac{E(y_{Th} - y_{Tg})^2 - E(y_R - y_R')^2}{E(y_R - y_R')^2/2} & \text{if } E(y_R - y_R')^2/2 \geq \sigma_0^2 \\[3mm] \dfrac{E(y_{Th} - y_{Tg})^2 - E(y_R - y_R')^2}{\sigma_0^2} & \text{if } E(y_R - y_R')^2/2 < \sigma_0^2, \end{cases} \qquad (10.5.2)$$

where y_{Th} and y_{Tg} are from test formulation h and g, respectively, y_R and y_R' are from the reference formulation, and y_{Th}, y_{Tg}, y_R and y_R' are independent. Note that we still use the mean squared error $E(y_R - y'_R)^2$ in the denominators in (10.5.2) so that the parameter $\theta_{h,g}$ is symmetric in h and g, i.e., $\theta_{h,g} = \theta_{g,h}$. Two test formulations are PBE when $\theta_{h,g} < \theta_{PBE}$, where θ_{PBE} is the PBE limit given by FDA (1999a).

Under the assumed model, $\theta_{h,g} < \theta_{PBE}$ if and only if $\lambda_{h,g} < 0$, where

$$\lambda_{h,g} = (\delta_h - \delta_g)^2 + \sigma_{Th}^2 + \sigma_{Tg}^2 - 2\sigma_{TR}^2 - \theta_{PBE} \max\{\sigma_0^2, \sigma_{TR}^2\}.$$

Hence, PBE between test formulations h and g can be claimed if $\hat{\lambda}_{h,g} < 0$, where $\hat{\lambda}_{h,g}$ is an approximate 95% upper confidence bound for $\lambda_{h,g}$. Using the method in §5.5, an approximate 95% upper confidence bound for $\lambda_{h,g}$ when $\sigma_{TR}^2 \geq \sigma_0^2$ is

$$\hat{\lambda}_{h,g} = (\hat{\delta}_h - \hat{\delta}_g)^2 + \hat{\sigma}_{TTh}^2 + \hat{\sigma}_{TTg}^2 - (2 + \theta_{PBE})\hat{\sigma}_{TR}^2 + z_{0.95}\sqrt{V},$$

where

$$V = \left(2(\hat{\delta}_h - \hat{\delta}_g), 1, 1, -(2 + \theta_{PBE})\right) D \left(2(\hat{\delta}_h - \hat{\delta}_g), 1, 1, -(2 + \theta_{PBE})\right)',$$

$\hat{\sigma}_{TR}^2$ is the combined estimator given by (10.5.1), and

$$D = \begin{pmatrix} \frac{\hat{\sigma}_{1,1,h}^2}{4}\left(\frac{1}{n_{1h}} + \frac{1}{n_{2h}}\right) + \frac{\hat{\sigma}_{1,1,g}^2}{4}\left(\frac{1}{n_{1g}} + \frac{1}{n_{2g}}\right) & (0,0,0) \\ (0,0,0)' & C_{h,g} \end{pmatrix},$$

and $C_{h,g}$ is an estimated variance-covariance matrix of $(\hat{\sigma}_{TTh}^2, \hat{\sigma}_{TTg}^2, \hat{\sigma}_{TR}^2)$. The elements of C, c_{ij}, can be obtained as follows. c_{11} is $(n_{1h} + n_{2h} - 2)^{-1}$ times the sample variance of $\{(y_{ijjh} - \bar{y}_{jjh})^2, j = 1, 2, i = 1, ..., n_{kh}\}$; c_{22} is $(n_{1g} + n_{2g} - 2)^{-1}$ times the sample variance of $\{(y_{ijjg} - \bar{y}_{jjg})^2, j = 1, 2, i = 1, ..., n_{kg}\}$; c_{33} is n_H^{-1} times the sample variance of $\{(y_{i21h} - \bar{y}_{21h})^2, (y_{i12h} - \bar{y}_{12h})^2, i = 1, ..., n_{kh}, h = 1, ..., H\}$; $c_{12} = c_{21} = 0$;

$$c_{13} = c_{31} = \frac{(n_{1h} - 1)c_{1,h}}{n_H(n_{1h} + n_{2h} - 2)} + \frac{(n_{2h} - 1)c_{2,h}}{n_H(n_{1h} + n_{2h} - 2)};$$

where $c_{t,h}$ is the off-diagonal element in C_t given by (5.5.2) but computed based on data in study h, $t = 1, 2$, $h = 1, ..., H$; and

$$c_{23} = c_{32} = \frac{(n_{1g} - 1)c_{1,g}}{n_H(n_{1g} + n_{2g} - 2)} + \frac{(n_{2g} - 1)c_{2,g}}{n_H(n_{1g} + n_{2g} - 2)}.$$

When $\sigma_{TR}^2 < \sigma_0^2$, the upper bound should be modified to

$$\hat{\lambda}_{h,g} = (\hat{\delta}_h - \hat{\delta}_g)^2 + \hat{\sigma}_{TTh}^2 + \hat{\sigma}_{TTg}^2 - 2\hat{\sigma}_{TR}^2 - \theta_{PBE}\sigma_0^2 + z_{0.95}\sqrt{V_0},$$

where

$$V_0 = \left(2(\hat{\delta}_h - \hat{\delta}_g), 1, 1, -2\right) D \left(2(\hat{\delta}_h - \hat{\delta}_g), 1, 1, -2\right)'.$$

The method discussed in the end of §5.6 can be applied to decide which bound should be used.

10.5.3   Meta-Analysis for IBE

For assessing IBE with the meta-analysis, we assume that the H independent data sets are obtained from a 2×4 crossover design as described in §5.2. Results for other designs, such as the 2×3 extra-reference design in §5.4, can be obtained similarly.

The assessment of IBE between a test formulation and the reference formulation with the meta-analysis is similar to that of PBE. By combining data from the H studies, we can obtain the following better estimator of the within-subject variance σ_{WR}^2:

$$\hat{\sigma}_{WR}^2 = \frac{1}{n_H} \sum_{h=1}^{H} (n_{1h} + n_{2h} - 2)\hat{\sigma}_{WRh}^2,$$

where $\hat{\sigma}_{WRh}^2$ is the $\hat{\sigma}_{WR}^2$ defined in §5.3.2 but is computed based on data from study h. The IBE test described in §5.3.2 can still be used with the quantities $n_1 + n_2 - 2$ and $\chi_{0.95;n_1+n_2-2}^2$ in (5.3.10) and (5.3.13) replaced by n_H and $\chi_{0.95;n_H}^2$, respectively.

The assessment of IBE between test formulations h and g, however, is more complicated. Similar to the case of PBE, we can define the IBE parameter as $\theta_{h,g}$ given by (10.5.2) but with y_{Th} and y_{Tg} from the same subject and y_R and y_R' from the same subject. Two test formulations are IBE when $\theta_{h,g} < \theta_{IBE}$, where θ_{IBE} is the IBE limit given by FDA (1999a). Under the assumed model,

$$\theta_{h,g} = \frac{(\delta_h - \delta_g)^2 + \sigma_{D,h,g}^2 + \sigma_{WTh}^2 + \sigma_{WTg}^2 - 2\sigma_{WR}^2}{\max\{\sigma_0^2, \sigma_{WR}^2\}},$$

where

$$\sigma_{D,h,g}^2 = \sigma_{BTh}^2 + \sigma_{BTg}^2 - 2\rho_{h,g}\sigma_{BTh}\sigma_{BTg}$$

and $\rho_{h,g}$ is the correlation coefficient between two observations from a single subject under test formulations h and g, respectively. Since each study has only one test formulation, it is not possible to estimate $\rho_{h,g}$ or $\sigma_{D,h,g}^2$ unless some assumptions are imposed. As an example, we assume that the random subject effects related to y_{Th}, y_{Tg} and y_R are respectively

$$S_{Th} = A + Z_{Th},$$

$$S_{Tg} = A + Z_{Tg},$$

and

$$S_R = A + Z_R,$$

where A, Z_{Th}, Z_{Tg}, and Z_R are independent random normal variables with means 0 and variances σ_A^2, σ_{ZTh}^2, σ_{ZTg}^2, and σ_{ZR}^2, respectively. Then

$$\sigma_{D,h,g}^2 = \text{Var}(S_{Th} - S_{Tg}) = \sigma_{ZTh}^2 + \sigma_{ZTg}^2$$

and

$$\sigma_{Dh}^2 + \sigma_{Dg}^2 = \text{Var}(S_{Th} - S_R) + \text{Var}(S_{Tg} - S_R)$$
$$= \sigma_{ZTh}^2 + \sigma_{ZTg}^2 + 2\sigma_{ZR}^2$$
$$= \sigma_{D,h,g}^2 + 2\sigma_{ZR}^2.$$

Let

$$\tilde{\theta}_{h,g} = \frac{(\delta_h - \delta_g)^2 + \sigma_{Dh}^2 + \sigma_{Dg}^2 + \sigma_{WTh}^2 + \sigma_{WTg}^2 - 2\sigma_{WR}^2}{\max\{\sigma_0^2, \sigma_{WR}^2\}},$$

which can be estimated using data from the H studies. Consider the hypotheses

$$H_0 : \tilde{\theta}_{h,g} \geq \theta_{IBE} \quad \text{and} \quad \tilde{\theta}_{h,g} < \theta_{IBE}. \tag{10.5.3}$$

If $\sigma_{ZR}^2 = 0$ (i.e., $Z_R \equiv 0$), then $\sigma_{D,h,g}^2 = \sigma_{Dh}^2 + \sigma_{Dg}^2$, $\theta_{h,g} = \tilde{\theta}_{h,g}$, and the IBE between test formulations h and g can be assessed by testing hypotheses (10.5.3). If $\sigma_{ZR}^2 > 0$, then $\sigma_{D,h,g}^2 < \sigma_{Dh}^2 + \sigma_{Dg}^2$, $\theta_{h,g} < \tilde{\theta}_{h,g}$, and testing hypotheses (10.5.3) provides a conservative approach for assessing the IBE between test formulations h and g, i.e., the hypothesis of $\tilde{\theta}_{h,g} < \theta_{IBE}$ implies that $\theta_{h,g} < \theta_{IBE}$.

It remains to construct an approximate 95% confidence bound for the parameter

$$\gamma_{h,g} = (\delta_h - \delta_g)^2 + \sigma_{Dh}^2 + \sigma_{Dg}^2 + \sigma_{WTh}^2 + \sigma_{WTg}^2 - 2\sigma_{WR}^2 - \max\{\sigma_0^2, \sigma_{WR}^2\}.$$

Applying the idea in §5.3.2, an approximate 95% upper confidence bound for $\gamma_{h,g}$ when $\sigma_{WR}^2 \geq \sigma_0^2$ is

$$(\hat{\delta}_h - \hat{\delta}_g)^2 + \hat{\sigma}_{0.5,0.5,h}^2 + \hat{\sigma}_{0.5,0.5,g}^2 + 0.5(\hat{\sigma}_{WTh}^2 + \hat{\sigma}_{WTg}^2) - (3 + \theta_{IBE})\hat{\sigma}_{WR}^2 + \sqrt{U},$$

where $\hat{\sigma}_{a,b,h}^2$ and $\hat{\sigma}_{WTh}^2$ are the same as those in §5.3.2 but are based on data from study h and U is the sum of the following six quantities:

$$\left[\left(|\hat{\delta}_h - \hat{\delta}_g| + z_{0.95} \sqrt{c_h \hat{\sigma}_{0.5,0.5,h}^2 + c_g \hat{\sigma}_{0.5,0.5,g}^2} \right)^2 - (\hat{\delta}_h - \hat{\delta}_g)^2 \right]^2,$$

$$\hat{\sigma}_{0.5,0.5,h}^4 \left(\frac{n_{1h} + n_{2h} - 2}{\chi_{0.05;n_{1h}+n_{2h}-2}^2} - 1 \right)^2,$$

$$\hat{\sigma}_{0.5,0.5,g}^4 \left(\frac{n_{1g} + n_{2g} - 2}{\chi_{0.05;n_{1g}+n_{2g}-2}^2} - 1 \right)^2,$$

$$0.5^2 \hat{\sigma}_{WTh}^4 \left(\frac{n_{1h} + n_{2h} - 2}{\chi_{0.05;n_{1h}+n_{2h}-2}^2} - 1 \right)^2,$$

$$0.5^2 \hat{\sigma}_{WTg}^4 \left(\frac{n_{1g} + n_{2g} - 2}{\chi_{0.05;n_{1g}+n_{2g}-2}^2} - 1 \right)^2,$$

and

$$(3 + \theta_{IBE})^2 \hat{\sigma}_{WR}^4 \left(\frac{n_H}{\chi_{0.95;n_H}^2} - 1 \right)^2, \qquad (10.5.4)$$

where $c_h = (n_{1h}^{-1} + n_{2h}^{-1})/4$ and $n_H = \sum_{h=1}^H (n_{1n} + n_{2h} - 2)$. When $\sigma_0^2 > \sigma_{WR}^2$, an approximate 95% upper confidence bound for $\gamma_{h,g}$ is

$$(\hat{\delta}_h - \hat{\delta}_g)^2 + \hat{\sigma}_{0.5,0.5,h}^2 + \hat{\sigma}_{0.5,0.5,g}^2 + 0.5(\hat{\sigma}_{WTh}^2 + \hat{\sigma}_{WTg}^2) - 3\hat{\sigma}_{WR}^2 + \theta_{IBE}\sigma_0^2 + \sqrt{U_0},$$

where U_0 is the same as U except that the factor $(3 + \theta_{IBE})^2$ in (10.5.4) should be replaced by 9. Again, the method discussed in the end of §5.3.2 can be applied to decide which bound should be used.

10.6   Discussion

In clinical research, a multicenter clinical trial is commonly employed because it expedites patient recruitment process within a desired time frame. The methods introduced in this chapter can be applied to multicenter clinical trials if centers in a multicenter clinical trial are treated as studies in a meta-analysis, in the investigation of drug effects and treatment-by-center (instead of treatment-by-study) interaction. However, in a multicenter clinical trial, all centers use the same the study protocol, inclusion/exclusion criteria, dosages and routes of administration, and trial procedure, and, consequently, the patient populations in different centers are likely to be more homogeneous than those in different studies of a meta-analysis. For example, v_h in §10.2-10.3 can be replaced by a pooled variance estimator v and the degrees of freedom m_h can be replaced by $\sum_h m_h$, which results in more efficient test procedures. Furthermore, when population variances are equal, there exist tests for qualitative treatment-by-center interaction with exact nominal sizes (Cheng, 2002).

In recent years, multinational multicenter trials have become very popular based on the implementation of international harmonization of regulatory requirements. Similarly, the methods introduced in this chapter can also be applied by treating a *country* as study in meta-analysis. In a multinational multicenter trial, each country may adopt a very similar but slightly different study protocol due to differences in culture and medical practice (Ho and Chow, 1998). In addition, patient populations in different countries may be ethnically different. Thus, patients in one country are more likely to be homogeneous for a meta-analysis.

Chapter 11

Quality of Life

In clinical trials, it has been a concern that the treatment of disease or survival may not be as important as the improvement of quality of life (QOL), especially for patients with chronic disease. Enhancement of life beyond absence of illness to enjoyment of life may be considered more important than the extension of life. The concept of QOL can be traced back to the mid-1920s. Peabody (1927) pointed out that the *clinical picture* of a patient is an impressionistic painting of the patient surrounded by his home, work, friend, joys, sorrows, hopes, and fears. In 1947, the World Health Organization (WHO) stated that health is a state of complete physical, mental, and social well-being and not merely the absence of disease or infirmity. In 1948, Karnofsky published *Performance Status Index* to assess the usefulness of chemotherapy for cancer patients. The New York Heart Association proposed a refined version of its functional classification to assess the effects of cardiovascular symptoms on performance of physical activities in 1964. In the past several decades, QOL has attracted much attention. Since 1970, several research groups have been actively working on the assessment of QOL in clinical trials. For example, Kaplan, Bush, and Berry (1976) developed the *Index of Well-Being* to provide a comprehensive measure of QOL; Torrance (1976, 1987) and Torrance and Feeny (1989) introduced the concept of utility theory to measure the health state preferences of individuals and quality-adjusted life year to summarize both quality of life and quantity of life; Bergner et al. (1981) developed the *Sickness Impact Profile* to study perceived health and sickness related QOL; Ware (1987) proposed a set of widely used scales for the Rand Health Insurance Experiment; and Williams (1987) studied the effects of QOL on hypertensive patients.

QOL not only provides information as to how the patients feel about drug therapies, but also appeals to the physician's desire for the best clinical practice. It can be used as a predictor of compliance of the patient. In addition, it may be used to distinguish between therapies that appear to be equally efficacious and equally safe at the stage of marketing strategy planning. The information can be potentially used in advertising for the promotion of the drug therapy.

QOL is usually assessed by a questionnaire, which may consists of a number of questions (items). We refer to such a questionnaire as a QOL instrument. A QOL instrument is a very subjective tool and is expected to have a large amount of variation. Thus, it is a concern whether the adopted QOL instrument can accurately and reliably quantify patients' QOL. In this chapter, we provide a comprehensive review of the validation of a QOL instrument, the use of QOL scores, statistical methods for assessment of QOL, and practical issues that commonly encountered in clinical trials.

In §11.1, we provide a brief definition of QOL and an introduction of some key performance characteristics such as validity and reliability that are commonly used for validation of a QOL instrument. Statistical indices for assessment of responsiveness and sensitivity of a validated QOL instrument are discussed in §11.2. In §11.3, the use of principal component analysis and factor analysis for grouping QOL items (subscales) to subscales (composite scores) are discussed. Statistical methods for assessment of QOL in clinical trials are given in §11.4. Also included in §11.4 is the analysis of parallel questionnaires. In §11.5, some statistical issues including multiplicity, sample size determination, calibration, and utility analysis are discussed.

11.1   Definition and Validation

11.1.1   Definition

It is recognized that there is no universal definition of QOL. Williams (1987) indicated that QOL may be defined as a collective term that encompasses multiple components of a person's social and medical status. Smith (1992), however, interpreted QOL as the way a person feels and how he or she functions in day-to-day activities. The definition of QOL may vary from one drug therapy to another and from one patient population to another. QOL may refer to a variety of physical and psychological factors. For example, for assessment of the effect of antihypertensive treatment on QOL, it is often of interest to quantitate patients' QOL in terms of the following indices: physical state, emotional state, performance of social roles, intellectual function and life satisfaction (Hollenberg, Testa, and Williams, 1991). For treatment of breast cancer, four aspects of the patients' QOL, namely mobility, side effects, pain, and psychological stress are usually considered (Zwinderman, 1990).

11.1.2   Validation

QOL is usually assessed by means of a number of questions that may be rated by patients, their spouses, or their physicians. In practice, it is expected that the responses will widely vary from patient to patient (or from rater to rater) and from time to time. Therefore, the validation of a given instrument is critical in order to have sound statistical inference for assessment of drug effects on a patient's QOL. Guilford (1954) discussed several methods such as Cronbach's α for measuring the reliability of internal consistency of QOL instruments. Guyatt et al. (1989) indicated that an instrument should be validated in terms of its reproducibility, validity, and responsiveness. However, there is no gold standard as to how an instrument should be validated. Hollenberg et al. (1991) discussed several methods of validation for an instrument, such as consensual validation, construct validity, and criterion-related validation. They also pointed out that these approaches to validations may be necessary, but not sufficient, because statistical validation of an effective instrument may involve more components such as precision and power. In this section, several performance characteristics that are commonly considered in validation of an instrument are described (Chow and Ki, 1996).

11.1.3   Validity

The validity of a QOL instrument is referred to as the extent to which the QOL instrument measures what is designed to measure. In other words, it is a measure of biasedness of the instrument. The biasedness of an instrument reflects the accuracy of the instrument.

In clinical trials, as indicated earlier, the QOL of a patient is usually quantified based on responses to a number of questions related to several components or domains of QOL. It is a concern that the questions may not be the right questions to assess the components or domains of QOL of interest. To address this concern, consider a specific component (or domain) of QOL that consists of k items (or subscales), i.e., x_i, $i = 1, ..., k$. Also, let y be the QOL component (or domain) of interest that is unobservable. Suppose that y can be quantified by x_i, $i = 1, ..., k$, i.e., there exists a function f such that

$$y = f(x_1, x_2, ..., x_k).$$

In practice, for convenience, the unknown function f is usually assumed to be the mean of x_i, i.e.,

$$f(x_1, x_2, ...x_k) = \frac{1}{k} \sum_{i=1}^{k} x_i.$$

Let $\mu_i = E(x_i)$ and $\mu = (\mu_1, \mu_2, ..., \mu_k)'$. If y is the average of x_i's, then

$$E(y) = \bar{\mu} = \frac{1}{k} \sum_{i=1}^{k} \mu_i$$

and it is desired to have the mean of x_i close to $\bar{\mu}$ As a result, we may claim that the QOL instrument is validated in terms of its validity if

$$|\mu_i - \bar{\mu}| < \delta, \quad i = 1, ..., k, \tag{11.1.1}$$

where δ is a given positive constant. To test the hypothesis H_1 in (11.1.1), we first consider the approach of confidence set (§8.2.1) that is based on a confidence set for

$$\mu_i - \bar{\mu} = a_i'\mu, \quad i = 1, ..., k,$$

where a_i is a k-vector whose ith component is $1 - k^{-1}$ and other components are $-k^{-1}$.

Suppose that the QOL questionnaire is administered to n patients. Let x_{ij} be the observed ith item (or subscale) from the jth patient, $X_j = (x_{1j}, ..., x_{kj})'$, $j = 1, ..., n$,

$$\hat{\mu} = \bar{X} = \frac{1}{n} \sum_{j=1}^{n} X_j,$$

and

$$S = \frac{1}{n-1} \sum_{j=1}^{n} (X_j - \bar{X})(X_j - \bar{X})'. \tag{11.1.2}$$

Assume that X_j's are independent and normally distributed with mean μ and covariance matrix Σ.

There are two ways to apply the confidence set approach. First, a level $1 - \alpha$ confidence rectangular for $\mu_i - \bar{\mu}$, $i = 1, ..., k$, is given by

$$[\zeta_{i-}, \zeta_{i+}], \quad i = 1, ..., k,$$

where

$$\zeta_{i\pm} = a_i'\hat{\mu} \pm \sqrt{\frac{k(n-1)}{n(n-k)} a_i' S a_i F_{1-\alpha;k,n-k}},$$

and $F_{1-\alpha;k,n-k}$ is the $(1-\alpha)$th quantile of the F-distribution with k and $n-k$ degrees of freedom. Second, we may consider Bonferroni's $1 - \alpha$ level simultaneous confidence intervals

$$[\xi_{i-}, \xi_{i+}], \quad i = 1, ..., k,$$

where

$$\xi_{i\pm} = a_i'\hat{\mu} \pm t_{1-\alpha/(2k);n-1}\sqrt{\frac{a_i'Sa_i}{n}}$$

and $t_{1-\alpha;n-1}$ is the $(1-\alpha)$th quantile of the t-distribution with $n-1$ degrees of freedom.

If the hypothesis in (11.1.1) is considered to be the null hypothesis and

$$|\mu_i - \bar{\mu}| \geq \delta \quad \text{for at least one } i \tag{11.1.3}$$

is taken as the alternative hypothesis, then we reject the null hypothesis and conclude that the QOL instrument is not validated at significance level α if and only if the intersection of the region defined by (11.1.1) and the confidence set for $a_i'\mu$, $i = 1, ..., k$, is empty.

If the hypothesis in (11.1.1) is considered as the alternative hypothesis to the null hypothesis given by (11.1.3), then the null hypothesis is rejected (i.e., the QOL instrument is considered validated) at the α level of significance if and only if all confidence intervals for $a_i'\mu$, $i = 1, ..., k$, are within the interval $(-\delta, \delta)$.

When the hypothesis in (11.1.3) is considered to be the null hypothesis, we may also apply the approach of two one-sided tests. For each fixed i, a size α test based on the two one-sided tests approach rejects the hypothesis that $|a_i'\mu| > \delta$ if and only if (η_{i-}, η_{i+}) is within $(-\delta, \delta)$, where

$$\eta_{i\pm} = a_i'\hat{\mu} \pm t_{1-\alpha;n-1}\sqrt{\frac{a_i'Sa_i}{n}}.$$

Then, using the approach of intersection-union, a size α test rejects the null hypothesis (11.1.3) and concludes that the QOL instrument is validated if and only if (η_{i-}, η_{i+}) is within $(-\delta, \delta)$ for all i.

11.1.4 Reliability

The reliability of a QOL instrument measures the variability of the instrument, which directly relates to the precision of the instrument. Therefore, the items are considered reliable if the variance of $y = f(x_1, ..., x_k)$ is small. To verify the reliability, we consider the following null hypothesis:

$$H_0 : \text{Var}(y) < \Delta \tag{11.1.4}$$

for some fixed Δ.

When $x_{1j}, ..., x_{kj}$, $j = 1, ..., n$, are observed, the variance of y can be estimated by

$$s_y^2 = \frac{1}{n-1}\sum_{j=1}^{n}(y_j - \bar{y})^2,$$

where $y_j = f(x_{1j}, ..., x_{kj})$ and $\bar{y}$ is the average of y_j's. If y_j's are normally distributed, then a $(1 - \alpha)$ lower confidence bound for $\text{Var}(y)$ is

$$\xi(y) = \frac{(n-1)s_y^2}{\chi_{1-\alpha;n-1}^2},$$

where $\chi_{1-\alpha;n-1}^2$ is the $(1-\alpha)$th quantile of the chi-square distribution with $n-1$ degrees of freedom. A test for reliability rejects the null hypothesis (11.1.4) if and only if $\xi(y) > \Delta$.

Since the items $x_1, x_2, ..., x_k$ are relevant to a QOL component (or domain), they are expected to be correlated. In classical validation, a group of items with high intercorrelations between items are considered to be internally consistent. The Cronbach's α defined below is often used to measure the intercorrelation (or internal consistency) between items:

$$\alpha_C = \frac{k}{k-1}\left(1 - \frac{\sum_{i=1}^k \sigma_i^2}{\sum_{i=1}^k \sigma_i^2 + 2\sum_{i<j}\sigma_{ij}}\right),$$

where σ_i^2 is the variance of x_i and σ_{ij} is the covariance between x_i and x_j. When the covariance between items is high compared to the variance of each item, the Cronbach's α is large. To ensure that the items are measuring the same component of QOL, the items under the component should be positively correlated, i.e., $\alpha_C \geq 50\%$. However, if the intercorrelations between items are too high, i.e., α_C is close to 1, it suggests that some of the items are redundant. When y is the average of x_i's, the variance of y,

$$\text{Var}(y) = \frac{1}{[k-(k-1)\alpha_C]k}\sum_{i=1}^k \sigma_i^2,$$

increases with α_C for fixed k and σ_i^2, $i = 1, ..., k$. By including redundant items we cannot improve the precision of the result. It is desired to have independent items reflect QOL component (or domain) at different perspective. However, in that case, it is hard to validate whether the items are measuring the same targeted component of QOL. Therefore, we suggest using items with moderate α_C between 50% and 80%.

11.1.5   Reproducibility

Reproducibility is defined as the extent to which repeat administrations of the same QOL instrument yield the same result, assuming no underlying changes have occurred. The assessment of reproducibility involves expected and/or unexpected variabilities that might occur in the assessment of QOL. It includes intertime point and inter-rater reproducibility. For the assessment of reproducibility, the technique of test-retest is often employed. The same QOL instrument is administered to patients who have reached stable conditions at two different time points. These two time points are generally separated by a sufficient length of time that is long enough to wear off the memory of the previous evaluation but not long enough to allow any change in environment. The Pearson's product moment correlation coefficient, ρ, of the two repeated results is then studied. In practice, a test-retest correlation of 80% or higher is considered acceptable. To verify this, the sample correlation between test and retest, denoted by r, is usually calculated from a sample of n patients. The following hypotheses are then tested:

$$H_0 : \rho \geq \rho_0 \quad \text{versus} \quad H_1 : \rho < \rho_0,$$

where ρ_0 is a given constant. When the sample size is large,

$$z(r) = \frac{1}{2} \ln \left(\frac{1+r}{1-r} \right)$$

is approximately normally distributed with mean $z(\rho)$ and variance $\frac{1}{n-3}$. The null hypothesis is rejected at an approximate significance level α if and only if

$$\sqrt{n-3}[z(r) - z(\rho_0)] < z_{1-\alpha},$$

where $z_{1-\alpha}$ is the $(1-\alpha)$th quantile of the standard normal distribution.

Note that a shift in means of the score at test-retest may be detected by using a simple paired t-test. The inter-rater reproducibility can be verified by the same method.

11.2 Responsiveness and Sensitivity

The responsiveness of a QOL instrument is usually referred to as the ability of the instrument to detect a difference of clinical significance within a treatment. The sensitivity is a measure of the ability of the instrument to detect a clinically significant difference between treatments. A validated QOL instrument should be able to detect a difference if there is indeed a difference and should not wrongly detect a difference if there is no difference. Chow and Ki (1994) proposed precision and power indices to assess the responsiveness and sensitivity of a QOL instrument when comparing the effect of drug on QOL between treatments under a time series model. The precision index measures the probability of not detecting a false difference and the power index reflects the probability of detecting a meaningful difference.

Suppose that a homogeneous group is divided into two independent groups A and B that are known to have the same QOL. A *good* QOL

instrument should have a small chance of *wrongly* detecting a difference.
Let

$$(y_{i1}, y_{i2}, ..., y_{ik})$$

and

$$(u_{j1}, u_{j2}, ..., u_{jk})$$

be the average scores observed on the ith subject in group A and jth subject
in group B at different time points over a fixed time period, respectively,
$i = 1, ..., n$, $j = 1, ..., m$. The objective is to compare mean average scores
between groups to determine whether the instrument reflects the expected
result statistically. Thus, the null hypothesis of interest is

$$H_0 : \mu_y = \mu_u \quad \text{versus} \quad H_1 : \mu_y \neq \mu_w, \tag{11.2.1}$$

where μ_y and μ_w are the mean average scores for groups A and B, respectively. Under the null hypothesis, the following statistic

$$z = \frac{\bar{y}_{..} - \bar{u}_{..}}{\sqrt{n^{-1}s_y^2 + m^{-1}s_u^2}}$$

is approximately distributed as a standard normal distribution when n and
m are both large, where $\bar{y}_{..}$ and s_y^2 are, respectively, the sample mean and
variance based on y_{ij}'s and $\bar{u}_{..}$ and s_u^2 are respectively the sample mean
and variance based on u_{ij}'s. Therefore, we reject the null hypothesis at an
approximate significance level α if and only if

$$|z| > z_{1-\alpha/2}.$$

The precision index, denoted by P_d, of an instrument is defined as the
probability of the interval estimator not detecting a difference when there
is no difference between groups, i.e.,

$$P_d = P\left(|\bar{y}_{..} - \bar{u}_{..}| \leq d | \mu_y = \mu_u\right),$$

which is approximately equal to $\Phi(d/\tau) - \Phi(-d/\tau)$, where Φ is the standard
normal distribution function and

$$\tau^2 = \text{Var}(\bar{y}_{..}) + \text{Var}(\bar{u}_{..}).$$

It can be seen that the precision index of an instrument is $(1 - \alpha)$ at
$d = z_{1-\alpha/2}\tau$ and increases as d increases. The precision index is related to a test of responsiveness (hypotheses in (11.2.1)) by using a fixed
d, i.e., a test rejecting H_0 in (11.2.1) if and only if $|\bar{y}_{..} - \bar{u}_{..}| < d$. If
$d = z_{1-\alpha/2}\sqrt{n^{-1}s_y^2 + m^{-1}s_u^2}$, then this procedure is exactly the same as

the previously discussed test. Although a large d leads to a high probability to capture the true difference between μ_y and μ_u, it has a too large probability of concluding a difference when $\mu_y = \mu_u$.

If the QOL instrument is administered to two groups of subjects who are known to have different QOL, then the QOL instrument should be able to correctly detect such a difference with a high probability. The power index of an instrument for detecting a meaningful difference, denoted by $\delta_d(\varepsilon)$, is defined as the probability of detecting a meaningful difference ε. That is,

$$\delta_d(\varepsilon) = P\left(|\bar{y}_{..} - \bar{u}_{..}| > d \,\big|\, |\mu_y - \mu_u| = \varepsilon\right).$$

When $d = z_{1-\alpha/2}\sqrt{n^{-1}s_y^2 + m^{-1}s_u^2}$, $\delta_d(\varepsilon)$ is the power of the previously discussed test. Note that for a fixed ε, $\delta_d(\varepsilon)$ decreases as d increases. We consider an instrument to be responsive in detecting a difference if both P_d and $\delta_d(\varepsilon)$ are above some reasonable limits for a given ε.

Note that the above precision index and power index for assessment of responsiveness and sensitivity of a QOL instrument were derived based on the total score across all subscales of each patient. In practice, some of these subscales may be positively correlated. Since two correlated subscales may contain the same information regarding QOL, they should not carry the same weights as other subscales in the total score approach. In this case, it is suggested a composite score be considered (see next section). In addition, the precision index and power index were derived for detecting a difference. Chow and Ki (1994) generalized the concept for detecting an equivalence in QOL between groups, which are useful in noninferiority/equivalence clinical trials.

11.3 QOL Scores

QOL is typically assessed by a QOL instrument, which consists of a number of questions (or items). To collect information on various aspects of QOL, a QOL instrument with a large number of questions/items is found necessary and helpful. For a simple analysis and an easy interpretation, these questions/items are usually grouped to form subscales, composite scores, or overall QOL. The items (or subscales) in each subscale (or composite score) are correlated. As a result, the structure of responses to a QOL instrument is multidimensional, complex and correlated. In addition, the following questions are of particular concern when subscales and/or composite scores are to be analyzed for the assessment of QOL.

1. How many subscales or composite scores should be formed?

2. Which items (subscales) should be grouped in each subscale (composite score)?

3. What are the appropriate weights for obtaining subscales (composite scores)?

These questions are important because the components and/or domains of QOL may vary from drug therapy to drug therapy. For example, for the assessment of the effect of antihypertensive treatment on QOL, it may be of interest to quantify the patient's QOL in terms of the following QOL components: physical state, emotional state, performance of social roles, intellectual function, and life satisfaction (Hollenberg, Testa, and Williams, 1991). For treatment of breast cancer, four aspects of QOL, namely, mobility, side effects, pain, and psychological stress are usually considered (Zwinderman, 1990). Olschewski and Schumacher (1990) proposed to use the standardized scoring coefficients from factor analysis as a criterion for selecting subscales for grouping of composite scores. The idea is to drop those subscales with small coefficients. This method of grouping is attractive because it is a selection procedure based on data-oriented weights. However, this method suffers the drawbacks that (i) the factorization of the correlation matrix is not unique, (ii) the standardization scoring coefficients used in combining subscales vary across different rotations of the factor system, (iii) each composite score is a linear combination of all the subscales (unless some subscales with small coefficients are dropped), and (iv) the resulting composite score does not have optimal properties. To overcome these drawbacks, Ki and Chow (1995) proposed an objective method for grouping subscales. The idea is to apply principal component analysis and factor analysis to determine (i) an appropriate number of composite scores, (ii) the subscales to be grouped in each composite score, and (iii) optimal weights for forming a composite score within each group. The method of grouping by Ki and Chow (1995) is outlined in the subsequent sections.

11.3.1 Number of Composite Scores

Suppose that there are p subscales, denoted by $X = (x_1, x_2, ..., x_p)'$, which are obtained by grouping a number of items (questions) from a QOL instrument. Assume that the subscales are in compatible scale. The x_i's follow a multivariate distribution with mean vector μ and covariance matrix Σ. The covariance matrix Σ can be estimated by the sample covariance matrix S defined in (11.1.2). The observed covariance matrix S contains not only information about the variation of the subscales but also the correlations among the subscales. Principal component analysis can be used to decompose the covariance of the subscales into uncorrelated (orthogonal) components which are a few linear combinations of the original subscales.

The solutions δ_i to the characteristic equation

$$|S - \delta_i I_p| = 0, \quad \delta_1 \geq \delta_2 \geq ... \geq \delta_p,$$

where $|M|$ denotes the determinant of a matrix M and I_p is the identity matrix of order p. The eigenvector $a_1 = (a_{11}, ..., a_{1p})'$ corresponding to the largest characteristic root δ_1 determines the first principal component given by

$$a_1' X = a_{11} x_1 + a_{12} x_2 + \cdots + a_{1p} x_p.$$

The sample variation explained by $a_1' X$ is then given by

$$\frac{\delta_1}{\text{trace}(S)}.$$

The first principal component is the linear combination of subscales such that its sample variance is maximum. In other words, the first principal component explains the majority of the total variation. The weights for combining subscales are uniquely determined under the constraint that the sum of the squares of weights equals unity. The other principal components are also linear combinations of subscales that explain progressively smaller portions of the total sample variation. Based on this idea, the first k ($k < p$) principal components (or k composite scores) are selected such that the k principal components can retain a predetermined desired portion $\Delta\%$ (say $\Delta = 80$) of the total variation. In this case, the p subscales can be replaced by the k principal components without losing much information. As a result, the original n measurements in a p-dimensional system are reduced to n measurements in a k-dimensional system. For example, if one single composite score (i.e., overall quality of life) is desired for making an overall conclusion, the first principal component, which retains maximum variation among all linear combinations of sunscales, can be used.

11.3.2 Subscales to Be Grouped in Each Composite Score

The ideal composite scores should not only retain most of the information of the data, but also reveal the underlying common factors which contribute to the correlations among the subscales. Therefore, it is useful to group highly correlated subscales to form a composite score that represents a single underlying factor. The results based on the composite score would then be more meaningful. The correlation structure among all the subscales can be assessed by factor analysis. In a factor analysis model, each subscale variate, x_i, can be expressed as in terms of a linear function of unobservable common factor variates, w_j, $j = 1, ..., k$, and a latent specific variate ϵ_i,

$i = 1, ..., p$, i.e.,

$$x_i = \lambda_{i1} w_1 + \lambda_{i2} w_2 + \cdots + \lambda_{ik} w_k + \epsilon_i, \quad i = 1, ..., p.$$

Let $X = (x_1, ..., x_p)'$, $W = (w_1, ..., w_k)'$, and $\epsilon = (\epsilon_1, ..., \epsilon_p)'$. Then

$$X = \Lambda W + \epsilon,$$

where

$$\Lambda = \begin{pmatrix} \lambda_{11} & \cdots & \lambda_{1k} \\ \cdots & \cdots & \cdots \\ \lambda_{p1} & \cdots & \lambda_{pk} \end{pmatrix}.$$

In the above model, it is assumed that the k common factor variates w_j's are independent with zero mean and unit variance and ϵ_i's are independently distributed with mean 0 and variances ϕ_i, that is,

$$\text{Var}(x_i) = \sigma_i^2 = \lambda_{i1}^2 + \lambda_{i2}^2 + \cdots + \lambda_{ik}^2 + \phi_i$$

and

$$\text{Cov}(x_i, x_j) = \sigma_{ij} = \lambda_{i1}\lambda_{j1} + \cdots + \lambda_{ik}\lambda_{jk}.$$

The covariance matrix of the subscales can be decomposed as

$$\Sigma = \Lambda'\Lambda + \Psi,$$

where Ψ is a diagonal matrix whose ith diagonal element is ϕ_i. The covariance between X and W is given by

$$\text{Cov}(X, Y') = E[(\Lambda W + \epsilon)W'] = \Lambda.$$

The common factors generate the correlations among the p subscales and the specific terms contribute the variances of the subscales. The goal is to find k uncorrelated common factors, which can explain all the correlation between subscale variates. The observed correlation matrix is decomposed and the coefficients (loadings) λ_{ij} of the factors for each subscales are estimated such that the sample partial correlations of the subscales controlling for the common factors should be as small as possible. The estimates of Λ and Ψ, denoted respectively by $\hat{\Lambda}$ and $\hat{\Psi}$, satisfy

$$\hat{\Lambda}(\hat{\Lambda}'\hat{\Psi}^{-1}\hat{\Lambda}) = S\hat{\Psi}^{-1}\hat{\Lambda} - \hat{\Lambda},$$

which can be solved numerically.

Usually the pattern of the loadings of the common factors is not easy to interpret. It is difficult to partition the subscales into distinct groups and identify them by the common factors to which they are highly correlated. The rotation of the factor space or rotation of the loadings is necessary to achieve a simple structure. Suppose that R is a $k \times k$ orthogonal matrix for rotation of the factors. The loadings of the rotated factors will be

$$\Gamma = \Lambda R$$

with γ_{ij} (the (i,j)th element of Γ) denoting the loading of the ith subscale on the jth rotated factor, where $i = 1, ..., p$ and $j = 1, ..., k$. The rotated factor system preserves the uncorrelation of the factors and the portion of variance x_i contributed by the k common factors, i.e.,

$$\sum_{j=1}^{k} \gamma_{ij}^2 = \sum_{j=1}^{k} \lambda_{ij}^2.$$

A simple factor structure should contain many large and zero loadings with minimal intermediate values. Kaiser (1958, 1959) proposed to maximize the variances of the squared loadings within each column of the factor matrix. The following varimax criterion for rotation was maximized

$$\nu = \frac{1}{p^2} \sum_{j=1}^{k} \left\{ p \sum_{i=1}^{p} z_{ij}^4 - \left(\sum_{i=1}^{p} z_{ij}^2 \right)^2 \right\},$$

where

$$z_{ij} = \frac{\gamma_{ij}}{\left(\sum_{j=1}^{k} \lambda_{ij}^2 \right)^{1/2}}, \quad i = 1, ..., p, \ j = 1, ..., k.$$

As a result, a few subscales, which have high loadings to a certain factor and low loadings to other factors, can be grouped together to form a composite score. The subscales within a composite score are highly correlated among themselves but have relatively small correlations with subscales in a different composite score.

11.3.3 Optimal Weights of Subscales

To determine the weights for combining subscales, Olschewski and Schumacher (1990) considered predicting the unobservable common factor by linear regression. Each factor score was predicted by a linear combination of all the subscales, and the weights were determined by the standardized scoring coefficients from regression. For simplicity, they ignored small coefficients in the linear combinations. A simplified expression for each factor, however, can only be obtained at the expense of losing some valuable information. In addition, since the factorization of the correlation matrix is not unique, the coefficients were not uniquely determined. As a result, it may be difficult to interpret the common factors when subscales participate in the estimation of more than one common factor. To overcome this drawback, Ki and Chow (1995) proposed to consider factor analysis to determine which subscales should be grouped and principal component analysis to determine the optimal weights for grouping. The first principal component of the subscales gives the optimal weights for grouping the subscales because it is the linear combination of the subscales that retained the most information from the subscales.

11.3.4 An Example

To illustrate the method of grouping described above, consider the study published by Testa et al. (1993). A QOL instrument was administered to 341 hypertensive patients before drug therapy. The instrument consists of 11 subscales as displayed in Table 11.3.1. Table 11.3.2 lists the three composite scores, which are established by psychologists and health experts, used in Testa et al. (1993). The sample covariance matrix and the correlation matrix of these 11 subscales are given in Tables 11.3.3 and 11.3.4,

Table 11.3.1. QOL Subscales

Subscale	QOL component	Number of items
1	GHS: General health status	3
2	VIT: Vitality	4
3	SLP: Sleep	4
4	EMO: Emotional ties	2
5	GPA: General positive affect	12
6	LIF: Life satisfaction	1
7	ANX: Anxiety	11
8	BEC: Behavioral/emotional control	3
9	DEP: Depression	10
10	SEX: Sexual functioning	5
11	WRK: Work well-being	11

Table 11.3.2. QOL Composite Scores

Composite Score	QOL dimension	Subscales
I	Psychological distress	7, 8, 9
II	General perceived health	1, 2, 3
III	Psychological well-being	4, 5, 6

Table 11.3.3. Covariance Matrix of the 11 QOL Subscales

Subscale	GHS	VIT	SLP	EMO	GPA	LIF	ANX	BEC	DEP	SEX	WRK
GHS	7133										
VIT	3790	6272									
SLP	3338	5205	8667								
EMO	2744	3736	3503	13333							
GPA	2801	4299	4169	6340	6566						
LIF	2201	2843	2415	3976	3672	5025					
ANX	2865	3615	3972	3828	4360	2418	5698				
BEC	1877	2397	2544	3334	3140	1931	3032	2608			
DEP	2767	3558	3551	4512	4370	2755	4198	2931	5031		
SEX	1364	2063	1231	1208	1148	1046	675	664	1190	23379	
WRK	2727	3777	3469	2949	3530	2592	2751	2006	2949	966	3875

Note: Only the lower triangular portion of the symmetric covariance matrix is given.

Table 11.3.4. Correlation Matrix of the 11 QOL Subscales

Subscale	GHS	VIT	SLP	EMO	GPA	LIF	ANX	BEC	DEP	SEX	WRK
GHS	1.00										
VIT	0.57	1.00									
SLP	0.42	0.71	1.00								
EMO	0.28	0.41	0.33	1.00							
GPA	0.41	0.67	0.55	0.68	1.00						
LIF	0.37	0.51	0.37	0.49	0.64	1.00					
ANX	0.45	0.60	0.57	0.44	0.71	0.45	1.00				
BEC	0.44	0.59	0.54	0.57	0.76	0.53	0.79	1.00			
DEP	0.46	0.63	0.54	0.55	0.76	0.55	0.78	0.81	1.00		
SEX	0.11	0.17	0.09	0.07	0.09	0.10	0.06	0.09	0.11	1.00	
WRK	0.52	0.77	0.60	0.41	0.70	0.59	0.59	0.63	0.67	0.10	1.00

Note: Only the lower triangular portion of the symmetric correlation matrix is given.

respectively. It is desirable to combine some subscales for simple analysis and easy interpretation. An overall QOL score combining the information of all subscales may be used to give a general summary of the results.

A principal component analysis was performed on the data. The coefficient of the principal components and the percentage of variation explained by each principal component are given in Table 11.3.5. It can be seen from Table 11.3.5 that three components could retain 80% of the total variation of the data. Most variation of the data could be captured by a three-dimensional space without much loss of information. If a one-dimensional summary score were used, the first principal component would give optimal weights for combining the subscales. The weights were close to the usual uniform weights. Thus, for simplicity, a simple average of the subscales might be used to summarize the information. Since principal component analysis suggested that the variation of the data could be appropriately explained by a three-dimensional space, a factor analysis model with three common factors is an appropriate statistical model for explaining the correlation matrix given in Table 11.3.4. All subscales are highly correlated with one another except for sexual functioning. The initial factor pattern and the partial correlation matrix controlling for the three common factors are summarized in Tables 11.3.6 and 11.3.7, respectively. The partial correlations between subscales controlling for the factors were very small, which indicated that three common factors could reasonably explain the correlations among the subscales. The initial factor loadings pattern in Table 11.3.6, however, were hard to interpret. All subscales except for Sexual Functioning (SEX) had heavy positive loadings on Factor 1 and a mix of positive and negative loadings for Factors 2 and 3. The loadings of all three common factors for SEX were very small. This is because the correlation between SEX and other subscales was low. Therefore, a rotation was necessary to produce a more easily understood factor pattern. The resulting factor pattern of an orthogonal varimax rotation is given in Table 11.3.8. The rotated factor patterns in Table 11.3.8 suggested that subscales Anxiety (ANX), Behavior/Emotional Control (BEC), and Depression (DEP) could be grouped together as a composite score named by Psychological Distress (PSD), the subscales Vitality (VIT), Work Well-Being (WRK), Sleep (SLP), and General Health Status (GHS) could be grouped together as a composite score named *General Perceived Health* (GPH), and the subscales Emotional Ties (EMO), General Positive Affect (GPA), and Life Satisfaction (LIF) could be grouped together as a composite score named Psychological Well-Being (PWB). Each subscale is grouped under the factor with which it has highest correlation. The subscale SEX, however, could be left as a single scale since it was not highly related to any factor.

Principal component analysis was performed on each group of subscales to determine the optimal weights for forming a composite score that can

Table 11.3.5. Principal Component Analysis on the 11 QOL Subscales

Total variance = 87587			
Principal component	Characteristic root	Proportion of variance explained	Cumulative proportion
1st	38558.2	0.440227	0.44023
2nd	22565.1	0.257630	0.69786
3rd	9064.0	0.103486	0.80134
4th	4590.8	0.052414	0.85376
5th	3954.2	0.045146	0.89890
6th	3181.3	0.036321	0.93522
7th	1913.5	0.021847	0.95707
8th	1178.9	0.013460	0.97053
9th	1134.5	0.012953	0.98348
10th	873.4	0.009972	0.99340
11th	537.1	0.006544	1.00000

Principal components: Coefficients for subscales					
	1st	2nd	3rd	4th	5th	6th
GHS	0.25996	-0.03631	0.31279	0.84650	-0.18158	-0.19230
VIT	0.32983	-0.03474	0.27734	-0.01468	-0.14728	0.22043
SLP	0.33798	-0.07828	0.41711	-0.47110	-0.55254	-0.00640
EMO	0.42090	-0.13232	-0.77033	0.07316	-0.39986	-0.10252
GPA	0.36113	-0.10014	-0.10921	-0.12033	0.22475	0.08725
LIF	0.24391	-0.05301	-0.07368	0.11839	0.30156	0.71953
ANX	0.29847	-0.09421	0.11942	-0.13877	0.40476	-0.46870
BEC	0.21121	-0.05872	-0.00691	-0.05977	0.21437	-0.17334
DEP	0.30210	-0.07183	0.01679	-0.06002	0.34750	-0.23264
SEX	0.23526	0.96977	-0.04375	-0.02314	0.01162	-0.02318
WRK	0.24906	-0.05537	0.15759	0.02174	0.08961	0.27232
	7th	8th	9th	10th	11th	
GHS	0.15898	-0.13396	0.04983	-0.03212	-0.00471	
VIT	-0.61165	0.25169	-0.46728	-0.27997	0.09167	
SLP	0.40113	-0.04580	0.12528	-0.00353	-0.02241	
EMO	-0.01775	0.14152	-0.04860	0.10925	-0.03928	
GPA	-0.16541	-0.82285	0.07980	-0.24557	-0.06259	
LIF	0.50087	0.15519	-0.18376	-0.02822	-0.00856	
ANX	0.14658	0.02992	-0.50937	0.38946	-0.22693	
BEC	0.06324	0.06815	0.11647	0.03354	0.92141	
DEP	-0.00208	0.43009	0.48014	-0.48225	-0.27701	
SEX	0.02122	-0.01407	0.00656	0.01944	-0.00297	
WRK	-0.36773	0.06857	0.46624	0.67957	-0.09115	

Table 11.3.6. Initial Factor Pattern

	Factor pattern loadings		
	Factor 1	Factor 2	Factor 3
GPA	0.88	-0.20	0.14
DEP	0.86	-0.15	-0.14
BEC	0.85	-0.21	-0.17
VIT	0.81	0.36	0.06
WRK	0.81	0.22	0.12
ANX	0.81	-0.09	-0.31
SLP	0.68	0.29	-0.09
LIF	0.65	-0.09	0.26
EMO	0.62	-0.32	0.21
GHS	0.57	0.24	0.00
SEX	0.13	0.09	0.07

Table 11.3.7. Partial Correlations Between Subscales Controlling
for the Three Factors

Subscale	GHS	VIT	SLP	EMO	GPA	LIF	ANX	BEC	DEP	SEX	WRK
GHS	1.00										
VIT	0.06	1.00									
SLP	-0.05	0.18	1.00								
EMO	0.02	0.03	0.03	1.00							
GPA	-0.13	0.08	0.07	0.15	1.00						
LIF	0.03	-0.04	-0.07	0.00	0.04	1.00					
ANX	0.03	-0.01	0.03	-0.07	0.11	-0.02	1.00				
BEC	0.01	-0.07	0.00	0.04	-0.04	0.01	0.11	1.00			
DEP	0.03	-0.03	-0.07	0.00	-0.06	0.02	0.10	0.09	1.00		
SEX	0.01	0.07	-0.03	0.00	-0.03	0.00	-0.03	0.02	0.05	1.00	
WRK	0.01	0.07	-0.03	-0.12	0.06	0.12	-0.06	0.03	0.07	-0.06	1.00

Note: Only the lower triangular portion of the symmetric correlation matrix is given.

Table 11.3.8. Results of Varimax Rotation on the Factor Loadings

	Orthogonal transformation matrix		
	1	2	3
1	0.61335	0.56976	0.54697
2	-0.16670	0.77032	-0.61548
3	-0.77202	0.28632	0.56746
	Rotated factor pattern loadings		
	Factor 1	Factor 2	Factor 3
ANX	0.76A	0.30	0.32
BEC	0.69A	0.28	0.50
DEP	0.67A	0.33	0.48
VIT	0.39	0.76B	0.26
WRK	0.37	0.67B	0.38
SLP	0.44	0.58B	0.15
GHS	0.31	0.50B	0.17
SEX	0.01	0.16	0.06
GPA	0.47	0.39	0.68C
EMO	0.27	0.16	0.66C
LIF	0.22	0.38	0.56C

The subscales can be grouped into three subgroups
as indicated by A, B, and C

retain as much information (sample variation) as possible. The results of principal component analysis are summarized in Table 11.3.9. The weights for grouping subscales in the first principal component were standardized such that the sum of weights equals unity and the composite scores were given by

$$PSD = 0.39 \text{ ANX} + 0.25 \text{ BEC} + 0.36 \text{ DEP}$$
$$GPH = 0.27 \text{ VIT} + 0.19 \text{ WRK} + 0.30 \text{ SLP} + 0.23 \text{ GHS}$$
$$PWB = 0.48 \text{ EMO} + 0.31 \text{ GPA} + 0.21 \text{ LIF}.$$

These three composite scores explained 76% of the total variation of the 10 subscales (excluding SEX). The results based on the analysis of these composite scores provide an easy interpretation compared to that from the analysis of the original subscales. These composite scores are similar to those used in Testa et al. (1993). The above analysis provided an objective justification of the use of composite scores, which were developed by psychologists, in the study population.

Table 11.3.9. Principal Component Analysis

I. On the subscales under psychological distress Total variance = 13337			
Principal component	Characteristic root	Proportion of variance explained	Cumulative proportion
1st	11561.2	0.86685	0.86685
2nd	1166.9	0.08749	0.95434
3rd	608.9	0.04566	1.00000
Principal components: Coefficients for subscales			
	1st	2nd	3rd
ANX	0.66190	-0.72185	-0.20203
BEC	0.42605	0.14053	0.89372
DEP	0.61674	0.67763	-0.40059

II. On the subscales under general perceived health Total variance = 25947				
Principal component	Characteristic root	Proportion of variance explained	Cumulative proportion	
1st	18064.8	0.69622	0.69622	
2nd	4493.0	0.17316	0.86936	
3rd	2308.0	0.08895	0.95833	
4th	1081.2	0.04167	1.00000	
Principal components: Coefficients for subscales				
	1st	2nd	3rd	4th
VIT	0.53385	-0.06452	0.52359	-0.66083
WRK	0.37739	-0.00091	0.55280	0.74296
SLP	0.59914	-0.57247	-0.54996	0.10416
GHS	0.46217	0.81739	-0.34323	0.02161

III. On the subscales under psychological well-being Total variance = 24924			
Principal component	Characteristic root	Proportion of variance explained	Cumulative proportion
1st	19135.9	0.76777	0.76777
2nd	3936.5	0.15794	0.92571
3rd	1851.6	0.07429	1.00000
Principal components: Coefficients for subscales			
	1st	2nd	3rd
EMO	0.78983	-0.57895	0.20245
GPA	0.50151	0.41964	-0.75657
LIF	0.35306	0.69909	0.62179

11.4   Statistical Methods

For the assessment of QOL, statistical analysis based on subscales, composite scores, and/or overall score are often performed for an easy interpretation. For example, Tandon (1990) applied a global statistic to combine the results of the univariate analysis of each subscale. Olschewski and Schumacher (1990), on the other hand, proposed to use composite scores to reduce the dimensions of QOL. However, due to the complex correlation structure among subscales, optimal statistical properties may not be obtained. As an alternative, to account for the correlation structure, the following time series model proposed by Chow and Ki (1994) may be useful.

11.4.1   Time Series Model

For a given subscale (or component), let x_{ijt} be the response of the jth subject to the ith question (item) at time t, where $i = 1, ..., k$, $j = 1, ..., n$, and $t = 1, ...T$. Consider the average score over k questions:

$$Y_{jt} = \bar{x}_{jt} = \frac{1}{k} \sum_{j=1}^{k} x_{ijt}.$$

Since the average scores $y_{j1}, y_{j2}, ..., y_{jT}$ are correlated, the following autoregressive time series model may be an appropriate statistical model for y_{jt}.

$$y_{jt} = \mu + \psi(y_{j(t-1)} - \mu) + e_{jt}, \quad j = 1, ..., n, \ t = 1, ..., T,$$

where μ is the overall mean, $|\psi| < 1$ is the autoregressive parameter, and e_{jt} are independent identically distributed random errors with mean 0 and variance σ_e^2. It can be verified that

$$E(e_{jt}, y'_{jt}) = 0 \quad \text{for all } t' < t.$$

The autoregressive parameter ψ can be used to assess the correlation of consecutive responses y_{jt} and $y_{j(t+1)}$. From the above model, it can be shown that the autocorrelation of responses with m lag times is ψ^m, which is negligible when m is large. Based on the observed average scores on the jth subject, $y_{j1}, y_{j2}, ..., y_{jT}$, we can estimate the overall mean μ and the autoregressive parameter ψ. The ordinary least-square estimators of μ and ψ can be approximated by

$$\hat{\mu}_j = \bar{y}_{j.} = \frac{1}{T} \sum_{t=1}^{T} y_{jt}$$

and

$$\hat{\psi}_j = \frac{\sum_{t=2}^{T}(y_{jt} - \bar{y}_{j.})(y_{j(t-1)} - \bar{y}_{j.})}{\sum_{t=2}^{T}(y_{jt} - \bar{y}_{j.})^2},$$

which are the sample mean and sample autocorrelation of consecutive observations. Under the above model, it can be verified that $\hat{\mu}_j$ is unbiased and that the variance of $\hat{\mu}_j$ is given by

$$\text{Var}(\bar{y}_{j.}) = \frac{\gamma_{j0}}{T}\left(1 + 2\sum_{t=1}^{T-1}\frac{T-t}{T}\psi^t\right),$$

where $\gamma_{j0} = \text{Var}(y_{jt})$. The estimated variance of $\hat{\mu}_j$ can be obtained by replacing ψ by $\hat{\psi}_j$ and γ_{j0} by

$$c_{j0} = \sum_{t=1}^{T}\frac{(y_{jt} - \bar{y}_{j.})^2}{T-1}.$$

Suppose that the n subjects are from the same population with the same variability and autocorrelation. The QOL measurements of these subjects can be used to estimate the mean average scores μ. An intuitive estimator of μ is the sample mean

$$\hat{\mu} = \bar{y}_{..} = \frac{1}{n}\sum_{j=1}^{n}\bar{y}_{j..}$$

Under the time series model, the estimated variance of $\hat{\mu}$ is given by

$$s^2(\bar{y}_{..}) = \frac{c_0}{nT}\left(1 + 2\sum_{t=1}^{T-1}\frac{T-t}{T}\hat{\psi}^t\right),$$

where

$$c_0 = \frac{1}{n(T-1)}\sum_{j=1}^{n}\left[\sum_{t=1}^{T}(y_{jt} - \bar{y}_{j.})^2\right]$$

and

$$\hat{\psi} = \frac{1}{n}\sum_{j=1}^{n}\hat{\psi}_j.$$

An approximate $(1-\alpha)100\%$ confidence interval for μ can then be obtained as follows:

$$\bar{y}_{..} \pm z_{1-\alpha/2}s(\bar{y}_{..}),$$

where $z_{1-\alpha/2}$ is the $(1-\alpha/2)$th quantile of a standard normal distribution.

Under the time series model, the method of confidence interval approach described above can be used to assess difference in QOL between treatments. Note that the assumption that all the QOL measurements over time are independent is a special case of the above model with $\psi = 0$. In practice, it is suggested that the above time series model be used to account for the possible positive correlation between measurements over the time period under study.

11.4.2   Parallel Questionnaire

Jachuck et al. (1982) indicated that QOL may be assessed in parallel by patients, their relatives, and physicians. The variability of the patient's rating is expected to be larger than those of the relatives' ratings and physicians' ratings. Although QOL scores can be analyzed separately based on individual ratings, they may lead to different conclusions. In that case, determining which rating should be used to assess the treatment effect on QOL is a concern. The question of interest is: "Should the individual ratings carry the same weights in the assessment of QOL?" If the patient's rating is considered to be more reliable than others, it should carry more weight in the assessment of QOL; otherwise, it should carry less weight in the analysis. Ki and Chow (1994) proposed a score function that combines the ratings with difference weights to account for different variabilities among these ratings. They developed a score function for the ratings between patients and their spouses (or significant others). The idea can be extended to the case where there are multiple parallel ratings. Ki and Chow (1994) considered the following weighted score function

$$z = ax + by,$$

where x and y denote the ratings of a patient and his/her spouse or significant other, respectively, and a and b are the corresponding weights assigned to x and y. When $a = 1$ and $b = 0$, the score function reduces to the patient's rating. On the other hand, when $a = 0$ and $b = 1$, the score function represents the spouse's rating. When $a = b = \frac{1}{2}$, the score function is the average of the two ratings. That is, the patient's rating and his/her spouse's rating are considered equally important. The choice of a and b determines the relative importance of the ratings in the assessment of QOL. Ki and Chow (1994) considered performing principal component analysis (as described in the previous section) to determine a and b based on the observed data, which are given by

$$a = \left[1 + \frac{(\lambda_1 - s_x^2)^2}{r^2 s_x^2 s_y^2}\right]^{-1/2}$$

and

$$b = \frac{(\lambda_1 - s_x^2)a}{r s_x s_y},$$

where s_x^2 and s_y^2 are sample variances of the patients' and spouses' ratings, respectively, r is the sample correlation coefficient between the two ratings, and

$$\lambda_1 = \left[s_x^2 + s_y^2 + \sqrt{(s_x^2 + s_y^2)^2 - 4 s_x^2 s_y^2 (1 - r^2)}\right]/2.$$

QOL assessment can then be performed based on z-scores following statistical methods described in §11.4.1.

11.5   Statistical Issues

11.5.1   Multiplicity

For assessment of QOL in many clinical trials, multiple comparisons based
on either subscales or composite scores are usually performed. In the interest of controlling the overall type I error rate at the α level, an adjustment
to the significance level of each individual comparison is necessary. In practice, however, it may be too conservative and not practical to adjust the α
level when there are too many subscales or composite scores or there are
too many comparisons to be made. As a rule of thumb, Biswas, Chan, and
Ghosh (2000) suggested that a multiplicity adjustment to the significance
level be made when at least one significant result (e.g., one of several QOL
components or domains or one of several pairwise comparisons) is required
to draw conclusion. On the other hand, a multiplicity adjustment is not
needed when (i) all results are required to be significant in order to draw
conclusion or (ii) the testing problem is closed. A test procedure is said to
be *closed* if the rejection region of a particular univariate null hypothesis at
a given significance α level implies the rejection of all higher dimensional
null hypotheses containing the univariate null hypothesis at the same significance α level (Marcus, Peritz, and Gabriel, 1976). When a multiplicity
adjustment is required, it is recommended that either the method of Bonferroni or the procedures described in Hochberg and Tamhone (1987) be
used.

11.5.2   Sample Size Determination

Under the time series model, Chow and Ki (1996) derived some useful
formulas for determination of sample size based on normal approximation.
For a fixed precision index $1 - \alpha$, to ensure a reasonable high power index δ
for detecting a meaningful difference ϵ, the sample size per treatment group
should not be less than

$$n_\delta = \frac{c[z_{1-1/2\alpha} + z_\delta]^2}{\epsilon^2} \quad \text{for } \delta > 0.5,$$

where

$$c = \frac{\gamma_y}{T}\left(1 + 2\sum_{t=1}^{T-1}\frac{T-t}{T}\psi_y^t\right) + \frac{\gamma_u}{T}\left(1 + 2\sum_{t=1}^{T-1}\frac{T-t}{T}\psi_u^t\right).$$

For a fixed precision index $1 - \alpha$, if the acceptable limit for detecting an
equivalence between two treatment means is $(-\Delta, \Delta)$, to ensure a reasonable high power ϕ for detecting an equivalence when the true difference in

treatment means is less than a small constant η, the sample size for each treatment group should be at least

$$n_\phi = \frac{c}{(\Delta - \eta)^2} [z_{1/2+1/2\phi} + z_{1-1/2\alpha}]^2.$$

If both treatment groups are assumed to have same variability and auto-correlation coefficient, the constant c can be simplified as

$$c = \frac{2\gamma}{T} \left(1 + 2 \sum_{t=1}^{T-1} \frac{T-t}{T} \psi^t \right).$$

When $n = max(n_\phi, n_\delta)$, it ensures that the QOL instrument will have precision index $1 - \alpha$ and power of no less than δ and ϕ in detecting a difference and an equivalence, respectively. It, however, should be noted that the required sample size is proportional to the variability of the average scores considered. The higher the variability, the larger the sample size that would be required. Note that the above formulas can also be applied to many clinical based research studies with time-correlated outcome measurements, e.g., 24-hour monitoring of blood pressure, heart rates, hormone levels, and body temperature.

To illustrate the use of the above sample size formulas, consider QOL assessment in two independent groups A and B. Suppose a QOL instrument containing 11 questions is to be administered to subjects at week 4, 8, 12, and 16. Denote the mean of QOL score of the subjects in group A and B by y_{it} and u_{jt}, respectively. We assume that y_{it} and u_{jt} have distributions that follow the time series model described in the previous section with common variance $\gamma = 0.5$ sq. unit and have moderate autocorrelation between scores at consecutive time points, say $\psi = 0.5$. For a fixed 95% precision index, 87 subjects per group will provide a 90% power for detection of a difference of 0.25 unit in means. If the chosen acceptable limits are $(-0.35, 0.35)$, then 108 subjects per group will have a power of 90% that the 95% confidence interval of difference in group means will correctly detect an equivalence with $\eta = 0.1$ unit. If sample size is chosen to be 108 per group, it ensures that the power indices for detecting a difference of 0.25 unit or an equivalence are not less than 90%.

11.5.3 Calibration with Life Event

In QOL assessment, an issue of particular interest is the interpretation of an identified significant change in QOL score. To provide a better interpretation, Testa, et al. (1993) considered the calibration of change in QOL against change in life events. A linear calibration curve was used to predict the relationship between the change in QOL score and change in life event index (only negative life events were considered) although the study was not designed for the calibration purpose and the changes in life events were collected as auxiliary information. The difficulty is that the effect of change of life event was confounded with the effect of medication. Since the impact of life events is subjective and varies from person to person, it is difficult to assign numerical scores/indices to life events. In addition, the relationship between QOL score and life event may not be linear. More complicated calibration functions or transformations may be required. In practice, we may expect that the QOL score has positive correlation with life event score. However, the correlation may not be strong enough to give a precise calibration curve. Besides, the calibration of the QOL score with the life event score, changes in the QOL score may be related to changes in disease status. Thus, if we wish to interpret the impact of change in QOL score by means of life events, further research in the design and analysis method for calibration is necessary.

11.5.4   Utility Analysis

Feeny and Torrance (1989) proposed a utility approach to measure the health-related QOL. Utility is a single summary score of the preference of an individual for a health state. The preference of health state is usually measured by some standard techniques, such as rating scale, standard gamble, and time tradeoff. A rating scale consists of a line with the least preferred state (e.g., death with score equals 0) on one end and the most preferred state (perfect health with score equals 1) on the other end. An individual will rate the disease state on the line between these two extreme states based on his/her experience of the disease or understanding of the hypothetical description of the disease. For the standard gamble technique, an individual is given the choice of remaining at the disease state for an additional t years or the alternative, which consists of perfect health for an additional t years with probability p and immediate death with probability $(1 - p)$. The probability p is varied until the individual is indifferent between the two alternatives. Then, the utility (or preference) of that disease state is p. For the method of time tradeoff, an individual is offered two alternatives: (i) at the disease state with life expectancy of t years, or (ii) in perfect health for x years. Then x is varied until the individual is indifferent between the two alternatives. The utility of the disease is then given by x/t. Although these methods are easy to understand, the utility values obtained from these values are expected to have high variability. As a result, it is strongly recommended that the utility values be validated for test and retest reproducibility before they are used to measure any change in health state.

Chapter 12

Medical Imaging

In recent years, the development of medical imaging agents has become increasingly important. Medical imaging agents can help not only make a diagnosis, but also alter patient management. In addition, medical imaging agents help ascertain the severity of a condition. In many cases, medical imaging agents are useful in determining the prognosis of an illness. Medical imaging agents are often used with many imaging modalities, and imaging data can be acquired, reconstructed, processed, stored, and displayed in numerous ways. Although medical imaging agents are generally governed by the same regulations as other drugs or biological products, FDA requires special considerations in clinical trials designed to establish or support the efficacy of a medical imaging agent. These special considerations include subject selection, imaging condition and image evaluation including appropriate blinded imaging evaluation procedures, the use of truth standards, comparison between groups, and appropriate statistical methods.

In the next section, we give a brief introduction to medical imaging drugs and agents. Also included in this section is regulatory requirement and statistical analysis for developing medical imaging drugs. Section 12.2 provides an overview of the receiver operating characteristic (ROC) analysis for evaluation of the performance of diagnostic medical products. Some basic design considerations and the analysis of reader agreement for blinded-reader studies are given in §12.3. Section 12.4 provides an overview of statistical methods for evaluating diagnostic accuracy without gold standard. Sample size calculation based on power for either reader to detect superiority is given in the last section.

12.1   Medical Imaging Drugs

Medical imaging drug products are drugs used with medical imaging methods such as radiography, computed tomography (CT), ultrasonography (US), magnetic resonance imaging (MRI), and radionuclide imaging to provide information on anatomy, physiology, and pathology. The term *image* can be used for films, likenesses, or other renderings of the body, body parts, organ systems, body functions, or tissues. For example, an image of the heart obtained with a diagnostic radiopharmaceutical or ultrasound contrast agent may in some cases refer to a set of images acquired from different views of the heart. Similarly, an image obtained with an MRI contrast agent may refer to a set of images acquired with different pulse sequences and interpluse delay times. In other words, medical imaging uses advanced technology to *see* the structure and function of the living body. Images are usually created from computerized acquisition of digital signals. The intention of a medical imaging drug is twofold. First, it is to delineate nonanatomic structures such as tumors or abscesses. Second, it is to detect disease or pathology within an anatomic structure. Therefore, the indications for medical imaging drugs may fall within the following general categories: (i) structure delineation (normal or abnormal), (ii) functional, physiological, or biochemical assessment, (iii) disease or pathology detection or assessment, and (iv) diagnostic or therapeutic patient management. Note that these categories need not be mutually exclusive.

The medical imaging drugs can be classified into the following two general categories.

12.1.1   Contrast Agents

Contrast agents are used to improve the visualization of tissues, organs, and physiologic processes by increasing the relative difference of imaging signal intensities in adjacent parts of the body. Contrast agents provide additional information in combination with an imaging device beyond the device alone. In other words, imaging with the contrast agent can add value when compared to imaging without the contrast agent. The most commonly used contrast agents that are in combination with medical imaging devices are summarized below:

Modality	Contrast Drug Products
X-ray and CT	Iodine agents (photon scattering)
MRI	Gadolinium, dysprosium, helium
Ultrasound	Liposomes, microbubbles
Suspensions nuclear	Tc-99m, TI-201, indium, samarium

12.1.2 Diagnostic Radiopharmaceuticals

Radiopharmaceuticals are used for a wide variety of diagnostic, monitoring, and therapeutic purposes. A diagnostic radiopharmaceutical is defined as either (i) an article that is intended for use in the diagnosis or monitoring of a disease or a manifestation of a disease in humans and that exhibits spontaneous disintegration of unstable nuclei with the emission of nuclear particles or photons, or (ii) any nonradioactive reagent kit or nuclide generator that is intended to be used in the preparation of such as article (FDA, 2000b). The FDA interprets this definition to include articles that exhibit spontaneous disintegration leading to the reconstruction of unstable nuclei and the subsequent emission of nuclear particles or photons. Diagnostic radiopharmaceuticals are radioactive drugs that contain a radioactive nuclide that may be linked to a ligand and carrier. These products are used in planar imaging, single photon emission computed tomography (SPECT), positron emission tomography (PET), or with other radiation detection probes.

As indicated in the 2000 FDA guidance on developing medical imaging drugs, diagnostic radiopharmaceuticals used for imaging typically have two distinct components, namely a radionuclide component and a nonradioactive component (FDA, 2000b). A radionuclide component can be detected through an *in vivo* testing such as technetium-99m, iodine-123, and indium-111. The radionuclide is a typical radioactive molecule with a relatively short half-life that emits radioactive decay photons having sufficient energy to penetrate the tissue mass of the patient. As a result, these photons can be detected with imaging devices. On the other hand, a nonradioactive component usually delivers the molecule to specific areas within the body. This nonradionuclidic portion of the diagnostic radiopharmaceutical often is an organic molecule such as a carbohydrate, lipid, nucleic acid, peptide, small protein, or antibody. The purpose of the nonradioactive component is to direct the radionuclide to a specific body location or process.

12.1.3 Regulatory Requirements

As indicated in the 2000 FDA guidance on developing medical imaging drugs, regulatory submission, review, and approval processes are generally governed by the same regulations as other drugs or biological products (medical imaging agents) such as investigational new drug applications (INDs), new drug applications (NDAs), biologics license applications (BLAs), abbreviated NDAs (ANDAs), and supplements to NDAs or BLAs. Since the techniques for evaluation of the performance of medical imaging drugs are very different from therapeutic pharmaceuticals and non-diagnostic devices, the FDA requires that specific considerations in the clinical evaluation of efficacy be followed to ensure that the information provided is valid and reliable. These specific considerations for evaluation of efficacy include the selection of subjects, appropriate blinding procedures, choices of appropriate endpoints, and use of suitable truth standards (or gold standards) and reference tests.

For selection of subjects, subjects should be representative of the population in which the medical imaging agent is intended to be used. In some cases, however, the 2000 FDA guidance indicates that subject selection for indications of structure delineation or functional, physiological, or biochemical assessment may be based on representative diseases that involve similar alterations in structure, function, physiology, or biochemistry if it appears that the results can be extrapolated to other unstudied disease states based on a known common process. To support the subsequent clinical use of the medical imaging agent, the FDA suggests the pretest odds and pretest probabilities of disease should be estimated for all subjects after enrollment but before any trial results are made available.

The FDA requires that blinded image evaluations by multiple independent readers be performed in the principal efficacy studies of diagnostic radiopharmaceuticals or contrast agents. The purpose of blinded image evaluation is to provide useful clinical information about its proposed indications for use. Appropriate blinding procedures can not only reduce possible confounding influences or biases but also increase the reliability of image evaluation. As indicated in the 2000 FDA guidance, readers should not have any knowledge of (i) treatment identity, (ii) the results of evaluation with the truth standard, the final diagnosis, or patient outcome, and (iii) any patient-specific information (e.g., history, physical examination, laboratory results, and results of other imaging studies) during a fully blinded image evaluation. In some cases, it is also suggested that general inclusion and exclusion criteria for patient enrollment, other details of the protocol, or anatomic orientation to the images should not be provided to the readers either.

As indicated in the 2000 FDA guidance, the primary endpoints in clinical trials designed to establish or support the efficacy of a medical imaging agent should be directly related to such clinically meaningful items, such as image interpretation, objective image features, subjective image assessments, and clinical outcomes. An image interpretation is the explanation or meaning that is attributed to objective image feature. In practice, image interpretations are usually supported by objective quantitative or qualitative information derived from the images. Image interpretations often have clinical implications and hence it is suggested that such interpretations be incorporated into the primary endpoint in clinical trials designed to establish or support the efficacy of a medical imaging agent. When the clinical implications of particular objective image features are apparent, the objective imaging features should also be incorporated in the primary endpoint. Subjective image assessments are assessments that are perceptible only to the reader, which are not visually perceptible and cannot be detected with instrumentation. The FDA guidance suggests that subjective image assessments, if included as endpoints in clinical trials intended to demonstrate or support efficacy of a medical imaging agent, should be linked to objective image features so that the objective basis for such assessments can be understood. In clinical trials, it is well recognized that clinical outcomes are among the most direct ways to measure clinical benefit. Accordingly, clinical outcomes can serve as primary endpoints in trials of medical imaging agents.

A truth standard (or gold standard) is defined as an independent method of measuring the same variable being measured by the investigational medical imaging agent that is known to give the true value of the measurement. Truth standards are used to demonstrate that the results obtained with the medical imaging agent are valid and reliable. For this purpose, the FDA suggests that the following general principles should be incorporated prospectively into the design, conduct, and analysis of the major efficacy trials for medical imaging agents. First, the true state of the subjects (e.g., diseased or nondiseased) should be determined with a truth standard without knowledge of the test results obtained with the medical imaging agent. On the other hand, test results obtained with the medical imaging agent should be evaluated without knowledge of the results obtained with the truth standard and without knowledge of outcome. In addition, truth standards should not include as a component any test results obtained with the medical imaging agent. Similarly, the truth standard for contrast agents should not incorporate the results of the unenhanced image obtained with the device alone. Finally, it is suggested that evaluation with the truth standard should be planned for all enrolled subjects and the decision to evaluate a subject with the truth standard should not be affected by the test results with the medical imaging under study.

12.1.4 Statistical Analysis

LaFrance (1999) pointed out that there are different considerations for designs of medical imaging studies. As indicated in the 2000 FDA guidance, since most of the imaging trials are designed to provide dichotomous or ordered categorical outcomes, the statistical tests for proportions and rates are commonly used, and the methods based on ranks are often applied to ordinal data (Fleiss, 1981; Woolson, 1987). The analyses based on odds ratios and the Mantel-Haenszel procedures are useful for data analysis. In addition, the use of model-based techniques, such as logistic regression models for binomial data, proportional odds models for ordinal data, and log-linear models for normal outcome variables are usually applied.

For evaluation of the performance of medical imaging drugs, the accuracy (or validity) is of common concern. The diagnostic validity can be assessed in many ways. For example, the pre- and postimages can be compared to the gold standard, and the sensitivity and specificity of the preimage compared to the postimage. Similarly, the same approaches can be used for two different active agents. The common methods used to test for differences in diagnosis are the McNemar test and Stuart-Maxwell test. The confidence intervals for sensitivity and specificity, and other measures can be also provided in the analysis. In addition, receiver operating characteristic (ROC) analysis is useful in assessing the diagnostic performance of medical imaging agents over a range of threshold values. Examples of products from which ROC analysis has been involved in FDA submission in Center for Devices and Radiological Health (CDRH) include ultrasound for breast cancer detection, ultrasound for bone mineral density to identify women prone to bone fracture, screening device for cervical cancer, mammography, and all sorts of clinical chemistry and other *in vitro* testing.

12.2   ROC Analysis

12.2.1   The ROC Curve

The receiver operating characteristics (ROC) curve is a graphical representation of pairs of values for true positive rate (TPR) and the corresponding false positive rate (FPR) for a diagnostic test. Each pair is established by classifying the test result as positive when the test outcome equals or exceeds the value set by a given threshold, and negative when the test outcome is less than this threshold value. For example, if a five-point ordinal scale is used to rate the likelihood of malignancy for a tumor (e.g., definitely benign, probably benign, equivocal, probably malignant, definitely malignant), setting the threshold at equivocal will classify tumors as malignant (i.e., a positive test result) when the test outcome is at this level or higher and will classify tumors as nonmalignant (i.e., a negative test result) when the test outcome is less than this level. To generate an ROC curve, the sensitivity and specificity of the diagnostic test are calculated and graphed for several thresholds (e.g., all values of the rating scale). In a typical ROC curve, values for TPR (or sensitivity) are plotted on the vertical axis, and the corresponding values for FPR (one minus specificity) are plotted on the horizontal axis.

In recent years, the receiver operating characteristic (ROC) analysis has become increasing important for evaluation of diagnostic performance. Not only because it is recommended in the 2000 FDA guidance, but also its advantage over more traditional measures of diagnostic performance (Metz 1986; Campbell, 1999). In the use of most diagnostic tests, test data do not necessarily fall into one of two obviously defined categories. Imaging studies usually require some confidence threshold be established in the mind of the decision maker. For example, if an image suggests the possibility of disease, how strong must the suspicion be in order for the image to be called positive? Therefore, the decision maker chooses between positive and negative diagnosis by comparing his/her confidence concerning with an arbitrary confidence threshold. Figure 12.2.1 is an example of the model that underlies ROC analysis. The bell-shaped curves represent the probability density distributions of a decision maker's confidence in a positive diagnosis that arises from actually positive patients and actually negative patients.

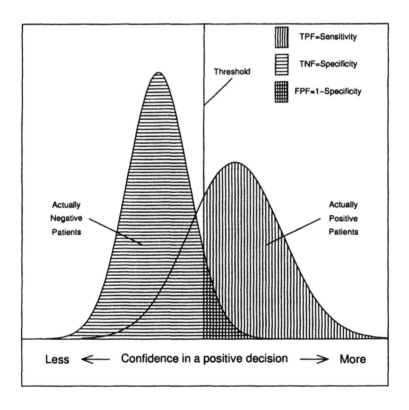

Figure 12.2.1. Model of ROC Analysis

The true negative fraction (TNF) is represented by the area to the left of the threshold under the curve for actually negative patients. Similarly, the true positive fraction (TPF) is represented by the area to the right of the threshold under the curve for actually positive patients. These imply that the sensitivity and specificity vary inversely as the confidence threshold is changed. In other words, TPF and FPF will increase or decrease together as the confidence threshold is changed. If we change the decision threshold several times, we will obtain several different pairs of TPF and FPF. These pairs can be plotted as points on a graph, such as that in Figure 12.2.2. We may conclude that better performance is indicated by an ROC curve that is higher to the left in the ROC space.

A practical technique for generating response data that can be used to plot a ROC curve is called the rating method. This method requires the

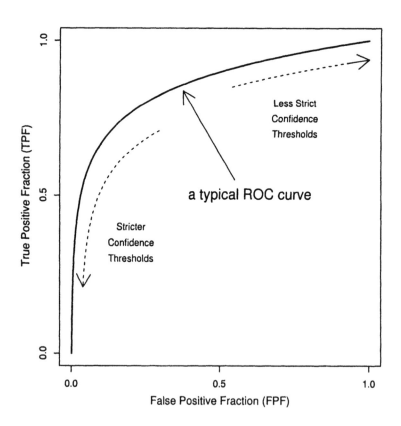

Figure 12.2.2. Typical ROC Curve

decision maker select a value from a continuous scale, such as

1 Definitely negative
2 Probably negative
3 Questionable
4 Probably positive
5 Definitely positive

An ROC plot has the following advantages. First, it displays all the information in terms of specificity and sensitivity at all cutoff points. It is a graphical way of displaying the complete performance of the device. Second, it allows the sponsors or the agency to consider for future reference other cutoffs than the one originally proposed. Third, one might use a different cutoff for different patients. Finally, it can facilitate better decision making. One could take a very different action close to some threshold than far away. The ROC plot helps one to see the performance at every threshold. It should be noted that the ROC plot does not depend on the prevalence of the disease.

However, ROC curves also suffer some drawbacks, including the determination of thresholds and numbers of subjects, which are usually not displayed on the graph. In addition, the appropriate software is not widely available. The ROC curve provides more information than just a single sensitivity and specificity pair to describe the accuracy of a diagnostic test. The curve depicts sensitivity and specificity levels over the entire range of decision thresholds. However, it would be helpful if the performance of a diagnostic test could be assessed by a single number.

One such measurement that can be derived from the ROC curve is the area under the curve (AUC). If a diagnostic test that discriminates almost perfect, then its ROC curve passes near the upper left corner. This makes an AUC approaching 1. On the other hand, if the curve of a test that discriminates almost randomly, then the curve would lie near the 45-degree diagonal line. This would turn an AUC close to 0.5. The AUC range is between 0.5 and 1. The AUC is calculated by summing the area of the trapezoids formed between the graph and the horizontal axis. This nonparametric method of calculation makes no assumptions regarding the underlying distributions of the diseased and nondiseased status. The meaning of AUC has been proved mathematically to be the probability that a random pair of positive/diseased and negative/nondiseased individuals would be identified correctly by the diagnostic test (Green and Swets, 1966). Also, it had been shown that the statistical properties of the Mann-Whitney-Wilcoxon statistics could be used to predict the statistical properties of AUC (Hanley and McNeil, 1982). For comparing corrected ROC curves, DeLong and DeLong (1988) suggested a nonparametric approach for comparing the AUCs. For the parametric approach, Swets and Pickett (1982) proposed a more exact method using the maximum likelihood estimation to estimate the AUC and its standard error. A comparison of nonparametric and binomial parametric areas has been made by Center and Schwartz (1985).

Receiver Operating Characteristic (ROC) analysis is very useful in the evaluation of medical devices and can be extremely useful in evaluating imaging drugs. In a diagnostic test, a commonly employed procedure is to diagnose *disease* if the test result z is greater than a threshold or cutoff value z_0, i.e., $z > z_0$, and *normal* otherwise. In practice, it matters how the gold standard is defined. In particular, the diagnostic test that is being evaluated cannot be part of the definition. In addition, it can be permissible to sample differentially from the normals and the disease population. The choice of what constitutes the normal population should mirror the way in which the test is to be utilized.

12.2.2 Characteristics of the ROC Curve

For evaluation of a medical device for diagnosing a specific disease, the outcomes are usually summarized in the following 2×2 contingency table.

	Present$(D+)$	Absent$(D-)$	Total
Positive$(T+)$	true positive $= a$	false positive $= b$	$a+b$
Negative$(T-)$	false negative $= c$	true negative $= d$	$c+d$
Total	$a+c$	$b+d$	$a+b+c+d$

The above 2×2 contingency table indicate that a (d) subjects are tested positive (negative) when in fact the disease is present (absent), while c (d) subjects are diagnosed negative (positive) when in fact the disease is present (absent). The sensitivity or the true positive rate (TPR) of the diagnostic test is given by

$$\text{Sensitivity} = \text{TPR}$$
$$= P(T+ \mid D+)$$
$$= \frac{a}{a+c}.$$

On the other hand, the specificity or one minus false positive rate (FPR) of the diagnostic test is

$$\text{specificity} = 1 - \text{FPR}$$
$$= 1 - P(T+ \mid D-)$$
$$= \frac{d}{b+d}.$$

The ROC plot can be obtained by plotting the (FPR,TPR) for all possible threshold values and connected with horizontal and vertical lines. Accuracy of the diagnostic test is defined as the proportion of cases, considering both positive and negative test results, for which the test results are correct (i.e., concordant with the truth standard or gold standard), which is given by

$$\text{Accuracy} = \frac{\text{true positive} + \text{true negative}}{\text{total}}$$

$$= \frac{a+d}{a+b+c+d}.$$

Likelihood ratio is a measure that can be interpreted as either (i) the relative odds of a diagnosis (e.g., being diseases or nondiseased) for a given test result, or (ii) the relative probabilities (i.e., relative risk or risk ratio) of a given test result in subjects with and without the disease. For tests with dichotomous results, the likelihood ratio of a positive test result can be expressed as

$$LR(+) = \frac{\text{Sensitivity}}{1 - \text{Specificity}}$$

$$= \frac{\text{TPR}}{\text{FPR}}$$

$$= \frac{a/b}{(a+c)/(b+d)}.$$

Similarly, the likelihood ratio of a negative test result is given by

$$LR(-) = \frac{1 - \text{Sensitivity}}{\text{Specificity}}$$

$$= \frac{\text{FNR}}{\text{TNR}}$$

$$= \frac{c/d}{(a+c)/(b+d)}.$$

The positive predictive value is defined as the probability that a subject has disease given that the test result is positive, while the negative predictive value is referred to as the probability that a subject doe not have the disease given that the test result is negative. Hence, the positive predictive value and the negative predictive value are given by

$$\text{Positive predicitive value} = \frac{a}{a+b}$$

and

$$\text{Negative predicitive value} = \frac{d}{c+d},$$

respectively. Note that the positive predictive value and the negative predictive value can also be expressed as the function of pretest probability of disease (p), sensitivity, and specificity as follows:

$$\text{Positive predicitive value} = \frac{(1-p)(\text{specificity})}{p(\text{sensitivity}) + (1-p)(1-\text{specificity})},$$

and

$$\text{Negative predicitive value} = \frac{p(\text{sensitivity})}{(1-p)(\text{specificity}) + p(1-\text{sensitivity})},$$

where pretest probability of disease in a subject before doing a diagnostic test can be obtained as

$$p = \frac{a+c}{a+b+c+d}.$$

Note that the pretest odds of disease in a subject can be obtained as $P(D+)/P(D-) = (a+c)/(b+d)$. Similarly, the post-test probability of disease is the probability of disease in a subject after the diagnostic test results are known. For subjects with a positive test result, the post-test probability of disease is then given by $P(D+|T+) = a/(a+b)$, while for subjects with a negative test result, the post-test probability of disease is $P(D+|T-) = c/(c+d)$. Consequently, the post-test odds of disease for subjects with a positive (negative) test result is given by a/b (c/d).

Note that ROC analysis can also be used to compare the performance of two tests or imaging systems that are on different scales. It facilitates the comparison of two tests even if each has a preselected cutoff and it can be more powerful for testing overall differences. It can be utilized to compare the performance of two or more readers because it minimizes the overcall/undercall difficulty since each reader can be operating on a (slightly) different scale.

12.2.3 Comparison of ROC Curves

For comparing different modalities, assume that there are N normal and N diseased subjects. The images from these subjects are processed under I modalities. Each of the resulting I sets of $2N$ images is rated independently K times by each of the J readers on an M-point scale. The M categories are determined by $M-1$ boundaries $K_1, K_2, ..., K_{M-1}$ which are fixed but unknown. Assume that the responses on a diseased subject, x_D's, follow a normal distribution with mean μ_D and variance σ_D^2, i.e., $N(\mu_D, \sigma_D^2)$, and those on normal subjects, x_N's, follow a normal distribution $N(\mu_N, \sigma_N^2)$. This model is usually referred to as a binormal model (Figure 12.3.1). Under the binormal model, define

$$a = \frac{\mu_D - \mu_N}{\sigma_D},$$

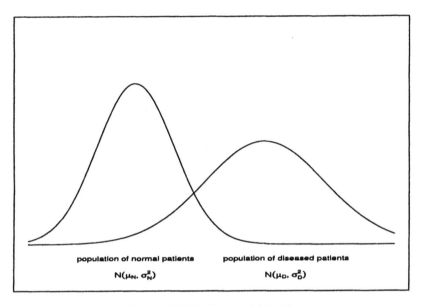

Figure 12.2.3. Binormal Model

and

$$b = \frac{\sigma_N}{\sigma_D}.$$

For an arbitrary point u,

$$\text{TPR} = P(x_D > u) = 1 - \Phi\left(\frac{u - \mu_D}{\sigma_D}\right),$$

and

$$\text{FPR} = P(x_N > u) = 1 - \Phi\left(\frac{u - \mu_N}{\sigma_N}\right),$$

where Φ is the distribution function of a standard normal variable. It follows that

$$u = \mu_N + \sigma_N \Phi^{-1}(1 - \text{FPR}).$$

Thus, we have

$$\text{TPR} = \Phi(a + b\Phi^{-1}(\text{FPR})),$$

which does not depend on the value of u. As a result, the ROC curve can be derived. For a given value of FPR, say FPR= x, the method of maximum likelihood can be used to obtain estimates of a and b from the observed counts in the M categories and thus provides an estimate of TPR. For comparing different modalities, it is suggested that the following be used:

$$\text{ZTPR}_x = \Phi^{-1}(\text{TPR}_x) = a + b\Phi^{-1}(x),$$

where
$$\mathrm{TPR}_x = \Phi(a + b\Phi^{-1}(x)).$$

Thompson and Zucchini (1989) introduced a new accuracy index for comparing ROC curves. The proposed accuracy index is the partial area under the binormal ROC graph over any specified region of interest. Denote by PA_c the partial area under the binormal ROC curve over the interval $(0, c)$. Then, we have

$$PA_c = \int_0^c \mathrm{TPR}_x dx = \int_0^c \Phi(a + b\Phi^{-1}(x))dx.$$

Letting $x_1 = \Phi(x)$ yields

$$PA_c = \int_{-\infty}^{\Phi^{-1}(c)} \Phi(a + bx_1)\phi(x_1)dx_1$$
$$= \int_{-\infty}^{\Phi^{-1}(c)} \int_{-\infty}^{a+bx_1} \phi(x_2)\phi(x_1)dx_2 dx_1,$$

where ϕ is the probability density function of a standard normal variable. Let

$$z_1 = \frac{x_2 - bx_1}{\sqrt{1 + b^2}}$$

and

$$z_2 = x_1.$$

Then,

$$PA_c = \int_{-\infty}^{\Phi^{-1}(c)} \int_{-\infty}^{a/\sqrt{1+b^2}} \frac{1}{\sqrt{1 - \rho^2}}\phi(z_2)\phi\left(\frac{z_1 - \rho z_2}{\sqrt{1 - \rho^2}}\right) dz_1 dz_2,$$

where $\rho = -b/\sqrt{1 + b^2}$. Note that the area under the entire binormal ROC curve can be obtained as a special case by setting $c = 1$. This yields

$$A = \int_{-\infty}^{a/\sqrt{1+b^2}} \phi(z_1)dz_2 = \Phi\left(\frac{a}{\sqrt{1 + b^2}}\right).$$

Let y denote a summary accuracy index, i.e., y may be TPR_x, PA_c, or A as described above. Thompson and Zucchini (1989) suggested the following analysis of variance model for the summary index y:

$$y_{ijk} = \mu + \alpha_i + b_j + (ab)_{ij} + c + e_{ijk},$$

where $i = 1, ..., I$, $j = 1, ..., J$, $k = 1, ..., K$, and the component $\mu + \alpha_i$ represents the mean level of y for the ith modality. The random variable

b_j, which has mean zero and variance σ_b^2, reflects the variation between readers, while $(ab)_{ij}$ is the effect due to the interaction between reader and modality. $(ab)_{ij}$ follows a distribution with mean zero and variance σ_{ab}^2. Note that the term c in the model is also a random variable with mean 0 and variance σ_c^2, which is common to all values of y. The term c reflects variation between groups of subjects of the same size. If a given experiment only involves a group of subjects, there is only a single value of the random variable c. However, if the experiment were repeated on a different set of subjects, then we would obtain a different estimate of c. Finally, the random error term e_{ijk} with mean zero and variance σ_e^2 reflects variation within readers, which is the variation of the index when a single reader repeatedly rates a given set of images. As pointed out by Thompson and Zucchini (1989), the interaction terms of ac, bc, and abc are ignored because these interactions are unlikely to be substantial when dealing with groups of subjects as opposed to individual subjects. As a result, an appropriate statistical test statistic for comparing the means of different modalities can be derived from the analysis of variance table as given in Table 12.2.1, which is given by $F = \text{MSA/MSAB}$. Under the null hypothesis H_0 that $\alpha_1 = \alpha_2 = \cdots = \alpha_I$ of no difference in the mean levels of the different modalities, F follows an F-distribution with $I - 1$ and $(I - 1)(J - 1)$ degrees of freedom.

Note that a similar ANOVA approach is applicable to the case of a single reader. McNeil and Hanley (1984) and Moise et al. (1985) discuss alternative methods for analysis of this case. Other approaches are also

Table 12.2.1. ANOVA Table for a Summary Accuracy Index

Source	Sum of squares	Degrees of freedom	Mean squares	Expected mean squares
Modality	SSA	$I - 1$	MSA	$\frac{JK}{I-1}\sum_i \alpha_i^2 + K\sigma_{ab}^2 + \sigma_e^2$
Reader	SSB	$J - 1$	MSB	$IK\sigma_b^2 + K\sigma_{ab}^2 + \sigma_e^2$
Interaction	SSAB	$(I - 1)(J - 1)$	MSAB	$K\sigma_{ab}^2 + \sigma_e^2$
Error	SSE	$IJ(K - 1)$	MSE	σ_e^2
Total	SST	$IJK - 1$		

SSA $= JK \sum_i (\bar{y}_{i..} - \bar{y}_{...})^2$
SSB $= IK \sum_j (\bar{y}_{.j.} - \bar{y}_{...})^2$
SSAB $= K \sum_i \sum_j (\bar{y}_{ij.} - \bar{y}_{i..} - \bar{y}_{.j.} + \bar{y}_{...})^2$
SSE $= \sum_i \sum_j \sum_k (y_{ijk} - \bar{y}_{ij.})^2$
SST $= \sum_i \sum_j \sum_k (y_{ijk} - \bar{y}_{...})^2$

available in the literature. For example, Wieand et al. (1989) consider nonparametric methods for comparing diagnostic markers with paired or unpaired data. Dorfman, Berbaum and Metz (1992) propose the concept of jackknifed pseudovalues for estimation of summary statistic for each modality and reader combination.

12.3   The Analysis of Blinded-Reader Studies

In order to demonstrate efficacy of a medical imaging drug, FDA suggests that evaluations of images should be performed by independent readers who are blinded. These independent and blinded image evaluations are intended to limit possible bias that could be introduced into the images evaluation by nonindependent or unblinded readers. This evaluation is then conducted in controlled setting with minimal clinical information provided to the reader. To provide a fair and unbiased evaluation of images, a valid design and the assessment of interrater agreement for blinded-reader studies are essential.

12.3.1   Design of Blinded-Reader Studies

Stevens (1999) introduced various designs for blinded-reader studies. For simplicity, consider two treatments (say A and B) and six patients per treatment group. Suppose there are three readers. The first design is the full design, in which each reader reads images from all of the patients. The full design is summarized below.

Patient	Treatment	Reader 1	Reader 2	Reader 3
1	A	X	X	X
2	A	X	X	X
3	A	X	X	X
4	A	X	X	X
5	A	X	X	X
6	A	X	X	X
7	B	X	X	X
8	B	X	X	X
9	B	X	X	X
10	B	X	X	X
11	B	X	X	X
12	B	X	X	X

For the full design, it is suggested that the readers be chosen from a pool
of homogeneous readers so that the readers can be treated as a repeated
measures factor. The distribution of degrees of freedom for the analysis of
variance of the full design is given by

Source	Degrees of Freedom
Treatment	1
Patient(Treatment)	10
Reader	2
Treatment × Reader	2
Patient (Treatment) × Reader	20

In the interest of reducing the number of tests, a fraction of the full design
may be considered. A commonly employed design is the so-called one-
third (1/3) design, in which each reader reads images from one-third of the
patients. The design layout of the one-third design is given below.

Patient	Treatment	Reader 1	Reader 2	Reader 3
1	A	X		
2	A		X	
3	A		X	
4	A			X
5	A			X
6	A	X		
7	B		X	
8	B	X		
9	B			X
10	B	X		
11	B			X
12	B		X	

The distribution of degrees of freedom for the analysis of variance of the
one-third design is given by

Source	Degrees of Freedom
Reader	2
Treatment	1
Error	8

Suppose there are n patients in blinded-reader studies under the study designs previously discussed. In general, there are $n-4$ degrees of freedom for testing the treatment effect in the one-third design, while there are $n-2$ degrees of freedom for testing the treatment effect in the full design. In practice, it may not be worthwhile spending triple amount of work for 2 degrees of freedom for testing the parameter of interest. Stevens (1999) proposed a compromised design, which is referred to as the overlap design. An overlap design is an incomplete block design, in which patients serve as blocks. The design layout of the overlap design is summarized below.

Patient	Treatment	Reader 1	Reader 2	Reader 3
1	A	X		X
2	A	X	X	
3	A	X		X
4	A		X	X
5	A		X	X
6	A	X	X	
7	B		X	X
8	B	X		X
9	B		X	X
10	B	X	X	
11	B	X	X	
12	B	X		X

As it can be seen from the above overlap design, each reader reads images from two-third of patients. The distribution of degrees of freedom of the analysis of variance of the design is given by

Source	Degrees of Freedom
Patient	11
Treatment	1
Reader	2
Treatment × Reader	2
Error	7

The above three designs allow for testing reader effects. The one-third design is preferred since it minimizes the work for testing treatment effect without loosing much degrees of freedom. In addition to the above designs, a design called miss-matched design is sometimes considered. In the miss-matched design, two readers read images from all of the patients while a third reader reads *disagreement* images. The design layout is given below.

Patient	Treatment	Reader 1	Reader 2	Reader 3
1	A	X	X	
2	A	X	X	X
3	A	X	X	
4	A	X	X	X
5	A	X	X	X
6	A	X	X	
7	B	X	X	
8	B	X	X	
9	B	X	X	X
10	B	X	X	
11	B	X	X	X
12	B	X	X	

In the miss-matched design, the distribution of random variables from reader 3 is conditional on the outcome of the first two readers. The distribution is generally unknown. As a result, the analysis is not clear.

12.3.2 Assessing Interreader Agreement

As indicated in the 2000 FDA guidance, at least two independent, blinded readers (and preferably three or more) are recommended for each study that is intended to demonstrate efficacy. The purpose is to provide a better basis for the findings in the studies. Therefore, the determination of interreader agreement and variability is the typical design issue to blinded read studies. For a diagnostic test, suppose there are k categories for the disease status. Let n_{ij} and $P_{ij}, i = 1, ..., k, j = 1, ..., k$, denote the number of patients and the proportion of patients diagnosed to be in the ith category by the first reader and diagnosed to be in the jth category by the second reader. Thus, $\{n_{ij}\}, i = 1, ..., k, j = 1, ..., k$ constitutes a $k \times k$ table. A simple measure for interreader agreement can be obtained as follows.

$$P_A = \sum_{i=1}^k P_{ii} = \sum_{i=1}^k \frac{n_{ii}}{n},$$

where $n = \sum_{i=1}^k \sum_{j=1}^k n_{ij}$. When $k = 2$, the following measures are usually considered. For example, if we assume category 1 is rare, we may consider

$$P_S = \frac{2n_{11}}{2n_{11} + n_{12} + n_{21}}$$

and

$$P_{S*} = \frac{2n_{22}}{2n_{22} + n_{12} + n_{21}}.$$

Rogot and Goldberg (1966) suggested the use of the average of P_S and P_{S*} as the measure of interreader agreement, i.e.,

$$P_{RG} = \frac{P_S + P_{S*}}{2}.$$

On the other hand, a classical approach is to consider the following measure

$$P_C = \frac{2n_{11} - (n_{12} + n_{21})}{2n_{11} + (n_{12} + n_{21})}.$$

In practice, the most commonly used statistical test to assess the interreader agreement is κ (kappa) statistics. The Cohen's kappa coefficient, introduced by Cohen (1960), is a measure of inter-reader agreement in terms of count data (see also Landis and Koch, 1977; Shrout and Fleiss, 1979; Kramer, 1980). It assumes that two response variables are two independent ratings of the n subjects. It should be noted that the kappa coefficient equals 1 when there is complete agreement of the readers. When the observed agreement exceeds chance agreement, kappa is positive. Also, the magnitude of kappa statistics reflects the strength of agreement. In a very unusual practice, kappa could be negative when the observed agreement is less than chance agreement. The total range of kappa is between -1 and 1. According to Fleiss at al. (1969),

$$\kappa = \frac{P_0 - P_e}{1 - P_e},$$

where

$$P_0 = \sum_{i=1}^{k} P_{ii},$$

$$P_e = \sum_{i=1}^{k} \sum_{j=1}^{k} P_{i.} P_{.j},$$

and $P_{i.}$ (or $P_{.j}$) is the average of P_{ij}'s with a fixed i (or j). It can be verified that the asymptotic variance of κ is given by

$$\text{Var}(\kappa) = \frac{1}{n(1 - P_e)^2}(A + B - C),$$

where

$$A = \sum_{i=1}^{k} P_{ii}[1 - (P_{i.} + P_{.j})(1 - \kappa)]^2,$$

$$B = (1 - \kappa)^2 \sum_{i \neq j} P_{ij}(P_{i\cdot} + P_{\cdot j})^2,$$

and

$$C = [\kappa - P_e(1 - \kappa)]^2.$$

As a result, an approximate 95% confidence interval for the kappa coefficient can be obtained.

Fleiss (1981) considered there is an excellent interreader agreement if $\kappa \geq 0.75$. The interreader agreement is considered poor when $\kappa \leq 0.40$. Landis and Koch (1977), on the other hand, provided different interpretation of the kappa coefficient. They conclude the agreement between readers is almost perfect if the kappa coefficient is within the range of (0.81, 1.00). The evidence of interreader agreement is substantial if the kappa coefficient falls within (0.61, 0.80). The interreader agreement is considered slight, fair or moderate if the kappa coefficient is within the ranges of (0.00, 0.20), (0.21, 0.40), or (0.41, 0.60), respectively. When the kappa coefficient falls below 0.00, the interreader agreement is considered poor and hence not acceptable.

Alternatively, we may consider a weighted kappa coefficient on the number of categories as follows (e.g., Brenner and Kleibsch, 1996):

$$\kappa_w = \frac{P_{0w} - P_{ew}}{1 - P_{ew}},$$

where

$$P_{0w} = \sum_{i=1}^{k} w_{ij} P_{ii},$$

$$P_{ew} = \sum_{i=1}^{k} \sum_{j=1}^{k} w_{ij} P_{i\cdot} P_{\cdot j},$$

and w_{ij}'s are some weights. It can be verified that the asymptotic variance of the weighted κ_w is given by

$$\text{Var}(\kappa_w) = \frac{D}{n(1 - P_e)^2}$$

where

$$D = \sum_{i=1}^{k} \sum_{j=1}^{k} P_{ij}[w_{ij} - (w_{i\cdot} + w_{\cdot j})(1 - \kappa_w)]^2 - [\kappa_w - P_{ew}(1 - \kappa_w)]^2,$$

$w_{i\cdot}$ is the average of w_{ij} over j, and $w_{\cdot j}$ is the average of w_{ij} over i. The commonly considered weight is the weight inversely proportional to distance from diagonal, which is given by

$$w_{ij} = 1 - \frac{|C_{1i} - C_{2j}|}{C_+ - C_-},$$

where C_{li} is the ith category of response from the lth reader, C_+ is the maximal category of responses, and C_- is the minimal category of responses. This weight is known as Cicchetti-Allison weight. If we consider the weight inversely proportional to squared distance from diagonal, it leads to the following Fleiss-Cohen weight:

$$w_{ij} = 1 - \frac{(C_{1i} - C_{2j})^2}{C_+ - C_-}.$$

Note that for measuring the inter-reader agreement in continuous data, the intraclass correlation proposed by Snedecor and Cochran (1967) is useful.

Example 12.3.1. To illustrate the use of simple measures and the kappa coefficient for interreader agreement, consider the example of patient diagnosis based on predose and postdose assessment of malignancy (Donovan, 1999). The results from two independent readers are summarized below.

Predose					
				Reader 1	
			Malignant	Benign	Unknown
		Malignant	22	6	2
	Reader 2	Benign	2	70	3
		Unknown	2	3	10
Postdose					
				Reader 1	
			Malignant	Benign	Unknown
		Malignant	28	6	0
	Reader 2	Benign	4	82	0
		Unknown	0	0	0

For simplicity, the unknown category was excluded. The results of the simple measures and the kappa coefficient for interreader agreement are summarized below.

Measure	Predose	Postdose
P_A	$92/100 = 0.920$	$110/120 = 0.917$
P_S	$44/52 = 0.846$	$56/66 = 0.848$
P_{S^*}	$140/148 = 0.946$	$164/174 = 0.943$
P_{RG}	$(0.846 + 0.946)/2 = 0.896$	$(0.848 + 0.943)/2 = 0.896$
P_C	$36/52 = 0.692$	$46/66 = 0.697$
κ	0.792	0.793

The results indicate that there is an excellent interreader agreement according to Fleiss' criterion (Fleiss, 1981) and the interreader agreement is considered substantial according to Landis and Koch (1977).

For another example, consider the example of predose and postdose leison detection using a test medical imaging agent (Donovan, 1999). The results of predose and postdose from two independent readers are summarized below:

Predose

		Reader 1						
		0	1	2	3	4	5	> 5
	0	40	21	9	8	0	1	0
	1	15	11	9	3	2	1	0
	2	12	9	10	3	2	1	0
Reader 2	3	5	5	4	7	3	3	0
	4	0	1	2	1	2	0	1
	5	0	2	1	1	2	0	0
	> 5	0	0	0	1	2	0	0

Postdose

		Reader 1						
		0	1	2	3	4	5	> 5
	0	9	8	2	7	2	0	0
	1	5	8	7	5	0	0	1
	2	7	4	7	10	8	3	1
Reader 2	3	1	5	10	8	8	2	4
	4	0	2	3	2	7	3	2
	5	0	1	2	3	6	5	9
	> 5	0	1	1	4	2	5	10

The results of the simple kappa and weighted kappa (i.e., Cicchetti-Allison κ and Fleiss-Cohen κ) coefficient for interreader agreement are summarized below.

Measure	Predose	Postdose
P_0	0.350	0.270
P_e	0.244	0.146
simple κ	0.140	0.145
Cicchetti-Allison κ	0.287	0.408
Fleiss-Cohen κ	0.441	0.598

According to Fleiss' criterion, the interreader agreement between the two independent reviewers is considered poor based on the simple kappa coefficient. On the other hand, according to the criterion proposed by Landis and Koch, the interreader agreement for detecting leisons between the two independent reviewers is considered fair to moderate and moderate based on Cicchetti-Allison weighted kappa and Fleiss-Cohen weighted kappa, respectively.

12.4   Diagnostic Accuracy

To determine how well a diagnostic imaging agent can distinguish disease subjects and nondiseased subjects, the outcome may often be classified into one of the four groups depending on (i) whether disease is present and (ii) the results of the diagnostic test of interest (positive or negative). The terms *positive* and *negative* concern some particular disease status, which must be specified clearly. The categories can be defined in any meaningful way to the problem. For example, patients could be classified as having one or more tumors (positive) or no tumor (negative); malignant (positive) or benign/no tumor (negative). It should be noted that the disease is often determined with a truth standard or gold standard. Truth standards are used to demonstrate that the results obtained with the medical imaging drug are valid and reliable. For example, for a MRI contrast agent intended to visualize the number of lesions in liver or determine whether a mass is malignant, the truth standard might include results from the pathology or long-term clinical outcomes. In diagnostic imaging studies, truth or gold standards are usually called as standard of reference (SOR). There are a number of possible choices of SOR in an imaging trail. These choices include histopathology, therapeutic response, clinical outcome, another validated imaging procedure (validated against a valid gold standard), and autopsy.

As indicated earlier, typical outcomes in the evaluation of a diagnostic test can be summarized in a 2 × 2 contingency table as described in §12.2. The simplest measure of diagnostic decision is the fraction of cases for which the physician is correct, which is often referred to as *accuracy*. In other words, the accuracy is the proportion of cases, considering both positive and negative test results, for which the test results are correct. However, accuracy is of limited usefulness as an index of diagnostic performance because two diagnostic modalities can yield equal accuracies but perform differently with respect to the types of decisions. Also, it can be affected by the disease prevalence strongly. Due to the limitation of the accuracy index, the sensitivity and specificity are used in the evaluation scheme. In effect, sensitivity and specificity represents two kinds of accuracy: the first is for actually positive cases and the second is for actually negative cases. However, very often a single pair of sensitivity and specificity measurements may provide a possibly misleading and even hazardous oversimplification of accuracy (Zweig and Campbell, 1993).

In what follows, we will discuss the assessment of accuracy in cases (i) where there is an imperfect reference test, and (ii) where there is no gold standards.

12.4.1 Diagnostic Accuracy with an Imperfect Reference Test

The conventional method for evaluating and comparing sensitivity and specificity for diagnostic tests is based on the assumptions that (i) diagnostic tests are independent given the disease status and (ii) the reference test is error free (i.e., the gold standard). However, the above assumptions are not always valid. In case where these assumptions are not valid, several statistical methods have been proposed. See, for example, Qu and Hadgu (1998 and 1999), Baker (1990), and Baker et al. (1998). Let y_i denote the response of the ith diagnostic test, i.e.,

$$y_i = \begin{cases} 1 & \text{nondisease} \\ 2 & \text{disease} \end{cases} \quad i = 1, ..., p, p+1,$$

where $y_1, ..., y_p$ are the diagnostic tests to be evaluated and y_{p+1} is the reference test. The true status of disease indicator is defined to be

$$D = \begin{cases} 1 & \text{nondisease} \\ 2 & \text{disease} \end{cases}$$

The sensitivity and specificity for the ith diagnostic test are then given by

$$\text{Sensitivity}(i) = P(y_i = 2|D = 2)$$

and

$$\text{Specificity}(i) = P(y_i = 1|D = 1),$$

where $i = 1, ..., p$. If no covariate is involved, the conventional method is just the 2×2 contingency table. We refer to the 2×2 contingency table as model 1. Suppose that the sensitivity depends on some covariate x. We may consider the following generalized linear model for sensitivity

$$g_1(P(y_{ki} = 2|D = 2, x_{ki})) = a_{i2} + b_{i2}x_{ki}, \quad i = 1, ..., p, k = 1, ..., n,$$

where $g_1(\cdot)$ is a link function, e.g., a logit or a probit link and $D = y_{p+1}$. Similarly, we may consider the following generalized model for specificity

$$g_2(P(y_{ki} = 1|D = 1, x_{ki})) = a_{i1} + b_{i1}x_{ki}, \quad i = 1, ..., p, k = 1, ..., n.$$

We refer to the above generalized model as model 2.

In practice, the accuracy may depend on unobserved variables, such as severity of the disease in the diseased population, which causes correlation between the diagnostic tests. In this case, Qu and Hadgu (1998) suggested the following random effects model for sensitivity

$$h(P(y_{ki} = 2|D = 2, x_{ki})) = a_{i2} + b_{i2}x_{ki} + \gamma_{k2}, \quad \gamma_{k2} \sim N(0, \sigma_2^2).$$

Similarly, in the nondiseased population,

$$h(P(y_{ki} = 2|D = 1, x_{ki})) = a_{i1} + b_{i1}x_{ki} + \gamma_{k1}, \quad \gamma_{k1} \sim N(0, \sigma_1^2).$$

The above model is referred to as model 3.

Qu and Hadgu (1998) indicated that model 2, which assuming conditional independence, is less efficient if the assumption of conditional independence is not true. On the other hand, model 3 is efficient in accuracy comparison since it incorporate the correlation between tests. Models 1-3 assume that the disease status is known. In practice, the disease status may be missing in a subset of patients. In this case, there is a uncertainty about D, i.e., either $D = 1$ or $D = 2$. As a result, the likelihood of $Y_k = (y_{k1}, ..., y_{kp}, y_{k(p+1)})'$ in this subset is given by

$$L_k = \tau_1 f(Y_k|D = 1) + \tau_2 f(Y_k|D = 2),$$

where τ_1 and τ_2 are the mixture proportions and $f(Y_k|D = 1)$ and $f(Y_k|D = 2)$ are two component densities. Qu and Hadgu (1998) recommended that a random effects model be used for correlated diagnostic tests and the above mixture model be considered for when there are missing disease status in a subset of patients (or imperfect gold standard). For both the random effects model and the mixture model, either the EM algorithm or Gibbs sampling is recommended for estimation (Qu and Hadgu, 1998, 1999).

12.4.2 Diagnostic Accuracy without Gold Standard

For simplicity, we only focus on the assessment of accuracy of TPR (or sensitivity) when the test is negative. The estimation of FPR (i.e., $1-$specificity) can be treated similarly. We first consider the case where there is no gold standard when the test is negative. In this case, commonly used statistical methods include (i) imputation based on follow-up data, (ii) the use of capture-recapture model, and (iii) the estimation of ratios.

Imputation Based on Follow-up Time

As indicated earlier, TPR in a 2×2 contingency table is given by

$$\text{TPR} = \frac{\text{number of subjects detected positive}}{\text{number of subjects with disease}}.$$

Let $i(t)$ be the number of subjects with disease (e.g., symptomatic cancer) within time t of the test. Then, TPR at time t can be expressed as follows

$$\text{TPR}(t) = \frac{a}{a + i(t)},$$

where a is the number of subjects detected with cancer on the screen and $i(t)$ is the number of subjects with follow-up cancers within time t of the screen. Baker, Connor, and Kessler (1998) suggest evaluating the accuracy at the optimal follow-up time. The optimal time is defined as the time at which TPR(t) has the smallest bias. Following the idea of Baker, Connor, and Kessler (1998), $i(t)$ can be partitioned into two parts as follows:

$$i(t) = i_{Miss}(t) + i_{New}(t),$$

where $i_{Miss}(t)$ is the number of subjects with follow-up cancers missed on screen and $i_{New}(t)$ is the number of subject with follow-up cancers arising after screen. Let N be the number of subjects at steady state who enter preclinical state at each time. Also, let $Q(y)$ be the probability of surviving y years in preclinical state. Then, TPR is the probability of a subject who is detected with cancer on screen given that he/she has preclinical cancer. As a result, we have

$$a = N\text{TPR}.P(\text{preclinical cancer at } s)$$

$$= N\text{TPR} \int_0^s Q(s-x)dx$$

$$= N\text{TPR}\mu,$$

where s is the maximum preclinical time such that $Q(s) = 0$ and μ is the mean preclinical duration. Similarly, we have

$$i_{Miss}(t) = N(1 - \text{TPR}) \left[\int_0^s P(\text{preclinical } s - x) \right.$$

$$- \int_0^s P(\text{preclinical } s+t-x)dx \Bigg]$$

$$= N(1-\text{TPR}) \int_0^s [Q(s-x) - Q(s+t-x)]dx$$

$$= N(1-\text{TPR}) \int_0^t Q(y)dy,$$

and

$$i_{New}(t) = N \int_s^{s+t} [1 - P(\text{preclinical at time } s+t-x)]dx$$

$$= N \int_s^{s+t} [1 - Q(s+t-x)]dx$$

$$= N \left[t - \int_0^t Q(y)dy \right].$$

As a result, TPR(t) is given by

$$\text{TPR}(t) = \frac{a}{a+i(t)}$$

$$= \frac{a}{a+i_{Miss}(t)+i_{New}(t)}$$

$$= \frac{\text{TPR}\mu}{\text{TPR}\mu + t - \text{TPR}\int_0^t Q(y)dy}.$$

It can be verified that when $t = 1$, TPR(t) is the same as that given in Day (1985).

Capture-Recapture Model

The use of capture-recapture model for estimation of TPR is to adopt the idea of capture-recapture for estimation of fish in a lake as introduced by Goldberg and Wittes (1978). The capture-recapture model is simply to estimate the proportion of subjects who are detected with disease on both tests. Suppose there are two tests say A and B, which operate through different mechanisms. It is assumed that Tests A and B are unrelated to the severity of disease. Test results can be summarized in the following 2×2 table.

	Test A - Positive (+)	Test A- Negative (−)
Test B - Positive (+)	a	b
Test B - Negative (−)	c	?

As a result, assuming that there is gold standard, we have

$$\frac{a}{N} = P(A+, B+ |GS+)$$
$$= P(A+ |GS+) P(B+ |GS+)$$
$$= \frac{a+c}{N}\frac{a+b}{N}.$$

Hence, N can be estimated as

$$\hat{N} = a+b+c+\frac{(a+b)(a+c)}{a}.$$

To illustrate the use of capture-recapture model, consider the example for diagnosis of cancer. Suppose test A is physical exam and test B is mammography and the test results are summarized below.

Physical Exam	M (+)	M (−)
P (+)	10	24
P (−)	21	?

Then, as discussed above, N can be estimated as

$$\hat{N} = 10+24+21+\frac{(10+24)(10+21)}{10} = 105.4.$$

Consequently, we have

$$P(M+ |cancer) = \frac{10+24}{105.4} = 0.29,$$

$$P(P+ |cancer) = \frac{10+24}{105.4} = 0.32,$$

and

$$P(M+ \text{ or } P+ |cancer) = \frac{10+21+24}{105.4} = 0.52.$$

Estimation of Ratios

Alternatively, we may estimate the ratio of TPR of the two tests as follows

$$r = \frac{P(A+ |GS+)}{P(B+ |GS+)} = \frac{(a+b)/N}{(a+c)/N} = \frac{a+b}{a+c}.$$

For obtaining a 95% confidence interval of r, Baker (1990) suggests a multinomial-Poisson transformation and delta method be used. In other words, the standard error of the estimate of r can be obtained as follows.

$$se(r) = \sqrt{a\left(\frac{\partial \log r}{\partial a}\right)^2 + b\left(\frac{\partial \log r}{\partial b}\right)^2 + c\left(\frac{\partial \log r}{\partial c}\right)^2}.$$

Thus, a 95% confidence interval for r, say (L, U), is given by

$$L = \exp\{r - 1.96\text{se}(r)\}$$

and

$$U = \exp\{r + 1.96\text{se}(r)\}.$$

To illustrate the estimation of TPR ratio, consider the same example as described in the previous subsection. The TPR ratio can be estimated as

$$r = \frac{P(P + |\text{cancer})}{P(M + |\text{cancer})} = \frac{34}{31} = 1.05$$

with a 95% confidence interval of (0.73, 1.64).

12.5   Sample Size

For power analysis for sample size calculation in blinded-reader studies, it is often of interest to ensure the study is powered to detect superiority with at least one reader (Makris, 1999). In practice, two designs are commonly employed. The first design requires only one read per patient using two or more readers. The second design is that all patients read by two or more readers. For the first design, we may split sample equally between readers, i.e., $N/2$ per reader per group. As a result, power for either reader to detect a clinically meaningful difference is given by

$$\omega = P(R_1 > C \text{ or } R_2 > C)$$
$$= P(R > C)[2 - P(R > C)].$$

For $\omega > 95\%$, it implies that $P(R > C) > 80\%$. For a given set of parameter assumptions, the sample size required for achieving a 95% power can be obtained. Similarly, for the second design that all patients read by two or more readers, we have N per reader per group. Power for either reader to detect superiority can be obtained as

$$\omega = P(R_1 > C \text{ or } R_2 > C)$$
$$= 2P(R > C) - P(R > C \text{ and } R > C).$$

For $\omega > 95\%$, $P(R > C)$ needs to be greater than 87%. For a given set of parameter assumptions, the sample size required for achieving a 95% power can be obtained.

It, however, should be noted that in practice, we may have only one read for a subset of patients using two readers. The remaining subset of patients read by both readers. In this case, sample size calculation based on power for either reader to detect a clinically meaningful difference is much more complicated.

Example 12.5.1. To illustrate the power analysis for sample size calculation, consider a blinded-reader study for cardiac ultrasound. The study design is a parallel group design comparing a test agent and an active control agent. The study endpoint is change from baseline in endocardial border delineation score. Suppose a difference of 3 in endocardial border delineation is considered of clinical importance. For the first design, a sample size of $N = 74$ per group is required to achieve a 95% power for either reader to detect superiority, i.e., a clinically meaningful difference of 3 in endocardial border delineation at the 5% level of significance, assuming that the active control agent has a mean response of 3 with a standard deviation of 4.5. Under the same assumptions, a sample size of $N = 45$ per group is required for the second design.

References

Adams, W.P., Singh, G.J.P., and Williams, R. (1998). Nasal inhalation aerosols and metered dose spray pumps: FDA bioequivalence issues. *Respiratory Drug Delivery*, VI.

Akaike, H. (1973). A new look at statistical model discrimination. *IEEE Trans Automat Control*, 19, 716-723.

Anderson, S. and Hauck, W.Ẇ. (1990). Considerations of individual bioequivalence. *Journal of Pharmacokinetics and Biopharmaceutics*, 8, 259-273.

Anderson-Sprecher, R. (1994). Model comparison and R^2. *The American Statistician*, 48, 113-116.

Atkinson, C.A. (1969). A test for discrimination between models. *Biometrika*, 56, 337-347.

Atkinson, C.A. (1970). A method for discriminating between models. *Journal of the Royal Statistical Society*, B, 32, 323-353.

Baker S.G. (1990). A simple EM algorithm for capture-recapture data with categorical covariates. *Biometrics*, 46, 1193-1200.

Baker S.G., Cannor R.J., and Kessler L.G. (1998). The partial testing design: a less costly way to test equivalence for sensitivity and specificity. *Statistics in Medicine*, 17, 2219-2232.

Bancroft, T.A. (1964). Analysis and inference for incompletely specified models involving the use of preliminary test(s) of significance. *Biometrics*, 20, 427-442.

Beal, S.L. (1987). Asymptotic confidence intervals for the difference between two binomial parameters for use with small samples. *Biometrics*, 43, 941-950.

Benet, L.Z. (1992). Narrow therapeutic index drugs. *Proceedings of the 1992 Open Conference on Dissolution on Bioavailability and Bioequivalence*, 35-39.

Berger, R.L. and Hsu, J.C. (1996). Bioequivalence trials, intersection-union tests and equivalence confidence sets (with discussion). *Statistical Science*, 11, 283-319.

Bergner, M., Bobbitt, R.A., Carter, W.B., Gilson, B.S. (1981). The sickness impact profile: development and final revision of a health status measure. *Medical Care*, 19, 787-805.

Bergum, J. S. (1990). Constructing acceptance limits for multiple stage tests. *Drug Develop Industrial Pharmacy*, 16, 2153-2166.

Bergum, J. and Utter, M.L. (2000). Process validation. In *Encyclopedia of Biopharmaceutical Statistics*, 422-439, Ed. S. Chow, Marcel Dekker, New York.

Biswas, N., Chan, I.S.F., and Ghosh, K. (2000). Equivalence trials: statistical issues. One-day short course at Joint Statistical Meetings, Indianapolis, Indiana, August 16, 2000.

Blackwelder, W.C. (1982). Proving the null hypothesis in clinical trials. *Controlled Clinical Trials*, 3, 345-353.

Blackwelder, W.C. (1993). Sample size and power for prospective analysis of relative risk. *Statistics in Medicine*, 12, 691-698.

Blackwell, D. and Hodges, J.L. Jr. (1957). Design for the control of selection bias. *The Annals of Mathematical Statistics*, 28, 449-460.

Bofinger, E. (1985). Expanded confidence intervals. *Communications in Statistics, Theory and Methods*, 14, 1849-1864.

Bofinger, E. (1992). Expanded confidence intervals, one-sided tests and equivalence testing. *Journal of Biopharmaceutical Statistics*, 2, 181-188.

Bohidar, N.R. (1983). Statistical aspects of chemical assay validation. *Proceedings of the Biopharmaceutical Section of the American Statistical Association*, 57-62.

Bohidar, N.R. and Peace, K. (1988). Pharmaceutical formulation development. Chapter 4 in *Biopharmaceutical Statistics for Drug Development*, 149-229, ed. Peace, K., Marcel Dekker, New York.

Borowiak, D.S. (1989). *Model Discrimination for Nonlinear Regression Models*. Marcel Dekker, New York.

Box, G.E.P. and Hill, W.J. (1967). Discrimination among mechanistic models. *Technometrics*, 9, 57-71.

Brenner, H. and Kleibsch, U. (1996). Dependence of weighted kappa coefficients on the number of categories. *Epidemiology*, 7, 199-202.

Brown, L.D., Casella, G., and Hwang, J.T.G. (1995). Optimal confidence sets, bioequivalence, and the limacon of pascal. *Journal of the American Statistical Association*, 90, 880-889.

Brown, L.D., Hwang, J.T.G. and Munk, A. (1997). An unbiased test for the bioequivalence problem. *The Annals of Statistics*, 25, 2345-2367 880-889.

Brownell, K.D. and Stunkard, A.J. (1982). The double-blind in danger: untoward consequences of informed consent. *American Journal of Psychiatry*, 139, 1487-1489.

Buonaccorsi, J.P. (1986). Design considerations for calibration. *Technometrics*, 28, 149-156.

Buonaccorsi, J.P. and Iyer, H.K. (1986). Optimal designs for ratios of linear combinations in the general linear model. *Journal of Statistical Planning and Inference*, 13, 345-356.

Campbell, G. (1999). Overview of ROC analysis. Presented at Drug Information Association symposium on Statistics in Diagnostic Imaging, Arlington, Virgina, March 1999.

Center, R.M. and Schwartz J.S. (1985). An evaluation of methods for estimating the area under the receiver operating characteristics (ROC) curve. *Medical Decision Making*, 5, 149-156.

Chein, Y.W. (1992). Nasal drug delivery and delivery systems. In *Novel Drug Delivery System*, 2nd Ed., 229-268, Marcel Dekker, New York.

Chen, K.W., Chow, S.C. and Li, G. (1997). A note on sample size determination for bioequivalence studies with higher-order crossover designs. *Journal of Pharmacokinetics and Biopharmaceutics*, 25, 753-765.

Chen, M.L. (1997). Individual bioequivalence — a regulatory update. *Journal of Biopharmaceutical Statistics*, 7, 5-11.

Cheng, B. (2002). *Statistical Tests in Clinical Studies*. Ph.D. Thesis, Department of Statistics, University of Wisconsin, Madison.

Chow, S.C. (1992). Statistical design and analysis of stability studies. Presented at the 48th Conference on Applied Statistics, Atlantic City, New Jersey.

Chow, S.C. (1997a). Good statistics practice in drug development and regulatory approval process. *Drug Information Journal*, 31, 1157-1166.

Chow, S.C. (1997b). Pharmaceutical validation and process controls in drug development. *Drug Information Journal*, 31, 1195-1201.

Chow, S.C. (1999). Individual bioequivalence—a review of the FDA draft guidance. *Drug Information Journal*, 33, 435-444.

Chow, S.C. (2000). *Encyclopedia of Biopharmaceutical Statistics*. Marcel Dekker, New York.

Chow, S.C. and Ki, F.Y.C. (1994). On statistical characteristics of quality of life assessment. *Journal of Biopharmaceutical Statistics*, 4, 1-17.

Chow, S.C. and Ki, F.Y.C. (1996). Statistical issues in quality-of-life assessment. *Journal of Biopharmaceutical Statistics*, 6, 37-48.

Chow, S.C. and Ki, F.Y.C. (1997). Statistical comparison between dissolution profiles of drug products. *Journal of Biopharmaceutical Statistics*, 7, 241-258.

Chow, S.C. and Liu, J.P. (1995). *Statistical Design and Analysis in Pharmaceutical Science*. Marcel Dekker, New York.

Chow, S.C. and Liu, J.P. (1997). Meta-analysis for bioequivalence review. *Journal of Biopharmaceutical Statistics*, 7, 97-111.

Chow, S.C. and Liu, J.P. (1998). *Design and Analysis of Clinical Trials*. Wiley, New York.

Chow, S.C. and Liu, J.P. (1999a). *Design and Analysis of Bioavailability and Bioequivalence Studies*, 2nd Edition. Marcel Dekker, New York.

Chow, S.C. and Liu, J.P. (1999b). *Design and Analysis of Animal Studies*. Marcel Dekker, New York.

Chow, S.C. and Shao, J. (1988). A new procedure for estimation of variance components. *Statistics and Probability Letters*, 6, 349-355.

Chow, S.C. and Shao, J. (1989). Test for batch-to-batch variation in stability analysis. *Statistics in Medicine*, 8, 883-890.

Chow, S.C. and Shao, J. (1990). On the difference between the classical and inverse methods of calibration. *Journal of Royal Statistical Society*, C, 39, 219-228.

Chow, S.C. and Shao, J. (1991). Estimating drug shelf-life with random batches. *Biometrics*, 47, 1071-1079.

Chow, S.C. and Shao, J. (1997). Statistical methods for two-sequence, three-period crossover designs with incomplete data. *Statistics in Medicine*, 16, 1031-1039.

Chow, S.C. and Shao, J. (1999). Bioequivalence review for drug interchangeability. *Journal of Biopharmaceutical Statistics*, 9, 485-497.

Chow, S.C. and Shao, J. (2001a). Shelf-life estimation with discrete responses. Manuscript submitted for publication.

Chow, S.C. and Shao, J. (2001b). Analysis of Clinical Data With Breached Blindness. Manuscript submitted for publication.

Chow, S.C., Shao, J., and Wang, H. (2001a). Probability lower bounds for USP/NF tests. Manuscript submitted for publication.

Chow, S.C., Shao, J., and Wang, H. (2001b). Statistical tests for population bioequivalence. Manuscript submitted for publication.

Chow, S.C., Shao, J., and Wang, H. (2001c). In vitro bioequivalence testing. Manuscript submitted for publication.

Chow, S.C., Shao, J., and Wang, H. (2002). Individual bioequivalence testing under 2 × 3 designs. *Statistics in Medicine*. In press.

Chow, S.C. and Tse, S.K. (1991). On variance estimation in assay validation. *Statistics in Medicine*, 10, 1543-1553.

Chow, S.C. and Wang, H. (2001). On sample size calculation in bioequivalence trials. *Journal of Pharmacokinetics and Pharmaccodynamics*, 28, 155-169.

Cohen, J. (1960). A coefficient of agreement for nominal scales. *Educational and Psychological Measurement*, 20, 37-46.

Cox, D.R. (1961). Tests of separate families of hypotheses. *Proceedings of 4th Berkeley Symposium*, 1, 105-123.

Cox, D.R. (1962). Further results on tests of separate families of hypotheses. *Journal of the Royal Statistical Society*, B, 24, 406-424.

Dawoodbhai, S., Suryanarayan, E., Woodruff, C. and Rhodes, C. (1991). Optimization of tablet formulation containing talc. *Drug Develop Industrial Pharmacy*, 17, 1343-1371.

DeLong E.R. and DeLong D.M. (1988). Comparing the areas under two or more correlated receiver operating characteristic curves: a nonparametric approach. *Biometrics*, 44, 837-845.

DerSimonian, R. and Laird, N. (1986). Meta-analysis in clinical trials. *Controlled Clinical Trials*, 7, 177-188.

Diggle, P.J. (1989). Testing for random dropout in repeated measurement data. *Biometrics*, 45, 1255-1258.

Diggle, P.J., Liang, K.Y. and Zeger, S. L. (1994). *Analysis of Longitudinal Data*. Oxford University Press, Oxford, UK.

Donovan, M. (1999). Measure for the evaluation of interreader agreement. Presented at Drug Information Association Symposium on Statistics in Diagnostic Imaging, Arlington, Virginia, March, 1999.

Dorfman, D.D., Berbaum, K.S., and Metz, C.E. (1992). ROC rating analysis: generalization to the population of readers and cases with the jackknife method. *Investigative Radiology*, 27, 723-731.

Dubey, S.D. (1988). Regulatory considerations on meta-analysis, dentifrice studies and multicenter trials. *Proceedings of the Biopharmaceutical Section of the American Statistical Association*, 18-27.

Dunnett, C.W. and Gent, M. (1977). Significant testing to establish equivalence between treatments with special reference to data in the form of 2×2 tables. *Biometrics*, 33, 593-602.

Durrleman, S. and Simon, R. (1990). Planning and monitoring of equivalence studies. *Biometrics*, 46, 329-336.

Eck, C.R., Chi, W.H., Christidis, G., Helm, M., Perlwitz, A.G., and Pilewski, S. (1998). Plume geometry and particle size measurements as a product development tool. *Respiratory Drug Delivery*, VI.

Efron, B. (1971). Forcing a sequential experiment to be balanced. *Biometrika*, 58, 403-417.

Esinhart, J.D. and Chinchilli, V.M. (1994). Extension to the use of tolerance intervals for assessment of individual bioequivalence. *Journal of Biopharmaceutical Statistics*, 4, 39-52.

Fahrmeir, L. and Tutz, G. (1994). *Multivariate Statistical Modeling Based on Generalized Linear Models*. Springer, New York.

Farrington, C.P. and Manning, G. (1990). Test statistics and sample size formulae for comparative binomial trials with null hypothesis of non-zero risk difference or non-unity relative risk. *Statistics in Medicine*, 9, 1447-1454.

FDA (1987a). *Guideline for Submitting Samples and Analytical Data for Methods Validation.* Center for Drug Evaluation and Research, Food and Drug Administration, Rockville, Maryland.

FDA (1987b). *Guideline for Submitting Documentation for the Stability of Human Drugs and Biologics.* Center for Drugs and Biologics, Office of Drug Research and Review, Food and Drug Administration, Rockville, Maryland.

FDA (1988). *Guideline for Format and Content of the Clinical and Statistical Sections of New Drug Applications.* Center for Drug Evaluation and Research, Food and Drug Administration, Rockville, Maryland.

FDA (1992). *Guidance on Statistical Procedures for Bioequivalence Studies Using a Standard Two-Treatment Crossover Design.* Office of Generic Drugs, Center for Drug Evaluation and Research, Food and Drug Administration, Rockville, Maryland.

FDA (1997a). *In Vivo Bioequivalence Studies Based on Population and Individual Bioequivalence Approaches. Division of Bioequivalence.* Office of Generic Drugs, Center for Drug Evaluation and Research, Food and Drug Administration, Rockville, Maryland.

FDA (1997b). *Draft Guidance for Industry — Clinical Development Programs for Drugs, Devices, and Biological Products for the Treatments of Rheumatoid Arthritis (RA).* Food and Drug Administration, Rockville, Martland.

FDA (1998). *Guidance for Industry on Providing Clinical Evidence of Effectiveness for Human Drug and Biological Products.* Food and Drug Administration, Rockville, Maryland.

FDA (1999a). *In Vivo Bioequivalence Studies Based on Population and Individual Bioequivalence Approaches. Division of Bioequivalence.* Office of Generic Drugs, Center for Drug Evaluation and Research, Food and Drug Administration, Rockville, Maryland.

FDA (1999b). *Guidance for Industry on Bioavailability and Bioequivalence Studies for Nasal Aerosols and Nasal Sprays for Local Action.* Center for Drug Evaluation and Research, Food and Drug Administration, Rockville, Maryland.

FDA (2000a). *Guidance for Industry on Bioavailability and Bioequivalence Studies for Orally Administered Drug Products - General Consideration.* Center for Drug Evaluation and Research, Food and Drug Administration, Rockville, Maryland.

FDA (2000b). *Guidance for Industry on Developing Medical Imaging Drugs and Biological Products.* Center for Drug Evaluation and Research and Center for Biologics Evaluation and Research, Food and Drug Administration, Rockville, Maryland.

FDA (2001). *Guidance for Industry on Statistical Approaches to Establishing Bioequivalence.* Center for Drug Evaluation and Research, Food and Drug Administration, Rockville, Maryland.

Feeny, D.H. and Torrance, G.W. (1989). Incorporating utility-based quality-of-life assessment measures in clinical trials. *Medical Care*, 27, S198-S204.

Fleiss, J.L. (1981). *Statistical Methods for Rates and Proportions.* Wiley, New York.

Fleiss, J.L., Cohen, J., and Everitt, B.S. (1969). Large-sample standard errors of kappa and weighted kappa. *Psychological Bulletin*, 72, 323-327.

Fleming, T.R. (1987). Treatment evaluation in active control studies. *Cancer Treatment Reports*, 71, 1061-1065.

Fleming, T.R. (1990). Evaluation of active control trials in AIDS. *Journal of Acquired Immune Deficiency Syndromes*, 3 (Suppl. 2), S82-S87.

Fuller, W.A. (1996). *Introduction to Statistical Time Series*, 2nd edition. Wiley, New York.

Gail, M.H. and Simon, R. (1985). Testing for qualitative interactions between treatment effects and patient subsets. *Biometrics*, 71, 431-444.

Ghosh, K., Chan, I., and Biswas, N. (2000). Equivalence Trials: Statistical Issues. One-day course at Joint Statistical Meeting, Indianapolis, Indiana, August 2000.

Gill, J.L. (1988). Repeated measurement: split-plot trend analysis versus analysis of first differences. *Biometrics*, 44, 289-297.

Goldberg, J.D. and Wittes, J.T. (1978). The estimation of false negative in medical screening. *Biometrics*, 34, 77-86.

Goodman, S.N. (1992). A comment on replication, p-values and evidence. *Statistics in Medicine*, 11, 875-879.

Graybill, F. and Wang, C.M. (1980). Confidence intervals on nonnegative linear combinations of variances. *Journal of American Statistical Association*, 75, 869-873.

Green, D.M. and Swets, J.A. (1966). *Signal Detection Theory and Psychophysics*. Wiley, New York.

Gui, R., Burdick, R.K., Graybill, F.A., and Ting, N. (1995). Confidence intervals on ratio of linear combinations for non-disjoint sets of expected mean squares. *Journal of Statistical and Planning Inference*, 48, 215-227.

Guilford, J.P. (1954). *Psychometric Methods*, 2nd Edition. McGraw-Hill, New York, New York.

Guyatt, G.H., Veldhuyen Van Zanten S.J.O, Feeny, D.H., Patric, D.L. (1989). Measuring quality of life in clinical trials: A taxonomy and review. *Canadian Medical Association Journal*, 140, 1441-1448.

Hanley, J.A. and McNeil, B.J. (1982). The meaning and use of the area under a receiver operating characteristic (ROC) curve. *Diagnostic Radiology*, 143, 29-36.

Hedges, L.V. and Olkin, I. (1985). *Statistical Methods for Meta-Analysis*. Academic Press, New York.

Helboe, P. (1992). New design for stability testing problems: matrix or factorial designs, authorities' viewpoint on the predictive value of such studies. *Drug Information Journal*, 26, 629-634.

Heyting, A., Tolboom, J.T.B.M., and Essers, J.G.A. (1992). Statistical handling of drop-outs in longitudinal clinical trials. *Statistics in Medicine* 11, 2043-2061.

Ho, C.H. and Chow, S.C. (1998). Design and analysis of multinational clinical trials. *Drug Information Journal*, 32, 1309-1316.

Ho, C.H., Liu, J.P. and Chow, S.C. (1992). On analysis of stability data. *Proceedings of the Biopharmaceutical Section of the American Statistical Association*, 198-203.

Hochberg, Y. and Tamhane, A.C. (1987). *Multiple Comparison Procedures*. Wiley, New York.

Hollenberg, N.K., Testa, M. and Williams, G.H. (1991). Quality of life as a therapeutic end-point — An analysis of therapeutic trials in hypertension. *Drug Safety*, 6, 83-93.

Howe, W.G. (1974). Approximate confidence limits on the mean of $X + Y$ where X and Y are two tabled independent random variables. *Journal of American Statistical Association*, 69, 789-794.

Hsu, J.C. (1984). Constrained two-sided simultaneous confidence intervals for multiple comparisons with the best. *The Annals of Statistics*, 12, 1136-1144.

Huque, M.F. and Dubey, S. (1990). Design and analysis for therapeutic equivalence clinical trials with binary clinical endpoints. *Proceedings of Biopharmaceutical Section of the American Statistical Association*, 91-97.

Hyslop, T., Hsuan, F. and Holder, D.J. (2000). A small sample confidence interval approach to assess individual bioequivalence. *Statistics in Medicine*, 19, 2885-2897.

ICH (1993). *Stability Testing of New Drug Substances and Products*. Tripartite International Conference on Harmonization Guideline.

ICH (1996). *Validation of Analytical Procedures: Methodology*. Tripartite International Conference on Harmonization Guideline.

ICH (1998a). *Ethnic Factors in the Acceptability of Foreign Clinical Data*. Tripartite International Conference on Harmonization Guideline, E5.

ICH (1998b). *Statistical Principles for Clinical Trials*. Tripartite International Conference on Harmonization Guideline, E9.

ICH (1999). *Choice of Control Group in Clinical Trials*. Tripartite International Conference on Harmonization Guideline, E10.

Jachuck, S.J., Brierley, H., Jachuck, S. and Wilcox, P.M. (1982). The effect of hypotensive drugs on the quality of life. *Journal of Ro. Coll. Gen. Practitioners*, 32, 103-105.

Jennison, C. and Turnball, B. (1993). Sequential equivalence testing and repeated confidence intervals, with application to normal and binary responses. *Biometrics*, 49, 31-44.

Johnson, R.A. and Wichern, D.W. (1998). *Applied Multivariate Statistical Analysis*. Prentice Hall, New Jersey.

Jones, B. and Kenward, M.G. (1989). *Design and Analysis of Cross-Over Trials*. Chapman & Hall, London.

Ju, H.L. and Chow, S.C. (1995). On stability designs in drug shelf-life estimation. *Journal of Biopharmaceutical Statistics*, 5, 201-214.

Ju, H.L. and Chow, S.C. (1996). A procedure for weight and model selection in assay development, *Journal of Food and Drug Analysis*, 4, 1-12.

Kaiser, H.F. (1958). The varimax criterion for analytic rotation in factor analysis. *Psychometrika*, 23, 187-200.

Kaiser, H.F. (1959). Computer program for varimax rotation in factor analysis. *Journal of Education Psycholog. Measure*, 27, 155-162.

Karlowski, T.R., Chalmers, T.C., Frenkel, L.D., Kapikian, A.Z., Lewis, T.L. and Lynch, J.M. (1975). Ascorbic acid for the common cold: A prophylactic and therapeutic trial. *Journal of American Medical Association*, 231, 1038-1042.

Kaplan, R.M., Bush, J.W., Berry, C.C. (1976). Health status: types of validity and Index of Well-Being. *Health Serv. Res.*, 4, 478-507.

Kervinen, L. and Yliruusi, J. (1993). Modeling S-shaped dissolution curves. *Int. J. Pharm.*, 92, 115-122.

Ki, F.Y.C. and Chow, S.C. (1994). Analysis of quality of life with parallel questionnaires. *Drug Information Journal*, 28, 69-80.

Ki, F.Y.C. and Chow, S.C. (1995). Statistical justification for the use of composite scores in quality of life assessment. *Drug Information Journal*, 29, 715-727.

Knickerbocker, R.K. (2000). Intention-to-treat analysis. In *Encyclopedia of Biopharmaceutical Statistics*, 271-275, Ed. S. Chow, Marcel Dekker, New York.

Kramer, H.C. (1980). Extension of the kappa coefficient. *Biometrics*, 36, 207-216.

L'Abbe, K., Detsky, A., and O'Rourke, K. (1987). Meta-analysis in clinical research. *Annals of Internal Medicine*, 107, 224-233.

Lachin, J.M. (1988a). Statistical properties of randomization in clinical trials. *Controlled Clinical Trials*, 9, 289-311.

Lachin, J.M. (1988b). Properties of simple randomization in clinical trials. *Controlled Clinical Trials*, 9, 312-326.

LaFrance, N.D. (1999). Developing new imaging agents and radiopharmaceuticals: where we're been, where we are and where we're going. Presented at Drug Information Association symposium on Statistics in Diagnostic Imaging, Arlington, Virgina, March 1999.

Landis, R.J. and Koch, G.G. (1977). The measurement of observer agreement for categorical data. *Biometrics*, 33, 159-174.

Langenbucher, F. (1972). Linearization of dissolution rate curves by the Weibull distribution. *J. Pharm. Pharmacol.*, 24, 979-981.

Leeson, L.J. (1995). In vitro/in vivo correlation. Drug *Information Journal*, 29, 903-915.

Lehmann, E.L. (1975). *Nonparametrics: Statistical Methods Based on Ranks.* Holden Day, San Francisco.

Lin, T.Y. D. (1994). Applicability of matrixing and bracketing approach to stability study design. Presented at the 4th ICSA Applied Statistics Symposium, Rockville, Maryland.

Lisook, A.B. (1990). FDA audits of clinical studies: policy and procedure. *Journal of Clinical Pharmacology*, 30, 296-302.

Little, R.J. and Rubin, D.B. (1987). *Statistical Analysis with Missing Data.* Wiley, New York.

Liu, H.K. (1990). Confidence intervals in bioequivalence. *Proceedings of the Biopharmaceutical Section of the American Statistical Association*, 51-54.

Liu, J.P. and Chow, S.C. (1992a). On the assessment of variability in bioavailability/bioequivalence studies. *Communications in Statistics, Theory and Methods*, 21, 2591-2608.

Liu, J.P. and Chow, S.C. (1992b). Sample size determination for the two one-sided tests procedure in bioequivalence. *Journal of Pharmacokinetics and Biopharmaceutics*, 20, 101-104.

Liu, J.P., Ma, M.C. and Chow, S.C. (1997). Statistical evaluation of similarity factor f_2 as a criterion for assessment of similarity between dissolution profiles. *Drug Information Journal*, 31, 1225-1271.

Ma, M.C., Lin, R.P. and Liu, J.P. (1999). Statistical evaluation of dissolution similarity. *Statistica Sinica*, 9, 1011-1028.

Ma, M.C., Wang, B.B.C., Liu, J.P. and Tsong, Y. (2000). Assessment of similarity between dissolution profiles. *Journal of Biopharmaceutical Statistics*, 10, 229-249.

Makris, L. (1999). Power and sample size considerations for the clinical study component vs. the blinded-reader study component. Presented at Drug Information Association symposium on Statistics in Diagnostic Imaging, Arlington, Virgina, March 1999.

Marcus, R., Peritz, E., and Gabriel, K.R. (1976). On closed testing procedures with special reference to ordered analysis of variance. *Biometrika*, 63, 655-660.

Matts, J.P. and Lachin, J.M. (1988). Properties of permuted-block randomization in clinical trials. *Controlled Clinical Trials*, 9, 327-344.

McNeil, B.J. and Hanley, J.A. (1984). Statistical approaches to the analysis of receiver operating characteristic curves. *Medical Decision Making*, 4, 137-150.

Mee, R.W. (1984). Confidence bounds for the difference between two probabilities. *Biometrics*, 40, 1175-1176.

Mellon, J.I. (1991). Design and analysis aspects of drug stability studies when the product is stored at several temperatures. Presented at the 12th Annual Midwest Statistical Workshop, Muncie, Indiana.

Metz, C.E. (1986). ROC methodology in radiologic imaging. *Investigative Radiology*, 21, 720-733.

Miettinen, O. and Nurminen, M. (1985). Comparative analysis of two rates. *Statistics in Medicine*, 4, 213-226.

Moise, A., Clement, B., Ducimetiere, P., and Bourassa, M.G. (1985). Comparison of receiver operating curves derived from the same population: a bootstrap approach. *Computers and Biomedical Research*, 18, 125-131.

Moore, J.W. and Flanner, H.H. (1996). Mathematical comparison of curves with an emphasis on dissolution profiles. *Pharma. Technol.*, 20, 64-74.

Murphy, J.R. and Weisman, D. (1990). Using random slopes for estimating shelf-life. *Proceedings of the Biopharmaceutical Section of the American Statistical Association*, 196-203.

Newcombe, R.G. (1998). Interval estimation for the difference between independent proportions: comparison of eleven methods. *Statistics in Medicine*, 17, 873-890.

Nordbrock, E. (1992). Statistical comparison of stability designs. *Journal of Biopharmaceutical Statistics*, 2, 91-113.

Nordbrock, E. (2000). Stability Matrix Design. In *Encyclopedia of Bio-pharmaceutical Statistics*, 487-492, Ed. S. Chow, Marcel Dekker, New York.

Olschewski, M. and Schumacher, M. (1990). Statistical analysis of quality of life data in cancer clinical trials. *Statistics in Medicine*, 9, 749-763.

Park, S. (2001). *Analysis of Longitudinal Data With Informative Missingness*. Ph.D. Thesis, Department of Statistics, University of Wisconsin, Madison.

Park, S., Palta, M., Shao, J. and Shen, L. (2002). Bias adjustment in analyzing longitudinal data with informative missingness. *Statistics in Medicine*. In press.

Peabody, F. (1927). The care of patient. *JAMA*, 88, 877.

Pena Romero, A., Caramella, C., Ronchi, M., Ferrari, F. and Chulia, D. (1991). Water uptake and force development in an optimized prolonged release formulation, *Int. J. Pharm.*, 73, 239-248.

Pledger, G. and Hall, D. (1986). Active control trials: Do they address the efficacy issue? *Proceedings of Biopharmaceutical Section of the American Statistical Association*, 1-7.

Pocock, S.J. (1983). *Clinical Trials: A Practical Approach*. Wiley, New York.

Pong, A. (2001). Comparing designs for stability studies and shelf life estimation for drug product with two components. Ph.D. Thesis, Temple University.

Qin, J., Leung, D. and Shao, J. (2002). Estimation with survey data under non-ignorable nonresponse or informative sampling. *Journal of the American Statistical Association*. In press.

Qu, Y. and Hadgu A. (1998). A model for evaluating sensitivity and specificity for correlated diagnostic tests in efficacy studies with an imperfect test. *Journal of the American Statistical Association*, 93, 920-928.

Qu, Y. and Hadgu A. (1999). A Bayesian approach to latent class analysis via data augmentation and Gibbs sampling. *Proceedings of the Bayesian Statistical Science Section of the American Statistical Association*.

Quiroz, J., Ting, N., Wei, G.C.G., and Burdick, R.K. (2000). A modified large sample approach in assessment of population bioequivalence. *Journal of Biopharmaceutical Statistics*, 10, 527-544.

Ridout, M.S. and Morgan, B.J.T. (1991). Modeling digit preference in fecundability studies. *Biometrics*, 47, 1423-1433.

Rosenburger, W.F. and Lachin, J.M. (1993). The use of response-adaptive designs in clinical trials. *Controlled Clinical Trials*, 14, 471-484.

Ruberg, S. and Hsu, J. (1992). Multiple comparison procedures for pooling batches in stability studies. *Technometrics*, 34, 465-472.

Ruberg, S. and Stegeman, J.W. (1991). Pooling data for stability studies: testing the equality of batch degradation slopes. *Biometrics*, 47, 1059-1069.

Schall, R. (1995). Assessing of individual and population bioequivalence using the probability that bioavailabilities are similar. *Biometrics*, 51, 615-626.

Schall, R. and Luus, H.G. (1993). On population and individual bioequivalence. *Statistics in Medicine*, 12, 1109-1124.

Schofield, T. (2000). Assay validation. In *Encyclopedia of Biopharmaceutical Statistics*, 21-30, Ed. S.C. Chow, Marcel Dekker, New York.

Schuirmann, D.J. (1987). A comparison of two one-sided tests procedure and the power approach for assessing the equivalence of average bioavailability. *Journal of Pharmacokinetics and Biopharmaceutics*, 15, 657-680.

Searle, S.R. (1971). *Linear Models*. Wiley, New York.

Shah, V.P., Midha, K.K., Dighe. S., McGilveray, I.J., Skelly, J.P., Yacobi, A., Layoff, T., Viswanathan, C.T., Cook, C.E., McDowall, R.D., Pittman, K.A. and Spector, S. (1992). Analytical methods validation: bioavailability, bioequivalence and pharmaceutical studies. *Pharmaceutical Research*, 9(4), 588-592.

Shah, V.P., Tsong, Y., Sathe, P. and Liu, J.P. (1998). *In vitro* dissolution profile comparison: statistics and analysis of the similarity factor f_2. *Pharmaceutical Research*, 15, 889-896.

Shao, J. (1999). *Mathematical Statistics*. Springer, New York.

Shao, J. and Chen, L. (1997). Prediction bounds for random shelf-lives. *Statistics in Medicine*, 16, 1167-1173.

Shao, J. and Chow, S.C. (1993). Two-stage sampling with pharmaceutical applications. *Statistics in Medicine*, 12, 1999-2008.

Shao, J. and Chow, S.C. (1994). Statistical inference in stability analysis. *Biometrics*, 50, 753-763.

Shao, J. and Chow, S.C. (2001a). Drug shelf-life estimation. *Statistica Sinica*, 11, 737-745.

Shao, J. and Chow, S.C. (2001b). Two-phase shelf-life estimation. *Statistics in Medicine*, 20, 1239-1248.

Shao, J. and Chow, S.C. (2002). Reproducibility probability in clinical trials. *Statistics in Medicine*. In press.

Shao, J., Chow, S.C. and Wang, B. (2000). The bootstrap procedure in individual bioequivalence. *Statistics in Medicine*, 19, 2741-2754.

Shao, J., Kübler, J. and Pigeot, I. (2000). Consistency of the bootstrap procedure in individual bioequivalence. *Biometrika*, 87, 573-585.

Shao, J. and Zhong, B. (2001). Last observation carry-forward and intention-to-treat analysis. Manuscript submitted for publication.

Sheiner, L.B. (1992). Bioequivalence revisited. *Statistics in Medicine*, 11, 1777-1788.

Shrout, P.E. and Fleiss, J.L. (1979). Intraclass correlations: uses in assessing rater reliability. *Psychological Bulletin*, 86, 420-428.

Simon, R. (1999). Bayesian design and analysis of active control clinical trials. *Biometrics*, 55, 484-487.

Smith, N. (1992). FDA perspectives on quality of life studies. Presented at DIA Workshop, Hilton Head, South Carolina.

Snedecor, G.W. and Cochran, W.G. (1967). *Statistical Methods*, sixth edition. The Iowa State University Press, Ames, Iowa.

Spilker, B. (1991). *Guide to Clinical Trials*. Raven Press, New York.

Stevens, G. (1999). Issues for the design of blinded-reader studies. Presented at Drug Information Association symposium on Statistics in Diagnostic Imaging, Arlington, Virgina, March 1999.

Sun, Y., Chow, S.C., Li, G. and Chen, K.W. (1999). Assessing distributions of estimated drug shelf lives in stability analysis. *Biometrics*, 55, 896-899.

SUPAC-IR (1995). *Guidance on Immediate Release Solid Oral Dosage Forms, Scale-up and Postapproval Changes: Chemistry, Manufacturing, and Controls, In Vitro Dissolution Testing, and In Vivo Bioequivalence Documentation,* U.S. Food and Drug Administration, Rockville, Maryland.

SUPAC-MR (1997). *Guidance on Modified Release Solid Oral Dosage Forms, Scale-up and Postapproval Changes: Chemistry, Manufacturing, and Controls, In Vitro Dissolution Testing, and In Vivo Bioequivalence Documentation,* U.S. Food and Drug Administration, Rockville, Maryland.

SUPAC-SS (1997). *Guidance on Nonsterile Semisolid Dosage Forms, Scale-up and Postapproval Changes: Chemistry, Manufacturing, and Controls, In Vitro Dissolution Testing, and In Vivo Bioequivalence Documentation,* U.S. Food and Drug Administration, Rockville, Maryland.

Swets, J.A. and Pickett, R.M. (1982). *Evaluation of Diagnostic System.* Academic Press, New York.

Tandon, P.K. (1990). Applications of global statistics in analyzing quality of life data. *Statistics in Medicine,* 9, 819-827.

Taves, D.R. (1974). Minimization: a new method of assigning patients to treatment and control groups. *Clin. Pharmacol. Ther.,* 15, 443-453.

Temple, R. (1983). Difficulties in evaluating positive control trials. *Proceedings of Biopharmaceutical Section of the American Statistical Association,* 1-7.

Testa, M., Anderson, R.B., Nackley, J.F., and Hollenberg, N.K. (1993). Quality of life and antihypertensive therapy in men: a comparison of captopril with enalapril. *New England Journal of Medicine,* 328, 907-913.

Thompson, M.L. and Zucchini, W. (1989). On the statistical analysis of ROC curves. *Statistics in Medicine,* 8, 1277-1290.

Ting, N. (2000). Carry-forward analysis. In *Encyclopedia of Biopharmaceutical Statistics,* 103-109, Ed. S. Chow, Marcel Dekker, New York.

Ting, N., Burdick, R.K., Graybill, F.A., Jeyaratnam, S. and Lu, T.-F.C. (1990). Confidence intervals on linear combinations of variance components that are unrestricted in sign. *Journal of Statistical Computation and Simulation,* 35, 135-143.

Tippett, L.H.C. (1931). *The Method of Statistics*. Williams and Norgate, London.

Torrance, G.W. (1976). Toward a utility theory foundation for health status index models. *Health Serv. Res.*, 4, 349-369.

Torrance, G.W. (1987). Utility approach to measuring health-related quality of life. *Journal of Chronice Dis.*, 40, 593-600.

Torrance, G.W. and Feeny, D.H. (1989). Utilities and quality-adjusted life years. *Journal of Technol. Assess Health Care*, 5, 559-575.

Tse, S.K. and Chow, S.C. (1995). On model selection for standard curve in assay development. *Journal of Biopharmaceutical Statistics*, 5, 285-296.

Tsong, Y., Hammerstrom, T. and Chen, J.J. (1997). Multiple dissolution specification and acceptance sampling rule based on profile modeling and principal component analysis. *Journal of Biopharmaceutical Statistics*, 7, 423-439.

Tsong, Y., Hammerstrom, T., Lin, K.K. and Ong, T.E. (1995). The dissolution testing sampling acceptance rules. *Journal of Biopharmaceutical Statistics*, 5, 171-184.

Tsong, Y., Hammerstrom, T., Sathe, P. and Shah, V.P. (1996). Statistical assessment of mean differences between two dissolution data sets. *Drug Information Journal*, 30, 1105-1112.

Tu, D. (1997). Two one-sided tests procedures in establishing therapeutic equivalence with binary clinical endpoints: fixed sample performances and sample size determination. *Journal of Statistical Computation and Simulation*, 59, 271-290.

USP/NF (2000). *The United States Pharmacopedia* XXIV *and the National Formulary* XIX. The United States Pharmacopedial Convention, Rockville, Maryland.

Ware, J.E. (1987). Standards for validating health measures definition and content. *Journal of Chronic Dis.*, 40, 473-480.

Wei, L.J. (1977). A class of designs for sequential clinical trials. *Journal of American Statistical Association*, 72, 382-386.

Wei, L.J. (1978). The adaptive biased-coin design for sequential experiment. *The Annals of Statistics*, 9, 92-100.

Wei, L.J. and Lachin, J.M. (1988). Properties of the urn randomization in clinical trials. *Controlled Clinical Trials*, 9, 345-364.

Wei, L.J., Smythe, R.T., Lin, D.Y., and Park, T.S. (1990). Statistical inference with data-dependent treatment allocation rules. *Journal of American Statistical Association*, 85, 156-162.

Westlake, W.J. (1976). Symmetric confidence intervals for bioequivalence trials. *Biometrics*, 32, 741-744.

Wieand, S., Gail, M.H., James, B.R., and James, K.L. (1989). A family of nonparametric statistics for comparing diagnostic markers with paired or unpaired data. *Biometrics*, 76, 585-592.

Williams, G.H. (1987). Quality of life and its impact on hypertensive patients. *American Journal of Medicine*, 82, 98-105.

Wilson, E.B. (1927). Probable inference, the law of succession, and statistical inference. *Journal of the American Statistical Association*, 22, 209-212.

Woolson, R. (1987). *Statistical Methods for the Analysis of Biomedical Data*. Wiley, New York.

Wu, M.C. and Carroll, R.J. (1988). Estimation and comparison of changes in the presence of informative right censoring by modeling the censoring process. *Biometrics*, 44, 175-188.

Zelen, M. (1969). Play the winner rule and the controlled clinical trial. *Journal of American Statistical Association*, 64, 131-146.

Zweig M.H. and Campbell G. (1993). Receiver-operating characteristic (ROC) plots: a fundamental evaluation tool in clinical medicine. *Clinical Chemistry*, 39(4), 561-577.

Zwinderman, A.H. (1990). The measurement of change of quality of life in clinical trials. *Statistics in Medicine*, 9, 931-942.

Index

363

Milton Keynes UK
Ingram Content Group UK Ltd.
UKHW031540071024
449327UK00034B/1380